James R. Mellberg/Louis W. Ripa

Fluoride in Preventive Dentistry

Fluoride in Preventive Dentistry

Theory and Clinical Applications

By

James R. Mellberg, BS, MS
Senior Scientist
Basic Dental Research
Research Center, Colgate-Palmolive Company
Piscataway, New Jersey

Louis W. Ripa, DDS, MS
Professor and Chairman
Department of Children's Dentistry, School of Dental Medicine
State University of New York at Stony Brook
Stony Brook, New York

With a special contribution by:

Gary S. Leske, DDS, MS, MPH
Professor
Department of Children's Dentistry
Assistant Dean for Student Affairs and Curriculum
School of Dental Medicine
State University of New York at Stony Brook
Stony Brook, New York

Quintessence Publishing Co, Inc
Chicago, Berlin, London, Tokyo, Paris, Barcelona, São Paulo, Moscow, Prague, and Warsaw

To the children of the world—for whom fluoride helps secure a legacy of good health

quintessence books

Quintessence Publishing Co, Inc
551 Kimberly Drive
Carol Stream, Illinois 60188

Printed in USA

ISBN: 0-86715-358-X

Table of Contents

Foreword

Except under the pressure of emergencies, such as war (which accelerated the use of penicillin), it takes about a quarter of a century for scientific discoveries to find their way into therapeutic use. Although more than 40 years have now passed since it was definitely established that fluoride in drinking water prevents caries in children, many people throughout the world still fail to enjoy the benefits that fluoride can provide.

There are several reasons for this situation. One is that there are definite limits to the number of people who can use fluoridated water supplies. According to a United Nations report, only 25% of the world's population obtain their drinking water from piped water systems. Even in advanced countries such as the United States, a considerable percentage of people, particularly in rural areas, still use private wells. This means that for years to come, the majority of the world's children cannot be helped even if all communal water supplies were to become fluoridated. In some countries, such as the Netherlands and Sweden, water fluoridation is prevented by law and other methods of fluoride therapy are being used. However, in newly developing countries there are usually neither trained health personnel nor sufficient funds to provide alternative caries prevention programs.

Despite the fact that diverse barriers to the use of fluoride exist, fluoride therapy presents a unique situation in that a wide choice of methods is available. Caries protection can be conferred by adding fluoride to drinking water; by consuming fluoride-containing tablets, drops, or other vehicles; or by applying fluoride topically to the teeth. These multiple techniques of fluoride therapy resulted, in part, from the studies of dental researchers in Rochester, New York, who determined that fluoride could impart resistance not only to developing teeth but also to teeth that were fully formed. In what stands in dentistry as a classic example of basic scientific research leading to practical therapy, it was shown that fluoride provided topical, as well as systemic, benefits and that the application of fluoride to erupted teeth in both humans and animals would inhibit decay. While at first there was some unwillingness to accept these findings, they have subsequently led to a variety of methods for using fluorides, which probably for years to come will continue to benefit people, as does water fluoridation.

The search for new fluoride agents and methods of delivery continues. However, the discovery of more efficient compounds and techniques will contribute nothing unless they are put into use. Thus, whether we have only existing fluoride preparations or new and more potent ones, the extent to which caries will be controlled will, in the last analysis, depend upon the dental profession. This means that if the benefits of fluoride are to be fully realized, dentists must be intelligently involved in their utilization. Additionally, dentists must be capable of instructing and guiding other professionals and nonprofessionals in the proper use of fluoride for caries prevention. This is not a simple undertaking, since the scientific reports dealing with fluoride appear in dozens of different journals, many of which are not readily available. This book by Mellberg and Ripa will greatly simplify the dentist's task.

In suggesting that dentists should offer leadership in this area, we are not making a new request of the profession. Dentistry has already won wide respect for its activities in promoting water fluoridation and other uses of fluorides, which thereby, in the eyes of laymen, imperils its very means of support. Even if fluoride therapy remains at its present level of effectiveness, it has already changed the epidemiology of the disease and altered the practice of dentistry. Whether or not individuals are exposed to fluoride in the drinking water, they usually have had fluoride contact of one type or another, such as from dentifrices. As a result, caries prevalence in some countries is decreasing, and dentists must modify their patient treatments accordingly. While researchers have, to date, offered only preliminary reports, it seems likely that as the effects of fluoride in retarding the progress of carious lesions accumulate, dentists may be justified in postponing the filling of early lesions or in using alternative nondestructive methods of treatment.

There is, unfortunately, a possibility that the caries resistance imparted by fluoride may be overwhelmingly challenged by the caries attack. It must be kept in mind, therefore, that while fluorides greatly increase the ability of teeth to resist a "normal" caries attack, they do not provide complete protection, especially against attacks of "unlimited" strength. To keep fluoride therapy in its proper perspective, the dentist must not lose sight of the role that foods play in the carious process and must ultimately devise a preventive strategy employing all appropriate modalities of prevention.

Basil G. Bibby
Rochester, New York

Preface

Although the use of fluoride in dentistry predates the twentieth century, the arousal of scientific interest in the dental benefits of the fluoride ion can be traced to the "Colorado Brown Stain" incident, which occurred early in this century. It was found that naturally occurring waterborne fluoride was responsible for this developmental enamel defect and, moreover, that teeth exposed to the fluoride were relatively immune to dental decay. This latter finding stimulated a virtual explosion of research activity, still going on today, into the multifaceted relationship between fluoride and dental health.

During the last 50 years, more articles have been published on fluoride than on any other area of dentistry. While no individual can be expected to completely master the voluminous and sometimes contradictory literature, an understanding of the field is essential for all who are concerned with preventive dentistry.

It is the purpose of *Fluoride in Preventive Dentistry* to review and organize the relevant literature in this broad field into a format that will be useful for both clinicians and researchers. Literature on both clinical and laboratory studies has been included in the hope that a more complete understanding of the nature of fluoride and how it can best be utilized will be provided. Because the subject matter is so extensive, it was thought this could best be accomplished by combining the experience of a laboratory researcher with that of a clinical researcher, each of whom has had some experience in the other field. Although contributions to all chapters were made by both authors, the principal author of those chapters oriented heavily toward laboratory science (Chapters 2, 3, 6, and 8) was JRM and those oriented toward clinical science (Chapters 1, 5, 7, and 9) was LWR. Because certain subjects fit naturally into more than one chapter some deliberate repetition was necessary, but it is hoped that this will enhance, rather than detract from, the merits of the book.

The authors wish to thank Dr. Gary Leske for authoring Chapter 4 and Linda Karabinchak, Charles Cooper, James Cucco, Robert Bauman, Robin Johnson, Kris Vandenberg, Kathleen Gebhardt, and Eugene McDermott for their invaluable assistance in the preparation of the manuscript and figures for this book.

James R. Mellberg
Louis W. Ripa

Chapter 1

Formation of Dental Caries

A rational approach to the control of dental caries requires an understanding of the nature of the disease itself. During this century, both clinical observation and active experimentation have produced a sufficiently detailed explanation of the etiology of dental decay to enable preventive therapy to be directed against its most vulnerable points.

Dental caries begins with the formation of acid by microorganisms in plaque overlying the enamel. It is a localized multifactorial disease requiring the simultaneous presence of three factors: (1) microorganisms, (2) a diet for the microorganisms, and (3) a susceptible host or tooth surface (Fig. 1-1). In the absence of any of these factors, caries will not develop.

Microorganisms

The "chemico-parasitic theory" of dental caries was proposed by *W. D. Miller* in 1890.[1] *Miller* showed that oral bacteria will ferment carbohydrates, producing lactic and other acids capable of dissolving tooth enamel. Direct experimental proof that bacteria are a primary requirement for caries development, however, was not furnished until 1954. At that time, *Orland* and co-workers demonstrated that germ-free laboratory rats fed a cariogenic diet did not develop caries. Conversely, feeding similar diets to conventional or gnotobiotic* rats resulted in the production of carious lesions.[2,3] Additional proof was furnished by *Fitzgerald* and *Keyes,*[4,5] who demonstrated that in laboratory animals dental decay was both infectious and transmissible, while *Shaw* and *Sweeney*[6] showed that suppression of oral microorganisms with antibiotics would eliminate caries. Subsequent experiments showed that although *all microorganisms that caused decay produced acid, not all microorganisms that produced acid would cause decay.*

Because lactobacilli are acidogenic (produce acid) and aciduric (grow under acidic conditions) and were found to proliferate when caries were present, they were once thought to be the major cause of decay. However, lactobacilli apparently lack the ability to form plaque and, therefore, their colonization on the enamel surface of the tooth is poor.[7,8] Animal experiments have generally been unsuccessful in producing caries using lactobacilli, particularly on smooth enamel surfaces, although some fissure caries in monoinfected gnotobiotic rats have been reported.[9,10]

The number of lactobacilli increases after caries have developed. *Loesche* and *Syed*[11] found that while lactobacilli averaged only 4% of the cultivable microorganisms in the

**Gnotobiotic animal* refers to one with a known (usually deliberately introduced) microbiota.

plaque covering proximal enamel lesions, in carious dentin they comprised an average of 21%. The low pH and available carbohydrate substrate associated with cavitated lesions favor the growth of lactobacilli, and they are now considered to be secondary invaders rather than initiators of the carious lesion. Since they increase in number as the lesion progresses, the acids produced by lactobacilli are believed to contribute to the growth of the lesion.[8]

Based upon the tooth surface on which they occur, carious lesions may be categorized into three types: root surface, smooth surface, and pit and fissure lesions. Although it is likely that caries formation is the result of complex interactions of many bacteria, *Keyes*[12] related the surface affected by caries to the predominant type of microorganism that he believed to be causative.

Root surface lesions

Caries of the root develop beneath plaque covering the exposed cementum of the tooth. Hence, root surface lesions are associated with microorganisms capable of producing a sticky extracellular polysaccharide (polyglucan) plaque from dietary carbohydrates, which will adhere to the root of the tooth.[12] The sticky plaque adheres both the causative microorganisms and the acids they produce to the root surface.

Actinomyces viscosus and *Actinomyces naeslundii* have been found to cause root caries in hamsters and gnotobiotic rats. In addition, they have also been associated with periodontal lesions and sometimes fissure cavities as well.[13-18] In humans, *Syed* and co-workers[19] found *Actinomyces viscosus* to be a dominant organism in all plaque samples that they recovered from root surfaces, comprising nearly 50% of the cultivable microorganisms.

The plaque overlying root surface lesions can also cover coronal portions of the tooth. Interestingly, while root surfaces may develop caries from plaque-forming microorganisms such as *Actinomyces viscosus* and *naeslundii,* the adjacent crown enamel remains free of caries. A possible explanation for this is that the rate of lactic acid produced by this species is very low, and thus better tolerated by the enamel.

Smooth surface lesions

The creation of lesions on smooth coronal surfaces also requires the presence of plaque to hold the microorganisms and acid against the teeth. Unlike the *Actinomyces* species, which produce root surface decay, the microorganisms that produce smooth surface enamel lesions are more rapid producers of acid. It must be recognized, however, that a microorganism that has the ability of adhering to a smooth enamel surface and is able to produce acid at a rate rapid enough to demineralize the underlying enamel can also demineralize less resistant cementum, exposed root dentin, and pits and fissures of occlusal surfaces.

The species that may be the major initiator of caries is *Streptococcus mutans.* It is an anaerobic facultative microorganism. It is acidogenic and aciduric, growing at an optimum pH of 6.2, which is somewhat lower than other streptococci.[20] *S. mutans* survives in the mouth only by adhering to solid surfaces such as teeth or dentures,[21,22] since they do not adhere to the oral epithelium or tongue.[23,24]

S. mutans produces large quantities of both intracellular and extracellular polyglucans and forms relatively voluminous quantities of adherent plaque. However, the types of polyglucan produced by streptococci can vary even when produced by the same organism.[25,26] This led *Gibbons* and *Banghart* to speculate that "individuals ingesting small amounts of dietary sucrose may harbor potentially cariogenic bacteria in an avirulent,

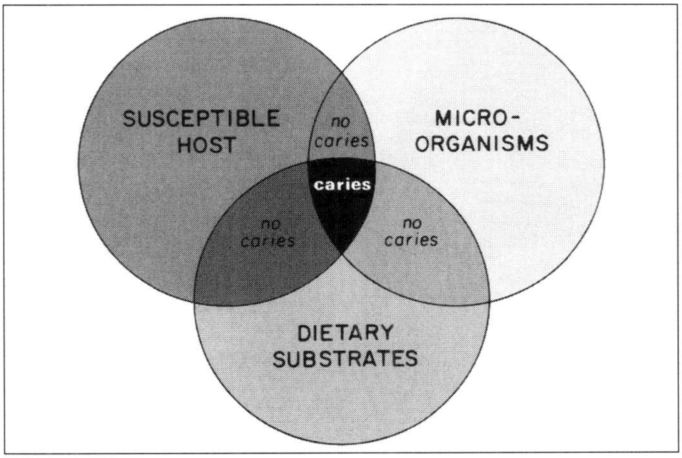

Fig. 1-1 Factors required for caries formation.

non-encapsulated phase."[27] That the virulence of cariogenic bacteria can be altered was shown by *Ikeda* and co-workers who included in the diet of laboratory rats certain coupling sugars that inhibited polyglucan production by streptococci.[26]

The association of organisms identified as *Streptococcus mutans* with dental caries has been shown in both animals[4,28] and humans.[8,25,29-36] *Keene* and *Shklair*[37] found that 17 of 21 caries-free military recruits were carriers of *S. mutans*. Within one year, ten of the carriers developed caries, whereas the noncarriers remained free of caries. *Ikeda* and co-workers[8] studied selected tooth surfaces in several children for a period of 18 months. *S. mutans* was found on 31 surfaces, of which 12 became carious over the study period. Conversely, five surfaces that were free of *S. mutans* did not develop caries. Recently, *Gibbons* and co-workers[38] reported a correlation between caries activity in schoolchildren and the degree of infection with *S. mutans*.

Human plaque studies indicate the worldwide distribution of *S. mutans*.[33,39,40] Other studies have shown that oral implantation can occur very early in the life of an individual. *Berkowitz* and co-workers have demonstrated the presence of *S. mutans* in infants soon after the eruption of the primary incisors, and additional evidence suggests that the infection may have been transmitted by the mother.[41-43] Nevertheless, it appears to be difficult to orally implant *S. mutans*, and, once established, it does not tend to spread throughout the mouth.[44] However, *Loesche* and co-workers[45] have suggested that normal dental examinations with an explorer may spread the organism in the mouth. A reduction in the number of *S. mutans* following restorative procedures has been reported by *Keene* and co-workers.[46]

Pit and fissure lesions

The deep occlusal pits and fissures provide protected areas for the retention of microorganisms and fermentable carbohydrates that are necessary for caries initiation (Fig. 1-2). These areas of the tooth are highly susceptible to decay, and actinomyces, *Streptococcus mutans*, and lactobacilli have all been implicated as potential initiators of carious lesions in pits and fissures.

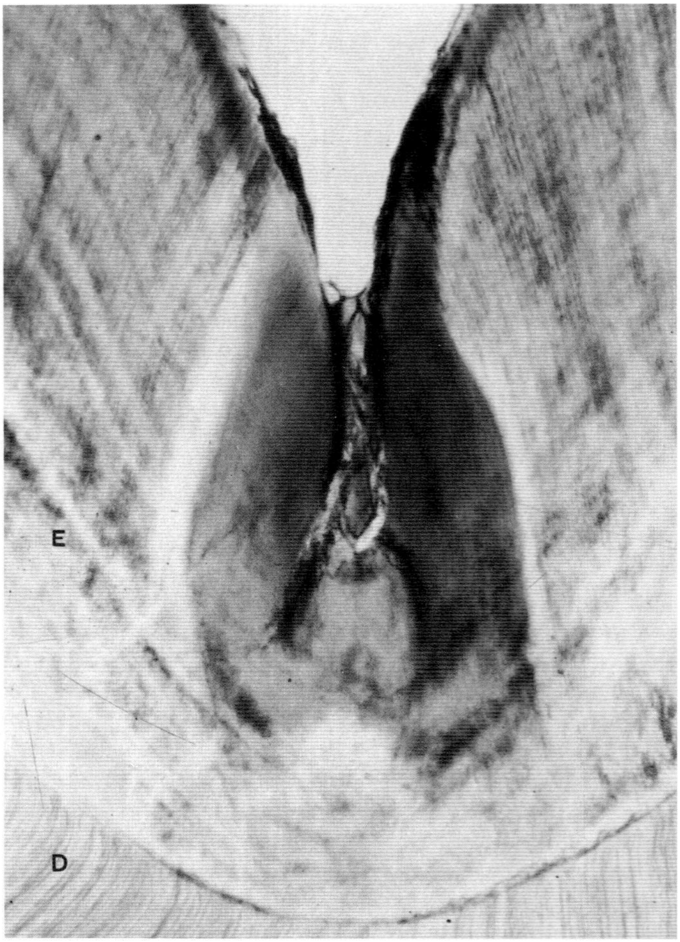

Fig. 1-2 Longitudinal section through an occlusal fissure. Note the debris present and the carious changes occurring around the fissure. The morphology of these areas makes them difficult to clean and they are very susceptible to caries. E = Enamel; D = Dentin
(Compliments of Dr. A. J. *Gwinnett*.)

Diet

It is the carbohydrate component of the diet that is associated with the formation of dental caries. Fats and protein either do not effect cariogenicity or are generally considered to be cariostatic.[47-49] Three factors influence the cariogenic potential of carbohydrates: (1) the type of carbohydrate, (2) the oral clearance of the carbohydrate or, conversely, its persistence on tooth surfaces, and (3) the frequency of consumption.

Type of carbohydrate

Sucrose, common table sugar, is believed to be the major cariogenic food factor in the human diet.[49-52] While glucose, fructose, galactose, lactose, maltose, dextrose, and starch have all been shown to form caries in experimental animals, sucrose invariably results in the greatest tooth destruction.[53-56]

Sucrose is utilized by oral microorganisms both in the formation of plaque matrix, which adheres the microorganisms to the tooth, and in the production of acids that dissolve the tooth.[57] Bacterial enzymes hydrolyze sucrose, a disaccharide, yielding glucose and fructose. These monosaccharides can be utilized as immediate sources of energy, yielding lactic and other organic acids that can dissolve the mineral of the tooth. Conversely, through the action of the enzymes dextran sucrase and levan sucrase, sucrose can be converted into long chain polymers of glucose, called dextran (polyglucan), or of fructose, called levan (polyfructan). Dextran promotes the adhesion of plaque bacteria to each other and of the plaque itself to the surface of the tooth.[58] Both dextran and levan also serve as extracellular substrates within the plaque that can be subsequently metabolized to their respective glucose and fructose moities with the further production of organic acids. The metabolic pathways of sucrose utilization by the plaque microorganisms is diagramed in Figure 1-3.

Because sucrose is utilized both in the formation of plaque matrix and in the production of acids that dissolve the tooth, its cariogenic potential is greatly enhanced above that of other sugars. For instance, while the amount of dental plaque is greatest when sucrose is the ingested carbohydrate, large quantities of plaque can also be formed in association with the ingestion of other carbohydrates such as sorbitol.[59] The cariogenicity of these plaques, however, is less than that formed in association with sucrose.

The adhesion produced by the polyglucans is especially important for the initiation of caries on smooth tooth surfaces where, in the absence of plaque, the saliva may be expected to wash away the microorganisms. The aggregation of *Streptococcus mutans, Streptococcus sanguis,* and *Actinomyces viscosus* is all mediated by polyglucans.[60] It has been demonstrated in both animals and humans that drastic reductions in the level of dietary sucrose can result in a decrease in the oral population of extracellular polysaccharide-forming streptococci.[61,62] Animal studies have also shown that while sucrose feeding will increase the population of *S. mutans,* that of *S. sanguis* will be reduced.[59] The opposite effect can be produced by replacing sucrose with sorbitol. While *S. sanguis* has been associated with caries formation, the intensity of the attack is much less than that associated with *S. mutans.*[63]

Because sucrose is a disaccharide, it is small enough to readily diffuse into the bacterial plaque. As long as it is a dietary constituent, therefore, it can continue to function as a precursor of the plaque matrix, as a direct source of acid that causes demineralization of the tooth, and as a raw material for plaque storage products, which can later be degraded to acids.[64]

Oral clearance

An important dietary factor in the formation of caries is the duration of time the carbohydrate remains in the mouth and is capable of interacting with the dental plaque. The duration is partly dependent upon the stickiness, or retentiveness, of the food consumed.

The physical form of the carbohydrate determines its retentiveness and thus appears to be a major factor in determining the cariogenicity of the diet. In the famous Vipeholm study, Swedish investigators rated the oral clearance of several sucrose-containing foods. They then selectively added them to the diet of institutionalized individuals and studied their caries activity for five years.[65] When the inmates' standard diet was supplemented with sugar in solution, which has a low retentive quality, there was a minimal caries increase. When sticky candies such as toffee and caramel were added to the diet, the subjects experienced a marked increase in caries activity. Sugar supplements with intermediate oral clearance were

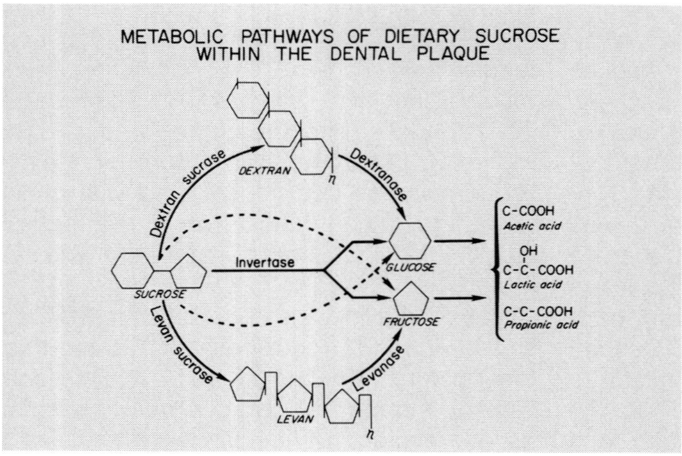

Fig. 1-3 Sucrose, a disaccharide consisting of glucose and fructose, is metabolized by plaque microorganisms to simple organic acids capable of dissolving the tooth and to complex polysaccharides that promote adhesion of the plaque or serve as future metabolites.

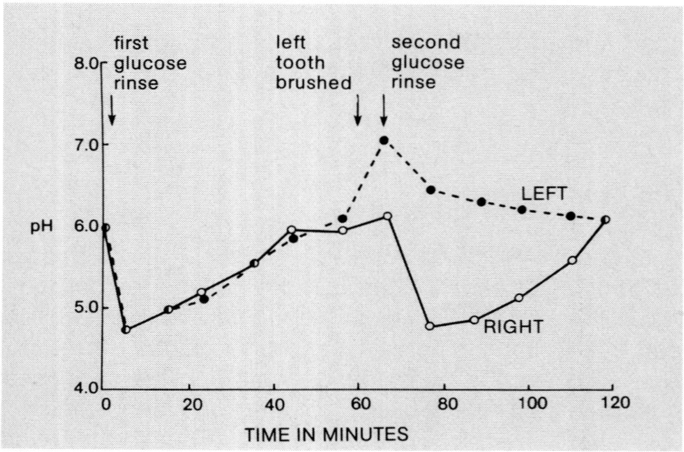

Fig. 1-4 Changes in pH of the dental plaque following rinsing with a 10% solution of glucose. The dispersal of plaque by brushing alters the pH curve.
(Modified from *Kleinberg*.[69])

associated with moderate levels of caries increase.

Frequency of eating

The third factor associated with the cariogenicity of foods is the frequency with which they are consumed.[66,67] A quantity of carbohydrate consumed during several snacking sessions is potentially more cariogenic than if the same amount were consumed at a single session. This is believed to be related to the change in plaque pH that accompanies ingestion of fermentable carbohydrates.

The pH of dental plaque is normally close to neutrality. When a fermentable carbohydrate is ingested, there is a rapid drop in pH to approximately 5.0 at which time acid dissolution of the tooth can occur.[68] The pH remains at this level for approximately 20 minutes and then gradually returns to its preingestion level. Frequent snacking results in repetitive drops of the plaque pH and, therefore, multiple attacks at the plaque-tooth surface interface.

The interaction between plaque and ingested carbohydrate is demonstrated in Figure 1-4. The resting pH of the plaque on the left and right maxillary incisors was measured. Rinsing with a 10% solution of glucose produced an immediate drop in pH followed by a gradual return to baseline levels. The left tooth was then brushed, removing most of the plaque, and the patient again rinsed. There was a minimal fall in pH on the tooth in which the plaque had been dispersed, whereas a low acid pH was again recorded for the plaque on the unbrushed tooth.[69]

Tooth and host

Clinical appearance of the incipient lesion

The acids produced in the plaque dissolve microchannels within the enamel to depths of approximately 20 to 50μ. At these depths, *subsurface* dissolution of the enamel occurs. As the carious lesion develops, the loss of mineral results in optical changes, which give the lesion an opaque white appearance, in contrast to the translucence of unaffected enamel. Thus, the initial carious lesion is referred to as a "white spot." At first, the surface of such a lesion is hard and resists penetration of an explorer tip. If the lesion continues to progress, however, the surface will become soft and chalky and cavitation will result.

Because plaque is required for caries formation, white spots are located on areas of the teeth that are covered by plaque in both humans and laboratory animals. Specifically, these are the proximal surfaces in association with the contact areas (Fig. 1-5a) and the gingival one-third of facial and lingual surfaces (Fig. 1-5b). While white spots also develop in pits and fissures (Fig. 1-5c), the initial lesion may go undetected clinically because of the presence of oral debris and stain.

The presence of a white opaque lesion on a tooth signifies a localized area of decreased mineral content, however all such areas are not the result of carious involvement. Some white areas are hypomineralized, having occurred during the period of tooth development. Mild fluorosis, for instance, is one example of a developmental white area.[70] Developmental *(hypomineralized)* areas can usually be clinically differentiated from carious *(demineralized)* areas because the former are more diffuse and are frequently found on areas of the teeth where there is relatively little plaque.[71,72]

Histological appearance of the incipient lesion

The histology of incipient carious lesions has been studied since the 1920s and most recently has been extensively reviewed by *Silverstone*.[73,74] Microscopic techniques have conclusively demonstrated the *subsurface* nature of the white spot.[75-78] Figure 1-6 is a longitudinal ground section of a white spot, or incipient carious lesion, viewed with polarized light. The appearance of the lesion under polarized light microscopy has been described as consisting of several zones. The appearance of these zones is believed to be due to a unique distribution and size of spaces, or pores, within the enamel caused by carious demineralization. From the surface inward, the principal zones of the lesion are as follows:

1. *The surface zone*—a relatively intact layer exhibiting only a slight degree of demineralization. Normal enamel consists of about 0.1% spaces or pores. The pore volume of the surface layer of the white spot is approximately 1 to 5%.

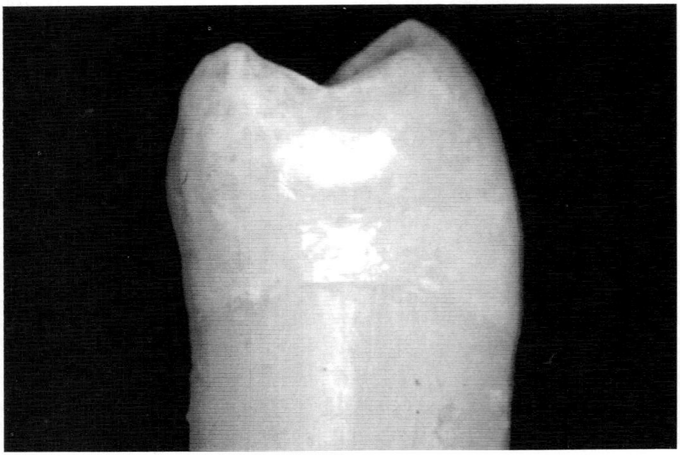

Fig. 1-5a Initial carious ("white spot") lesion on the proximal surface of a human premolar.

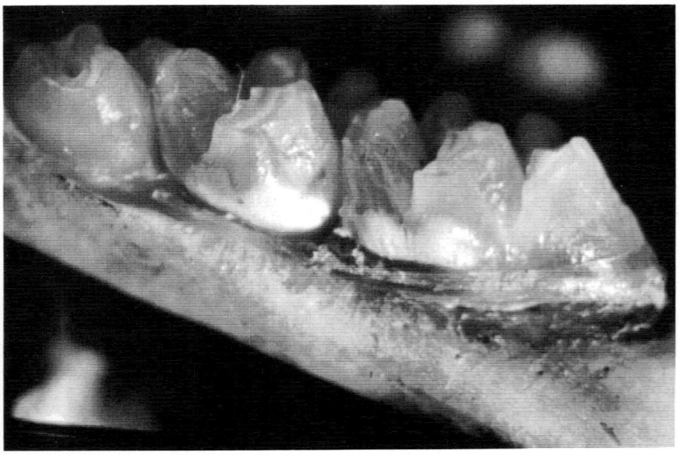

Fig. 1-5b Initial carious ("white spot") lesions on the buccal surfaces of the molars of a laboratory rat fed a cariogenic diet.

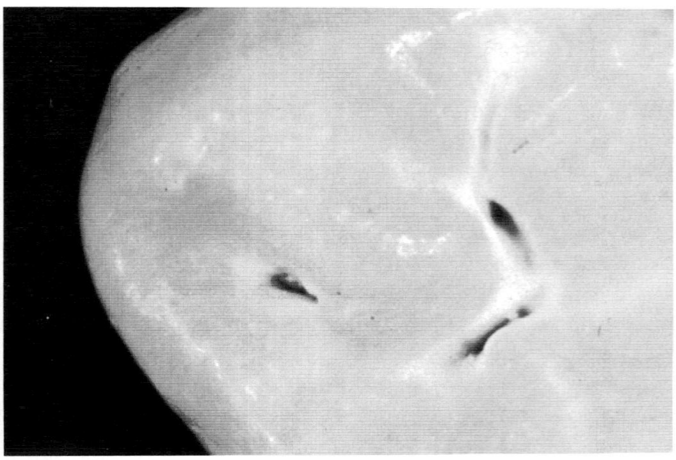

Fig. 1-5c Initial carious ("white spot") lesions on the occlusal surface of a human molar.
(Compliments of Dr. A. J. *Gwinnett.*)

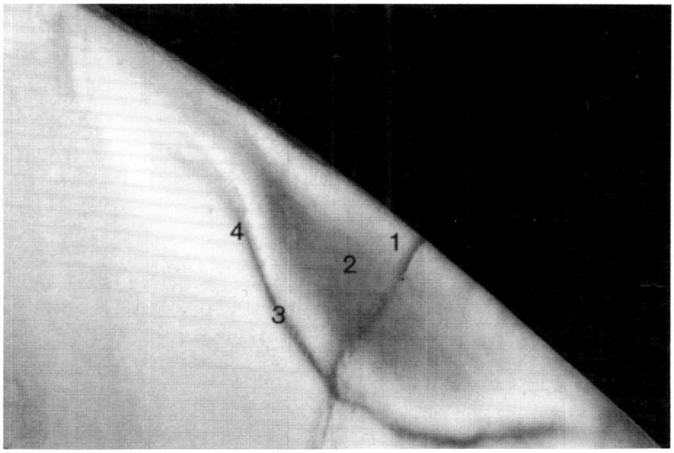

Fig. 1-6 Polarized light view of a longitudinal ground section through a white spot on the proximal surface of a permanent tooth. A relatively intact surface layer (1) overlies the body of the lesion (2) where the greatest demineralization has occurred. The positive zone (3) and translucent zone (4) are other histologic features of the early carious lesion. (Original magnification X100.)

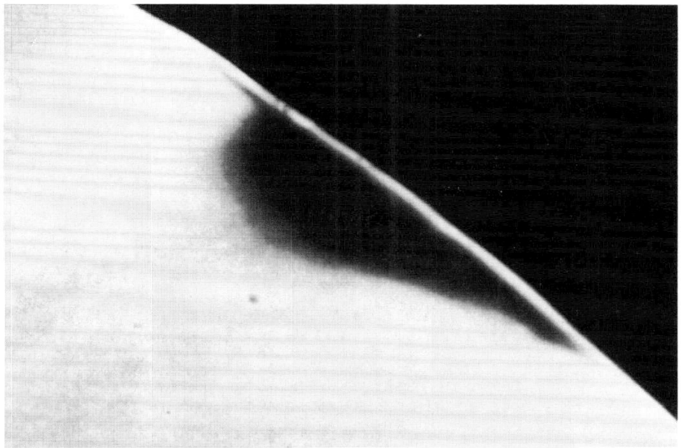

Fig. 1-7 Microradiograph of a longitudinal ground section through a white spot on the proximal surface of a primary tooth. Note the relatively intact surface layer, which is radiopaque, and the subsurface area of demineralization, which is radioluscent. (Original magnification X80.)

2. *The body of the lesion*—the largest zone in the lesion and the one that exhibits the greatest degree of demineralization. The pore volume in this zone is between 5 to 25%. The extent of demineralization present in this area allows the lesion to be detected radiographically.
3. *The dark or positive zone*—contains approximately 2 to 4% of spaces. Most of these are extremely small and therefore remain filled with air when placed in different liquids for viewing beneath polarized light. The difference in refractive index between the air-filled spaces and enamel crystals produces what is called positive form birefringence—hence the term positive zone.
4. *The translucent zone*—though not present in all lesions, is located at the advancing front of the cariously altered enamel. It contains approximately 1% of spaces, the size of which appears to be larger than that of spaces found in unaffected enamel or the positive zone.

Figure 1-7 is a typical microradiograph (radiograph of a microscopic section) of a white spot or incipient carious lesion demonstrating the radiopaque, relatively intact surface layer overlying a radiolucent area of subsurface demineralization.

Incipient lesion formation

Theories of formation

There is no universally accepted theory for the formation of a lesion consisting of a relatively intact surface layer overlying a demineralized subsurface except for the agreement that acid is necessary. Some suggested mechanisms (reviewed by *Brown*[79]) are described below.

Membrane effects Two types of membrane effects have been proposed: the permselective type and the Donnan type. The permselective membrane theory, proposed by *Brown,*[79] suggests that only cations can pass through the outer enamel and plaque. Within the interior of the tooth, calcium will be lost and will be replaced by hydrogen ions, a process that facilitates dissolution of subsurface enamel. According to the Donnan membrane theory, cationic proteins are not able to penetrate beyond the enamel surface. The pH within the enamel can, therefore, be lower than at the surface, resulting in greater subsurface dissolution.[80]

Protective coatings The enamel surface contains organic integuments or films.[81,82] It has been proposed that these materials protect the outer surface from dissolution while allowing penetration of acid into the subsurface enamel. *Pearce* and *Bibby*[83] have suggested insoluble proteins; *Francis* and coworkers[84] have suggested polyphosphates and polyphosphonates, while *Gray* has suggested organic compounds in plaque as protective coatings.[85]

Solubility differences The enamel surface is more mineralized and consists of larger crystals than the underlying enamel; it contains many trace elements, a higher concentration of fluoride, and a lower concentration of carbonate.[86-89] These physical and chemical differences decrease the acid solubility of the outer enamel surface. The greater acid resistance of the surface layer can contribute to the development of a lesion with a more intact surface.

Diffusion rate differences *Moreno* and *Zahradnik*[90] suggested that, under appropriate conditions, a slight acid dissolution of the surface enamel occurs with dicalcium phosphate dihydrate and fluorapatite precipitating within the surface region. Since the chemical potential of phosphoric acid and acid buffer outside the surface enamel is higher than the solution filling the pores of the underlying subsurface enamel, the acid will diffuse into the enamel and the basic component, $Ca(OH)_2$, will diffuse in the opposite direction. Diffusion of the basic solution into the surface region results in its precipitation. If the rate of this precipitation is greater than the rate of diffusion of ions away from the surface, the surface layer will remain relatively intact. Support for this concept is found in the demonstration that the surface layer of artificially formed lesions actually increased in width as subsurface dissolution progressed.[91,92]

Brown[79] summarized his review of incipient lesion formation by stating that the factors controlling events within the subsurface enamel, including the body of the lesion, translucent and dark zones, appear to be *thermodynamic* in nature, involving variations in solubility. Conversely, the dominant factors at the relatively intact surface and plaque interface are *kinetic* in nature and involve restricted diffusion.

Rate of formation The rate of demineralization depends upon the rate at which acid

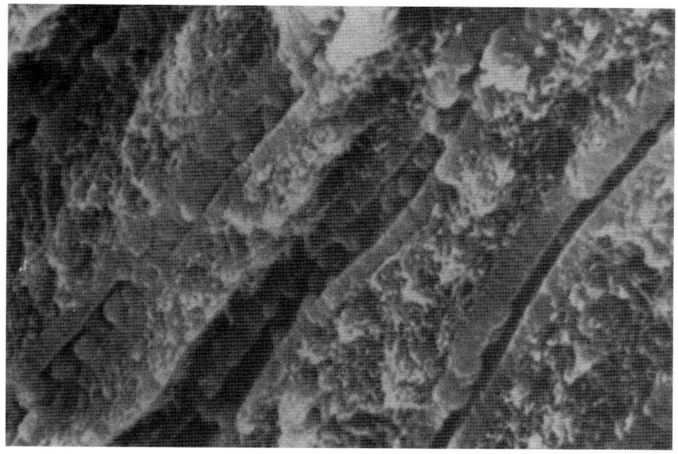

Fig. 1-8 Bacteria within the dentinal tubules of a tooth with a carious lesion. (SEM; original magnification X5,000.)
(Compliments of Dr. A. J. *Gwinnett.*)

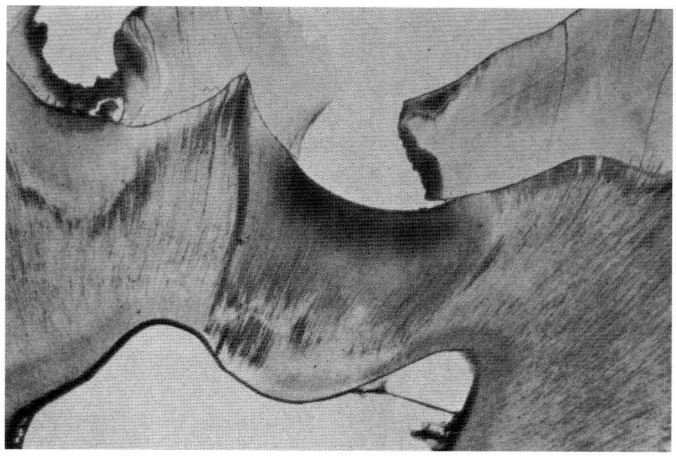

Fig. 1-9 Separate areas of cavitation of occlusal lesions on the same tooth. Notice the progression into the dentin. (Original magnification X4.)
(Compliments of Dr. A. J. *Gwinnett.*)

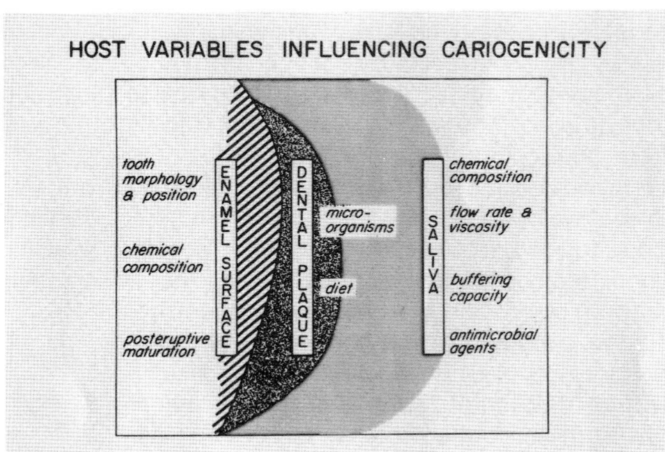

Figure 1-10

can diffuse into the enamel and dissolved mineral can leave. *Holly* and *Gray*,[93] using a plaque-free enamel surface, demonstrated that the rate of development of an artificial lesion was dependent principally on the rate of diffusion through the relatively intact surface layer. It is likely that in the more complex oral environment, the plaque, in addition to the surface enamel layer, will control the rate of development of the initial lesion.[79] For instance, the thickness and density of the plaque can influence the degree of calcium-phosphate saturation in it. This, in turn, will affect the pH at which the enamel dissolves. Any barrier to diffusion, such as an increased plaque solution viscosity, should slow the demineralization process. Conversely, agents that are able to maintain ions in solution at a higher pH, such as chelating agents, will enhance demineralization because of the longer time available for outward diffusion.

Bacterial invasion

The initial carious changes in the tooth and the advancing front of the lesion are believed to involve acid dissolution, with microorganisms invading the tooth secondarily (Fig. 1-8). Nevertheless, as reported by *Brannstrom* and co-workers,[94] microorganisms can be early invaders of demineralized tissue. These investigators placed 20 intact permanent teeth in the upper dentures of four patients. The patients wore the dentures from one to three years, following which the teeth were retrieved and the carious lesions that developed in the teeth were studied. They found bacteria in the enamel and dentin of teeth with white spots, as well as in teeth in which the lesions had cavitated.

As the carious process continues, cavitation occurs (Fig. 1-9). In addition to the dissolution of calcium-phosphate salts, the enamel's organic matrix is also removed. Likewise, carious destruction of the dentin involves an attack upon both the organic and inorganic components. Some of the organic matrix is simply dissolved by acid; however, the remainder is broken down by the proteolytic activity of the bacteria that have invaded the tooth.[94-96]

Tooth and host variables

The important host factors that influence the tooth's susceptibility to decay are diagramed in Figure 1-10. Such factors as diet, plaque, and bacterial flora have already been discussed. These are environmental factors and are generally alterable by a change in the behavior of the host. The other factors, relating to the tooth and the saliva, are intrinsic to the host. Nevertheless, under the proper circumstances, these are also modifiable.

Morphology and position

The relative position of teeth and their morphology influence caries susceptibility. The surfaces of the teeth that are most caries susceptible, the occlusal and proximal surfaces, are also the areas that are least easily cleaned by toothbrushing and are least accessible to the saliva.[97-99] These areas provide protective enclaves for the retention of plaque and food debris. The proximal surfaces of teeth that are crowded and have tight contact areas are considered to be more susceptible to decay because of their greater propensity to harbor plaque. Conversely, teeth with proximal spacing, in which the surfaces are more amenable to physical cleaning and are accessible to the saliva, are less prone to develop caries.

Chemical composition

Normal enamel consists of approximately 96% mineral by volume (hydroxyapatite, a form of calcium-phosphate), 1% organic material, and 3% water. It is porous, allowing many ions to pass through at measurable rates, but it is also quite dense, having a specific gravity of almost 3.0.

The enamel surface reflects its environment. It acquires trace elements from the saliva and from the tissue fluids in which it is bathed prior to eruption.[100,101] Some of the elements reduce the tooth's susceptibility to decay, whereas others increase it. The presence of fluoride in enamel correlates with a low susceptibility to dental decay. Other elements that may have a caries-inhibitory effect due to their incorporation into enamel or their presence in plaque include molybdenum, vanadium, strontium, copper, boron, lithium, and gold.[47] Some elements that appear to favor the formation of caries are selenium, magnesium, cadmium, platinum, and lead.[47]

Fluoride is more concentrated at the enamel surface than in deeper enamel. Conversely, carbonate, a compound that increases enamel solubility and, presumably, caries susceptibility, is less concentrated at the surface.[102] *Nikiforuk* and *Grainger*[103] studied the interrelationship between fluoride and carbonate in enamel using primary teeth obtained from fluoridated and fluoride-deficient communities. The ratio of carbonate to fluoride was markedly different between carious and noncarious teeth in both areas (Table 1-1). The CO_3/F ratio was lowest in the enamel of caries-free teeth from a fluoridated community and highest in the enamel of carious teeth from a fluoride-deficient community. Fluoride can replace carbonate in enamel. While the data presented in Table 1-1 indicate that a low CO_3/F ratio results in a more caries-resistant enamel, the role of carbonate in caries susceptibility still requires further research.

Table 1-1 Ratio of carbonate to fluoride (CO_3/F) in enamel from fluoridated and fluoride-deficient communities

	F in water (ppm)	
Caries status of teeth	0.1	1.0
Caries-free	1.52	0.53
Carious	2.45	0.93

Adapted from Nikiforuk and Grainger.[103]

Posteruptive maturation

Maturation is generally referred to as the deposition of mineral into the enamel during pre- and posteruptive periods. During the preeruptive phase, minerals, including trace elements, are derived from the tissue fluid bathing the tooth. After eruption, minerals are derived from food and saliva.

During the initial stages of enamel mineralization, the enamel matrix is relatively porous, allowing a rather uniform deposition of mineral. However, as mineralization progresses, ionic movement becomes progressively restricted until only the outer surface is readily accessible. This results in the surface accumulating higher concentrations of trace elements.

Posteruptive maturation occurs as calcium and phosphate from saliva are deposited in the remaining available sites on the enamel surface.[104-106] All enamel, however, cannot be considered "normal" upon eruption. Developmental faults are frequently present and may be more susceptible to caries,[71] a condition that has been well documented in rat and hamster enamel. One hundred percent of newly erupted rat molars have been shown to contain areas of hypomineralization.[107,108] These areas increase in number and severity when the animals are placed on a cariogenic diet.[107] (This change could result from either an increase in size of already existing areas or from demineralization of previously sound areas.) In the presence of a noncariogenic diet, or of one lack-

ing cariogenic microorganisms, the hypomineralized areas will mineralize (mature) within 60 days.[108-110]
Studies on laboratory animals have shown that newly erupted teeth are more susceptible to decay than teeth that have been exposed to the oral environment.[105,111] Maturation of the hypomineralized areas is believed to be the reason why fewer caries develop in animals as they become older.
Von der Fehr[112] suggested that in humans mineral deposition, or maturation, continues throughout the life of the tooth. *Von der Fehr* also found that maturation can occur rapidly. He removed the enamel surface by abrasion and then measured the amount of ^{32}P acquired at intervals after the abrasion. He concluded that maturation of abraded enamel was complete within 7 to 14 days. The rate of maturation, however, may vary and is not necessarily the same for all surfaces.[113] For instance, *Fitzgerald* and *Larson*[111] found that the smooth surfaces of rat molars mature more rapidly than fissure surfaces. Materials that interfere with crystal growth (such as phosphonates) may inhibit maturation of hypomineralized areas,[113] whereas crystallization promoters (such as fluoride) will promote the rate of maturation.[106,113]
The influence of maturation on demineralization of human enamel was demonstrated on extracted teeth by *Yonan* and *Fosdick*.[114] These investigators applied acid to longitudinal sections prepared from first molars of individuals of varying ages. They found that the area of relatively acid-resistant surface enamel was wider in sections prepared from older individuals. *Carlos* and *Gittelsohn*[115] have shown that the probability of human permanent teeth decaying is greatest during the first two to three years after eruption and decreases thereafter. This substantiates the clinical impression that the susceptibility of teeth to decay decreases with age. Experiments with rat and hamster molars do not establish either the rate of maturation of human enamel or the relative importance of hypomineralized areas in human caries formation. However, the work of *Yonan* and *Fosdick* suggests that chemical changes of the enamel with age may influence the caries susceptibility of human teeth.

Saliva

Saliva consists of the secretions of the major salivary glands—the sublingual, submandibular, and parotid—and the minor salivary glands. Cervicular exudate also contributes to the fluid in the mouth generally referred to as "saliva."
The importance of saliva as a mediating factor in caries development has been demonstrated in both animals and humans. Extirpation of the salivary glands in animals significantly increases caries incidence.[116] Similarly, any condition that causes xerostomia in humans, such as irradiation of the salivary glands, prolonged use of anticholinergic drugs, pathological conditions like Sjögren's syndrome in which the quantity of saliva is reduced, usually is associated with the development of rampant caries.[117-119]
Physical, chemical, and biological properties of the saliva have been implicated in providing protection against caries.[120-122] The physical properties of saliva that have been studied are its viscosity and flow rate. These factors affect the saliva's ability to physically wash adherent particles from the teeth. Chemical properties include composition, such as calcium and phosphate concentrations, pH, and salivary buffering capacity. These factors alter the cariogenicity of the plaque. Biological properties include the presence of antibacterial factors (e.g., lysozyme—an enzyme found in both saliva and tears; immunoglobulins—especially salivary IgA; and the peroxidase system—enzymes released by the parotid and submandibular glands), proline-rich peptides and statherin (which stabilize high calcium

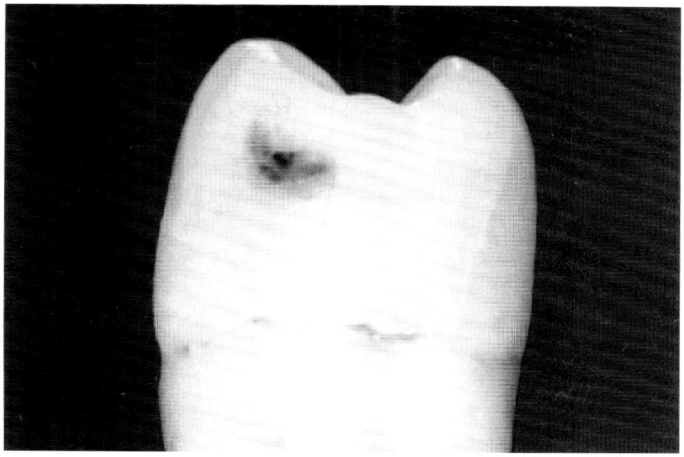

Fig. 1-11 A "brown spot" lesion on the proximal surface of a human permanent tooth. The brown spot is an area of altered enamel that is believed to signify an arrested lesion.

concentrations in saliva), and lactoferrin (which interferes with bacterial metabolism). Recently, *Kleinberg* and co-workers[123] isolated a salivary peptide, which they call sialin, and which they believe has anticariogenic properties.

Caries resistance and repair

Destruction of enamel, principally through acid dissolution, is no longer regarded as the only dynamic process that occurs within the carious lesion. In the last 20 years, the concept that resistance and reparative mechanisms occur concomitantly with the process of dissolution has gained acceptance.[124-128] This theory is consistent with the clinical findings that some lesions not only arrest, but also reverse to their previously sound state.[71]

Acquisition of organic material

As previously described, white spots represent the earliest macroscopic evidence of caries. They are characterized by porosity in which the intercrystalline spaces, normally present in enamel, increase in both volume and number. These microspaces do not remain empty, but rather fill with water and organic material.[129,130]

A white spot may arrest or may fail to advance to the stage of cavitation. White spot lesions that undergo arrestment often appear clinically as "brown spots" (Fig. 1-11). The brown color is from the accumulation into the enamel pores of organic material originating from the overlying plaque, saliva, and food.[131-134]

The presence of brown spots in areas of known caries predilection was recognized by *Miller* nearly 100 years ago.[1] *Miller* noted that the discoloration occurred when the decay process was very slow or had arrested. Others have equated the degree of discoloration to the age of the lesion and have also found a direct relationship between the number of brown spots on proximal surfaces and the patient's age.[135] *Bibby*[128] has suggested that the accumulated organic material may act to increase the resistance of these arrested areas to further demineralization.

Acquisition of fluoride

Weatherell and co-workers[136] have demonstrated that porous or slightly demineralized enamel, such as the white spot lesion, has a greater capacity to acquire fluoride than adjacent sound enamel. This finding agrees with the series of reports by *Little* and co-workers[134,137,138] in which they found three to five times as much fluoride in altered (white or brown spot) enamel compared to sound enamel. Using microtechniques, *Weatherell* and co-workers were able to map the fluoride distribution within the several zones of white spot lesions.[136] As seen in Figure 1-12, the highest concentration of fluoride is in the relatively intact surface layer.

While the increased concentration of fluoride in white spot enamel is probably due to the greater capacity of demineralized enamel to absorb fluoride, the unequal distribution within the lesion may be partially due to a preferential dissolution of enamel crystallites as the lesion develops.[139,140] In any event, the greater fluoride concentration of the white spot lesion imparts a degree of chemical resistance to acid dissolution, which is not enjoyed by adjacent sound enamel, thus potentially altering the rate of progress of the lesion.

Remineralization

Remineralization is the deposition of calcium, phosphate, and other ions into areas previously demineralized by caries or other causes. While remineralization and posteruptive maturation are similar phenomena, they differ in that the former involves deposition of mineral into *de*mineralized, as distinct from *hypo*mineralized, areas. In the process, the enamel prism structure or the enamel crystals are not necessarily reconstructed in their original forms. Instead, the quantity of mineral in the altered area is increased by growth on existing crystals or by precipitation into the enamel pores.

Saliva has been thought to be the natural remineralizing solution.[141-143] However, since most lesions are covered by plaque, the available concentrations of calcium and phosphate in plaque fluid and the effect of plaque on ionic diffusion are important factors in the remineralization process.

Reversals

A *reversal* occurs when a tooth surface initially diagnosed as carious is, at a subsequent examination, found to be sound. While this difference can be the result of an error in examination or recording, there is now general acceptance of the concept that changes in the enamel can occur whereby an initially carious lesion (e.g., a white spot) can revert to a sound status.[72,144,145]

Reversals are the result of enamel remineralization. The likelihood of white spots undergoing remineralization depends upon such factors as their location, the duration of the lesion and age of the patient, and changes within the oral cavity that affect cariogenic conditions at the tooth surface.

White spots on smooth surfaces appear to remineralize under natural conditions more easily than lesions on pit and fissure surfaces. *Backer-Dirks*[71] observed the fate of 72 white spot lesions on the buccal surfaces of first permanent molars in 8-year-old children. After several years, nine of the lesions had advanced to the stage of cavitation, while 26 still remained white spots; however, 37 of the surfaces were diagnosed as sound. *Backer-Dirks* stated that the white spot always preceded cavitation by about two years. If a white spot had been present for two years without becoming a cavity, there was little probability that cavitation would occur within the age group studied.

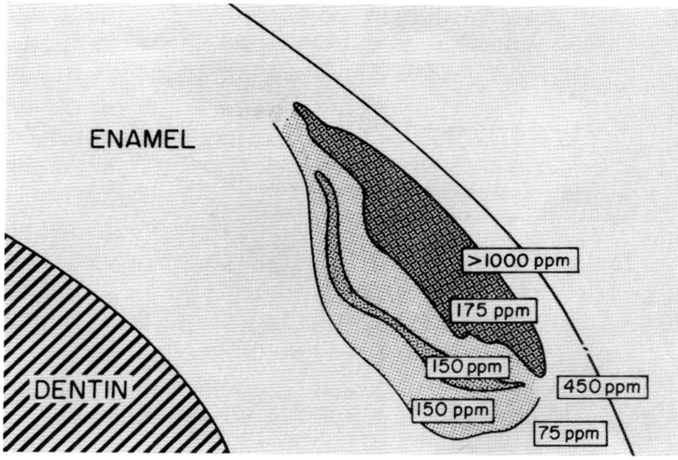

Fig. 1-12 A typical distribution of fluoride within a white spot lesion. The relatively intact surface layer has a higher fluoride content (> 1,000 ppm) than sound surface enamel (450 ppm). The body of the lesion, positive zone, and translucent zone have higher fluoride levels (175, 150, and 150 ppm, respectively) than sound inner enamel (75 ppm). Concentrations approximate.
(Modified from *Weatherell* et al.[136])

In the same study, *Backer-Dirks* found that only half of early carious lesions, diagnosed radiographically on the proximal surfaces of 8- to 15-year-old children, progressed to cavitation; whereas white spots in fissures cavitated rapidly.[71] Conversely, in a study by *Hyde,*[146] it was reported that 82% of radiographically diagnosed proximal surface lesions in 10-year-old children progressed to the dentin within two years. It should be remembered, however, that when a proximal lesion is large enough to be detected radiographically, the lesion has actually advanced histologically to the dentoenamel junction or beyond.[147]

Kolehmainen and *Rytomaa*[148] studied the two-year caries increment in Finnish dental students. Cavitation of occlusal white spots did not occur as rapidly as was reported by *Backer-Dirks.* While the dental students' oral hygiene practices may have altered the rate of development and progression of the carious lesions, it is highly likely that, in this older age group, the investigators were evaluating teeth that were more resistant to decay.

Reversals of white lesions were also reported in the Turku xylitol studies.[149] Chalky lesions that were present at the baseline examination reverted to a clinically sound status when xylitol (a sweet pentose alcohol not readily metabolized by plaque microorganisms) was substituted for sucrose in the diet.

Experimentally induced caries in humans were also reported to undergo reversal.[150] Subjects rinsed nine times daily with a 50% sucrose solution and refrained from oral hygiene practices. As a result, white spot areas in the enamel resembling early carious lesions developed within 23 days. With the cessation of the sucrose rinses, reestablishment of oral hygiene practices, and institution of daily mouthrinses of 0.2% sodium fluoride, the incipient lesions entirely disappeared and the enamel regained its normal appearance.

Rehardening

Indirect evidence of remineralization comes from microhardness studies. Softening of the enamel is presumptive evidence of acid dissolution and caries development, while *rehardening* of previously softened areas suggests remineralization.

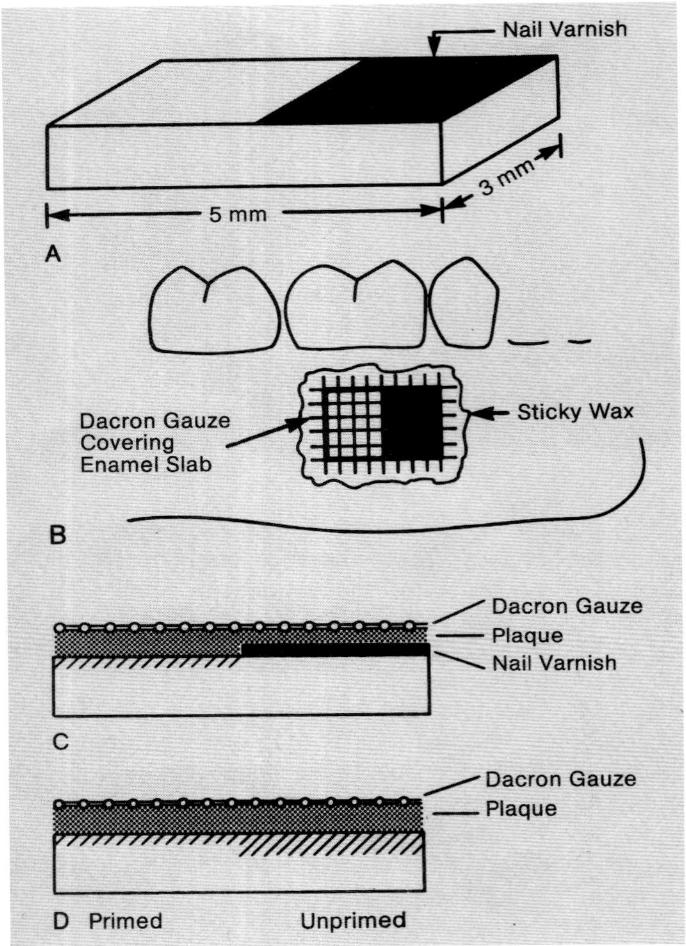

Fig. 1-13 Steps in cariogenic priming experiment. A) A slab of human enamel with one-half of the surface protected with a coating of nail varnish. B) Prepared slab attached to denture base and covered with Dacron gauze. C) Cross section through enamel slab showing relationship of plaque to nail varnish-protected and unprotected sides. After 1 week intraorally beneath the Dacron gauze, the unprotected half undergoes slight cariogenic demineralization (becomes "primed"). D) Cross section through enamel slab after the nail varnish was removed and the entire surface treated with topical fluoride solution. After 1 month intraorally beneath the Dacron gauze, the primed side exhibits less demineralization. (After the method of *Koulourides* et al.[156])

Koulourides induced the development of cariogenic changes on blocks of enamel that were mounted in removable acrylic insets on fixed bridges worn in patients' mouths.[125] To allow plaque to form, the enamel surfaces were covered with protective Teflon patches. Within a week, the Teflon-covered enamel surfaces showed softening as demonstrated by microhardness tests. When the patches were removed, exposing the enamel to the saliva, a rehardening, consistent with a precipitation of calcium-phosphate salts on the previously softened enamel, occurred.

Controlled etching

Controlled application of phosphoric acid to tooth enamel is the principal step in *acid-etch* dentistry techniques. Clinically, a one-minute treatment with 50% phosphoric acid will impart a dull opaque appearance to the tooth surface. Histologically, the surface appears pitted from preferential prism-end demineralization patterns.[151] If left untreated, such areas return to their normal translucency and surface texture in a matter of days.[152,153] Presumably, the treated enamel has been remineralized by the deposition of calcium-phosphate salts from the saliva.

Subsurface precipitation

Since fermentable carbohydrates are not present continuously, the formation of acid at the plaque-tooth surface interface or its presence within the lesion is not continuous. The pH of the microenvironment of the lesion, therefore, fluctuates. As the pH falls, mineral dissolves, but with a rise in pH some of the mineral reprecipitates. In a broad sense, this reprecipitation is part of remineralization.

The type of inorganic crystals precipitated at different points during the rise in pH toward neutrality will depend on the proportions of inorganic ions present and will be influenced considerably by the presence of trace elements. For example, a very small amount of fluoride will enhance reprecipitation of apatite crystal structures such as hydroxyapatite and fluoroapatite.[154,155]

The fluctuations in pH, with its concomitant dissolution and reprecipitation, may explain some of the histological features of the early carious lesion. Reprecipitation of previously dissolved mineral may account for the occurrence of areas of smaller pore size (the dark or positive zone) than is found in either the body of the lesion or unaffected enamel. Since mineral dissolved from the interior of the lesion must diffuse out, during its passage some mineral may reprecipitate at the enamel surface.[87] This reprecipitation is likely related to the persistence of the relatively more intact surface layer of the white spot.

Cariogenic priming

Koulourides and co-workers[156] have demonstrated experimentally that areas of carious demineralization, when treated with topical fluoride solutions, are more resistant to further demineralization than noncarious enamel similarly treated with fluoride. The investigators refer to this as "cariogenic priming" of the enamel.

In their experiment, small slabs of human enamel were attached to dentures worn by test subjects. Half of each enamel surface was protected with nail varnish and the entire surface was covered with a Dacron gauze before intraoral insertion (Fig. 1-13a and b). Plaque accumulated between the Dacron and test enamel surfaces causing demineralization of the halves that were unprotected by the nail varnish (Fig. 1-13c). The cariously demineralized portions of the enamel slabs constituted the "primed" surfaces. The slabs were removed from the dentures after one week, and the accumulated plaque and nail varnish were removed. The primed and unprimed surfaces were treated for four minutes with either 2% sodium fluoride or 8% stannous fluoride solution. The slabs were again covered with the Dacron gauze, reattached to the dentures, and worn for one month (Fig. 1-13d).

The recovered slabs were examined for visual changes and for changes in surface hardness. The unprimed halves exhibited an opaque whiteness typical of subsurface demineralization to a greater extent than the primed halves; additionally, the surfaces of the unprimed halves were softer than the primed ones.

Thin sections were prepared from the enamel slabs and were evaluated microradiographically. Figure 1-14 shows the microradiographic appearance of two enamel slabs. In both, the side that received the initial cariogenic challenge (the primed surface) suffered less enamel demineralization from one month's exposure beneath the Dacron gauze than the side that was initially protected by the nail varnish (unprimed surface), despite the fact that both received the same fluoride treatment.

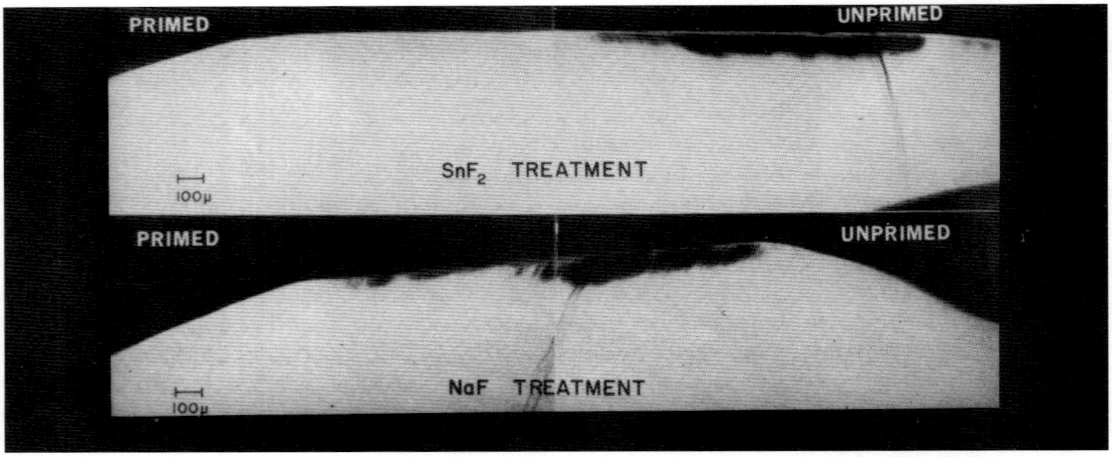

Fig. 1-14 Microradiographs of sections of enamel slabs demonstrating the less demineralized subsurface lesions of the primed sides compared to the unprimed sides. Both sides were similarly treated with topical fluoride solutions.
(With the compliments of Dr. T. *Koulourides* and *Caries Research.*)

The investigators' conclusion that minor cariogenic alterations of the enamel may be beneficial for remineralization and increased resistance to subsequent cariogenic attacks has important clinical implications. It further strengthens the concept that fluoride intervention can not only prevent the initiation of new carious lesions, but can also alter the progress of already existing ones.

Summary

Dental caries is a dynamic process of demineralization and proteolysis, the continuation of which leads to the ultimate destruction of the tooth. If caries are to initiate, the occurrence will usually be during the first two to three years after a tooth's eruption. Caries can only develop, however, by the favorable confluence of three factors: (1) microorganisms that adhere to the tooth surface, (2) carbohydrates that the microorganisms can readily metabolize to acid, and (3) a tooth surface that will dissolve in the acid. Several bacterial species have been indicated as cariogenic. *Streptococcus mutans* has been especially implicated in the initiation of lesions on the smooth coronal surfaces, while *Actinomyces viscosus* and *naeslundii* have been associated with the development of root caries. *Lactobacilli* appear to proliferate once the lesion has cavitated and are believed to aid in its progression, but usually not in its initiation. Because the morphology of pits and fissures offers a favorable site for colonization of microorganisms, streptococci, actinomyces, and lactobacilli have all been associated with lesions on the occlusal surface.

Many carbohydrates can be metabolized by oral microorganisms. Nevertheless, sucrose has been labeled the most cariogenic carbohydrate in the human diet. It is readily diffusable into plaque; it serves as a substrate for acid production; and it is a precursor of the polyglucans that give the plaque its adherent properties. Dietary habits, however, can influence cariogenicity. The choice of carbohydrate foods whose physical properties make them retentive and frequent snacking are both habits that increase a diet's capability to induce dental decay.

The teeth themselves differ in their susceptibility to decay. Their morphology, position in the arch, chemical composition, and degree of maturation are all factors that affect their fate after eruption. In addition, the teeth react with their posteruptive environment acquiring both organic and inorganic materials that further affect their ultimate disease course.

While caries is generally regarded as destructive, the chemical interaction occurring between the affected tooth surface and the oral environment can, under the proper circumstances, render a tooth *less* susceptible to acid dissolution. Teeth that develop initial white spot lesions need not cavitate. Not only can a lesion cease to progress (i.e., it arrests), but it can also reverse to a clinically sound state. The role that fluoride plays in these processes was briefly mentioned in this chapter and will be discussed in more detail later.

References

1. Miller, W.D. 1890. Micro-organisms of the human mouth. S.S. White Dental Mfg. Co.
2. Orland, F.J.; Blayney, R.; Harrison, R.W.; Reyniers, J.A.; Trexler, P.C.; Wagner, M.; Gordon, H.A.; and Luckey, T.D. 1954. Use of the germ-free animal technic in the study of experimental dental caries. I. Basic observations on rats reared free of all microorganisms. *J. Dent. Res.* 33:147-74.
3. Orland, F.J.; Blayney, J.R.; Harrison, R.W.; Ervin, R.F.; Reyniers, J.A.; Trexler, P.C.; Gordon, H.A.; and Wagner, M. 1955. Experimental caries in germ-free rats inoculated with enterococci. *J. Amer. Dent. Assoc.* 50:259-72.
4. Fitzgerald, R.J., and Keyes, P.H. 1960. Demonstration of the etiologic role of streptococci in experimental caries in the hamster. *J. Amer. Dent. Assoc.* 61:9-19.
5. Keyes, P.H. 1960. Infectious and transmissible nature of experimental dental caries — findings and implications. *Arch. Oral Biol.* 1:304-20.
6. Shaw, J.H., and Sweeney, E.A. 1957. Studies on the influence of antibiotic substances in dental caries in the white and cotton rat. *J. Dent. Res.* 36:349-60.
7. van Houte, J.; Gibbons, R.J.; and Pulkkinen, A.J. 1972. Ecology of human oral lactobacilli. *Infect. Immun.* 6:723-29.
8. Ikeda, T.; Sandham, H.J.; and Bradley, E.L., Jr. 1973. Changes in *Streptococcus mutans* and lactobacilli in plaque in relation to the initiation of dental caries in Negro children. *Arch. Oral Biol.* 18:555-66.
9. Fitzgerald, R.J.; Jordan, H.V.; and Archard, H.O. 1966. Dental caries in gnotobiotic rats infected with a variety of *Lactobacillus acidophilus*. *Arch. Oral Biol.* 11:473-76.
10. Rosen, S.; Lenney, W.S.; and O'Malley, J.E. 1968. Dental caries in gnotobiotic rats inoculated with *Lactobacillus casei*. *J. Dent. Res.* 47:358-63.
11. Loesche, W.J., and Syed, S.A. 1973. The predominant cultivable flora of carious plaque and carious dentine. *Caries Res.* 7:201-16.
12. Keyes, P.H. 1968. Research in dental caries. *J. Amer. Dent. Assoc.* 76:1357-73.
13. Llory, H.; Guillo, B.; and Frank, R.M. 1971. A cariogenic *Actinomyces viscosus* — a bacteriological and gnotobiotic study. *Helv. Odontol. Acta* 15:134-38.
14. Frank, R.M.; Guillo, B.; and Llory, H. 1972. Caries dentaires chez le rat gnotobiote inoculé avec *Actinomyces viscosus* et *Actinomyces naeslundii*. *Arch. Oral Biol.* 17:1249-53.
15. Jordan, H.V., and Hammond, B.F. 1972. Filamentous bacteria isolated from human root surface caries. *Arch. Oral Biol.* 17:1333-42.
16. Jordan, H.V.; Keyes, P.H.; and Bellack, S. 1972. Periodontal lesions in hamsters and gnotobiotic rats infected with actinomyces of human origin. *J. Periodont. Res.* 7:21-26.
17. Guillo, B.; Klein, J.P.; and Frank, R.M. 1973. Fissure caries in gnotobiotic rats infected with *Actinomyces naeslundii* and *Actinomyces israelii*. *Helv. Odontol. Acta* 17:27-30.
18. van der Hoeven, J.S.; Mikx, F.H.M.; Konig, K.G.; and Plasschaert, A.J.M. 1974. Plaque formation and dental caries in gnotobiotic and SPF Osborne-Mendel rats associated with *Actinomyces viscosus*. *Caries Res.* 8:211-23.
19. Syed, S.A.; Loesche, W.J.; Pape, H.L., Jr.; and Grenier, E. 1975. Predominant cultivable flora isolated from human root surface caries plaque. *Infect. Immun.* 11:727-31.
20. Drucker, D.B. 1970. Optimum pH values for

growth of various plaque streptococci, *in vitro.* In *Dental plaque,* ed. W.D. McHugh, pp. 241-48. Dundee, Scotland: D.C. Thompson.

21. Carlsson, J. 1967. Presence of various types of non-haemolytic streptococci in dental plaque and in other sites in the oral cavity in man. *Odont. Rev.* 18:55-74.
22. Carlsson, J.; Soderholm, G.; and Almfeldt, I. 1969. Prevalence of *Streptococcus sanguis* and *Streptococcus mutans* in the mouth of persons wearing full dentures. *Arch. Oral Biol.* 14:243-49.
23. Gibbons, R.J., and van Houte, J. 1971. Selective bacterial adherence to oral epithelial surfaces and its role as an ecological determinant. *Infect. Immun.* 3:567-73.
24. van Houte, J.; Gibbons, R.J.; and Pulkkinen, A.J. 1971. Adherence as an ecological determinant for streptococci in the human mouth. *Arch. Oral Biol.* 16:1131-41.
25. Guggenheim, B., and Schroeder, H.E. 1967. Biochemical and morphological aspects of extracellular polysaccharides produced by cariogenic streptococci. *Helv. Odontol. Acta* 11:131-52.
26. Ikeda, T.; Shiota, T.; McGhee, J.R.; Otake, S.; Michalek, S.M.; Ochiai, K.; Hirasawa, M.; and Sugimoto, K. 1978. Virulence of *Streptococcus mutans:* comparison of the effects of coupling sugar and sucrose on certain metabolic activities and cariogenicity. *Infect. Immun.* 19:477-80.
27. Gibbons, R.J., and Banghart, S. 1968. Variation in extracellular polysaccharide synthesis by cariogenic streptococci. *Arch. Oral Biol.* 13:697-701.
28. Fitzgerald, R.J.; Jordan, H.V.; and Stanley, H.R. 1960. Experimental caries and gingival pathologic changes in the gnotobiotic rat. *J. Dent. Res.* 39:923-35.
29. Zinner, D.D.; Aran, A.P.; Saslaw, M.S.; Jablon, J.M.; and Fitzgerald, R.J. 1967. Induction of dental caries in gnotobiotic rats by streptococci of human origin. *Nature* 213:200-201.
30. Zinner, D.D.; Jablon, J.M.; Aran, A.P.; and Saslaw, M.S. 1965. Experimental caries induced in animals by streptococci of human origin. *Proc. Soc. Exp. Biol.* 118:766-70.
31. Zinner, D.D.; Jablon, J.M.; Aran, A.P.; Saslaw, M.S.; and Fitzgerald, R.J. 1966. Comparative pathogenicity of streptococci of human origin in hamster caries. *Arch. Oral Biol.* 11:1419-20.
32. Gibbons, R.J.; Berman, K.S.; Knoettner, P.; and Kapsimalis, B. 1966. Dental caries and alveolar bone loss in gnotobiotic rats infected with capsule forming streptococci of human origin. *Arch. Oral Biol.* 11:549-60.
33. Gibbons, R.J., and Loesche, W.J. 1967. Isolation of cariogenic streptococci from Guatemalan children. *Arch. Oral Biol.* 12:1013-14.
34. Krasse, B. 1966. Human streptococci and experimental caries in hamsters. *Arch. Oral Biol.* 11:429-36.
35. Hoerman, K.C.; Keene, H.J.; Shklair, I.L.; and Burmeister, J.A. 1972. The association of *Streptococcus mutans* with early carious lesions in human teeth. *J. Amer. Dent. Assoc.* 85:1349-52.
36. Shklair, I.L.; Keene, H.J.; and Simonson, L.G. 1972. Distribution and frequency of *Streptococcus mutans* in caries-active individuals. *J. Dent. Res.* 51:882.
37. Keene, H.J., and Shklair, I.L. 1974. Relationship of *Streptococcus mutans* carrier status to the development of carious lesions in initially caries-free recruits. *J. Dent. Res.* 53:1295.
38. Gibbons, R.J.; DePaola, P.F.; Spinell, D.M.; and Skobe, Z. 1974. Interdental localization of *Streptococcus mutans* as related to dental caries experience. *Infect. Immun.* 9:481-88.
39. Schamschula, R.G., and Charlton, G. 1971. A study of caries aetiology in New South Wales school children. I. The streptococcal flora of plaque and caries prevalence. *Aust. Dent. J.* 16:77-82.
40. de Stoppelaar, J.D.; van Houte, J.; and Backer-Dirks, O. 1969. The relationship between extracellular polysaccharide-producing streptococci and smooth surface caries in 13-year-old children. *Caries Res.* 3:190-99.
41. Berkowitz, R.J. 1976. *Streptococcus mutans* — establishment and transmission in infants. *J. Dent. Child.* 43:192-95.
42. Berkowitz, R.J., and Jordan, H.V. 1975. Similarity of bacteriocins of *Streptococcus mutans* from mother and infant. *Arch. Oral Biol.* 20:725-30.
43. Berkowitz, R.J.; Jordan, H.V.; and White, G. 1975. The early establishment of *Streptococcus mutans* in the mouths of infants. *Arch. Oral Biol.* 20:171-74.
44. Edman, D.C.; Keene, H.J.; Shklair, I.L.; and Hoerman, K.C. 1975. Dental floss for implantation and sampling of *Streptococcus mutans* from approximal surfaces of human teeth. *Arch. Oral Biol.* 20:145-48.
45. Loesche, W.J.; Walenga, A.; and Loos, P. 1973. Recovery of *Streptococcus mutans* and *Streptococcus sanguis* from a dental explorer after clinical examination of single human teeth. *Arch. Oral Biol.* 18:571-75.
46. Keene, H.J.; Shklair, I.L.; and Hoerman, K.C. 1976. Partial elimination of *Streptococcus*

mutans from selected tooth surfaces after restoration of carious lesions and SnF_2 prophylaxis. *J. Amer. Dent. Assoc.* 93:328-33.
47. Navia, J.M. 1970. Effect of minerals on dental caries. In *Dietary chemicals vs. dental caries,* ed. R.S. Harris, pp. 123-60. Washington, D.C.: American Chemical Society.
48. Pigman, W. 1970. Carbohydrates, fats and dental caries. In *Dietary chemicals vs. dental caries,* ed. R.S. Harris, pp. 7-22. Washington, D.C.: American Chemical Society.
49. Barenie, J.T., and Bibby, B.G. 1977. Food-caries interrelationships. In *Oral hygiene in oral health,* eds. H.J.V. Goldberg and L.W. Ripa, pp. 256-82. Springfield, Ill.: Charles Thomas.
50. Makinen, K.K. 1972. The role of sucrose and other sugars in the development of dental caries; a review. *Int. Dent. J.* 22:363-86.
51. Newbrun, E. 1969. Sucrose, the arch criminal of dental caries. *J. Dent. Child.* 36:239-48.
52. Shannon, I.L. 1977. Sucrose—the tooth's mortal enemy; fluoride—the tooth's best friend. *J. Dent. Child* 44:429-37.
53. Green, R.M. and Hartles, R.L. 1969. The effect of diets containing different mono- and disaccharides on the incidence of dental caries in the albino rat. *Arch. Oral Biol.* 14:235-41.
54. Frostell, G.; Keyes, P.H.; and Larson, R.H. 1967. Effect of various sugars and sugar substitutes on dental caries in hamsters and rats. *J. Nutr.* 93:65-76.
55. Shaw, J.H.; Krumins, I.; and Gibbons, R.J. 1967. Comparison of sucrose, lactose, maltose, and glucose in the causation of experimental oral diseases. *Arch. Oral Biol.* 12:755-68.
56. Guggenheim, B.; Konig, K.G.; Herzog, E.; and Mühlemann, H.R. 1966. The cariogenicity of different dietary carbohydrates tested on rats in relative gnotobiosis with a streptococcus producing extracellular polysaccharide. *Helv. Odontol. Acta* 10:101-13.
57. Kleinberg, I. 1974. The role of dental plaque in caries and inflammatory periodontal disease. *J. Canad. Dent. Assoc.* 40:56-66.
58. Guggenheim, B. 1970. Extracellular polysaccharides and microbial plaque. *Int. Dent. J.* 20:657-78.
59. Cornick, D.E.R., and Bowen, W.H. 1972. The effect of sorbitol on the microbiology of the dental plaque in monkeys *(Macaca Irus). Arch. Oral Biol.* 17:1637-48.
60. Bourgeau, G., and McBride, B.C. 1976. Dextran-mediated interbacterial aggregation between dextran-synthesizing streptococci and *Actinomyces viscosus. Infect. Immun.* 13:1228-34.
61. Bowen, W.H., and Cornick, D.E. 1967. Effects of carbohydrate restriction in monkeys (*M. Irus*) with active caries. *Helv. Odontol. Acta* 11:27-31.
62. van Houte, J. 1964. Relationship between carbohydrate intake and polysaccharide-storing micro-organisms in dental plaque. *Arch. Oral Biol.* 9:91-93.
63. Shklair, I.L.; Hoffman, S.; and Tow, H.D., Jr. 1970. The cariogenic potential of some streptococci in relatively gnotobiotic Osborne-Mendel rats. *IADR Abst.* 48th general meeting, Abst. 24, p. 54. New York.
64. Schachtele, C.F.; Loken, A.E.; and Schmitt, M.K. 1972. Use of specifically labeled sucrose for comparison of extracellular glucan and fructan metabolism by oral streptococci. *Infect. Immun.* 5:263-66.
65. Gustafsson, B.E.; Quensel, C.E.; Lanke, L.S.; Lundquist, C.; Grahnen, H.; Bonow, B.E.; and Krasse, B. 1954. The Vipeholm dental caries study. The effect of different levels of carbohydrate intake on caries activity in 436 individuals observed for five years. *Acta Odontol. Scand.* 11:232-364.
66. Weiss, R.L., and Trithart, A.H. 1960. Between-meal eating habits and dental caries experience in preschool children. *Am. J. Pub. Health* 50:1097-1104.
67. Dunay, L.F.; Zinner, D.D.; and Jablon, J.M. 1972. Epidemiologic studies of caries-free and caries-active students: II. Diet, dental plaque, and oral hygiene. *J. Dent. Res.* 51:727-33.
68. Stephan, R.M. 1940. Changes in hydrogen-ion concentration in tooth surfaces and in carious lesions. *J. Amer. Dent. Assoc.* 27:718-23.
69. Kleinberg, I. 1970. Formation and accumulation of acid on the tooth surface. *J. Dent. Res.* 49:1300-1316.
70. Fejerskov, O.; Thylstrup, A.; and Larsen, M.J. 1977. Clinical and structural features and possible mechanisms of dental fluorosis. *Scand. J. Dent. Res.* 85:510-34.
71. Backer-Dirks, O. 1966. Post-eruptive changes in dental enamel. *J. Dent. Res.* 45:503-11.
72. Groeneveld, A., and Purdell-Lewis, D.J. 1977. The origin and behavior of white spot enamel lesions. *Netherlands Dent. J.* 85 (Suppl. 15):6-18.
73. Silverstone, L.M. 1977. Structural alterations of human dental enamel during the incipient lesion development. In *Proceedings of a symposium on incipient caries of enamel,* ed. N.H. Rowe, pp. 3-50. Ann Arbor: Univ. of Michigan Press.
74. Silverstone, L.M. 1973. Structure of carious enamel, including the early lesion. *Oral Sci. Rev.*

3:100-160.
75. Gustafson, G. 1957. The histopathology of caries of human dental enamel with special reference to the division of the carious lesion into zones. *Acta Odontol. Scand.* 15:13-55.
76. Guzman, C.I.; Brudevold, F.; and Mergamen, H. 1957. A soft roentgen ray study of early carious lesions. *J. Amer. Dent. Assoc.* 55:509-15.
77. Darling, A.I. 1956. Studies on the early carious lesion of enamel with transmitted light, polarized light, and radiography. *Brit. Dent. J.* 101:289-97, 329-41.
78. Soni, N., and Brudevold, F. 1959. Microradiographic and polarizing microscopic study of sound enamel. *J. Dent. Res.* 38:1181-86.
79. Brown, W.E. 1974. Physiochemical mechanisms of dental caries. *J. Dent. Res.* 53 (Suppl. to no. 2):204-16.
80. von Bartheld, F. 1961. Membrane phenomena in carious dissolution of the teeth. *Arch. Oral Biol.* 6:284-303.
81. Meckel, A.H. 1965. The formation and properties of organic films on teeth. *Arch. Oral Biol.* 10:585-97.
82. Meckel, A.H. 1968. The nature and importance of organic deposits on dental enamel. *Caries Res.* 2:104-11.
83. Pearce, E.I.F., and Bibby, B.G. 1966. Effects of time, surface area, pH, and some ions on protein adsorption by bovine enamel. *Arch. Oral Biol.* 11:825-32.
84. Francis, M.D.; Briner, W.W.; and Gray, J.A. 1973. Chemical agents in the control of calcification processes in biological systems. In *Hard tissue growth, repair, and remineralization,* pp. 56-90. Ciba Foundation, Symposium 11.
85. Gray, J.A. 1966. Kinetics of enamel dissolution during formation of incipient caries-like lesions. *Arch. Oral Biol.* 11:397-421.
86. Gwinnett, A.J. 1966. Histology of normal enamel. IV. Microradiographic study. *J. Dent. Res.* 45:870-73.
87. Weatherell, J.A; Robinson, C.; and Hallsworth, A.S. 1974. Variations in the chemical composition of human enamel. *J. Dent. Res.* 53 (Suppl. to no. 2):180-92.
88. Brudevold, F. 1962. Chemical composition of the teeth in relation to caries. In *Chemistry and prevention of dental caries,* ed. R.F. Sognnaes. Springfield, Ill.: Charles C. Thomas.
89. Ingraham, G. 1973. The role of carbonate in dental mineral. *Caries Res.* 7:217-30.
90. Moreno, E.C., and Zahradnik, R.T. 1974. Chemistry of enamel subsurface demineralization *in vitro. J. Dent. Res.* 53:226-35.
91. Featherstone, J.D.B. 1977. Diffusion phenomena during artificial carious lesion formation. *J. Dent. Res.* 56:D48-D52.
92. Groeneveld, A., and Arends, J. 1975. Influence of pH and demineralization time on mineral content, thickness of surface layer, and depth of artificial caries lesions. *Caries Res.* 9:36-44.
93. Holly, F.J., and Gray, J.A. 1968. Mechanism for incipient carious lesion growth utilizing a physical model based on diffusion concepts. *Arch. Oral Biol.* 13:319-34.
94. Brannstrom, M.; Friskopp, J.; Isacsson, G.; and Wictorin, L. 1977. Experimental caries in young human permanent teeth implanted in removable dentures. *Arch. Oral Biol.* 22:571-78.
95. Johnson, N.W.; Taylor, B.R.; and Berman, D.S. 1969. The response of deciduous dentine to caries studied by correlated light and electron microscopy. *Caries Res.* 3:348-68.
96. Frank, R.M. 1967. The ultrastructure of the tooth from the point of view of mineralization, demineralization, and remineralization. *Int. Dent. J.* 17:661-83.
97. Mandel, I.D. 1978. Effectiveness of biomedical and biosocial research on improving oral health. *J. Public Health Dent.* 38:312-23.
98. Grainger, R.M.; Paynter, K.J.; and Shaw, J.H. 1959. Differences in morphology and size of the teeth of a caries susceptible and a caries resistant strain of rats. *J. Dent. Res.* 38:105-20.
99. Grainger, R.M.; Paynter, K.J.; Honey, L.; and Lewis, D. 1966. Epidemiologic studies of tooth morphology. *J. Dent. Res.* 45:693-702.
100. Brudevold, F.; Steadman, L.T.; and Smith, F.A. 1960. Inorganic and organic components of tooth structure. *Ann. N.Y. Acad. Sci.* 85:110-32.
101. Retief, D.H.; Cleaton-Jones, P.E.; Turkstra, J.; and DeWet, W.J. 1971. The quantitative analysis of sixteen elements in normal human enamel and dentine by neutron activation analysis and high-resolution gamma spectrometry. *Arch. Oral Biol.* 16:1257-67.
102. Sobel, A.E.; Shaw, J.H.; Hanok, A.; and Nobel, S. 1960. Calcification. XXVI. Caries susceptibility in relation to composition of teeth and diet. *J. Dent. Res.* 39:462-72.
103. Nikiforuk, G., and Grainger, R.M. 1965. Fluoride-carbonate-citrate interrelations in enamel. In *Tooth enamel,* eds. M.V. Stack and R.W. Fernhead, pp. 26-31. Bristol, England: John Wright & Sons.
104. Fanning, R.J.; Shaw, J.H.; and Sognnaes, R.F. 1954. Salivary contribution to enamel maturation and caries resistance. *J. Amer. Dent. Assoc.* 49:668-71.
105. Larson, R.H., and Fitzgerald, R.J. 1964. Caries development in rats of different ages with con-

trolled flora. *Arch. Oral Biol.* 9:705-12.

106. Speirs, R.L. 1967. Factors influencing "maturation" of developmental hypomineralized areas in the enamel of rat molars. *Caries Res.* 1:15-31.
107. Francis, M.D., and Brinner, W.W. 1966. The development and regression of hypomineralized areas of rat molars. *Arch. Oral Biol.* 11:349-54.
108. Fitzgerald, R.J., and Konig, K.G. 1968. Maturation of dental enamel in germ-free and monoinfected Sprague-Dawley rats. *Helv. Odontol. Acta* 12:55-61.
109. Briner, W.W., and Rosen, S. 1967. Effect of fluoride on hypomineralized areas in the molars of rats fed a cariogenic diet. *Arch. Oral Biol.* 12:1077-84.
110. Yonan, T.; Nicolau, J.; and Fosdick, L.S. 1966. The posteruptive maturation of teeth. II. Normal posteruptive maturation of hamster teeth. *J. Dent. Res.* 45:1701-5.
111. Fitzgerald, R.J., and Larson, R.H. 1967. Age and caries susceptibility in gnotobiotic rats. *Helv Odontol. Acta* 11:49-52.
112. von der Fehr, E.R. 1965. Maturation and remineralization of enamel. *Adv. Fluorine Res.* 3:83-95.
113. Briner, W.W.; Francis, M.D.; and Widder, J.S. 1971. Factors affecting the rate of posteruptive maturation of dental enamel. *Calcif. Tissue Res.* 7:249-56.
114. Yonan, T., and Fosdick, L.S. 1964. The degree of etching as a function of the age of the teeth. *J. Dent. Res.* 43:629.
115. Carlos, J.P., and Gittelsohn, A.M. 1965. Longitudinal studies of the natural history of caries—II. A life-table study of caries incidence in the permanent teeth. *Arch. Oral Biol.* 10:739-51.
116. Finn, S.B.; Klapper, C.E.; and Volker, J.F. 1955. Intraoral effects upon experimental hamster caries. In *Advances in experimental caries research,* ed. R.F. Sognnaes, pp. 152-68. Washington, D.C.: Amer. Assoc. for the Advancement of Science.
117. Karmiol, M., and Walsh, R.F. 1975. Dental caries after radiotherapy of the oral regions. *J. Amer. Dent. Assoc.* 91:838-45.
118. Dreizen, S.; Daly, T.E.; Drane, J.B.; and Brown, L.R. 1977. Oral complications of cancer radiotherapy. *Postgrad Med.* 61:85-92.
119. Bahn, S.L. 1972. Drug-related dental destruction. *Oral Surg.* 33:49-54.
120. Levine, R.S. 1977. The aetiology of dental caries—an outline of current thought. *Int. Dent. J.* 27:341-48.
121. Newbrun, E. 1978. Current concepts of caries etiology. In *Cariology,* pp. 15-43. Baltimore: Williams & Wilkens.
122. Kleinberg, I.; Ellison, S.A.; and Mandel, I.D. 1979. *Saliva and dental caries: a special supplement to microbiology abstracts.* New York: Information Retrieval.
123. Kleinberg, I.; Kanapka, J.A.; and Craw, D. 1977. The effect of saliva and salivary factors on the metabolism of the mixed oral flora. In *Microbial aspects of dental caries,* eds. H.M. Stiles, W.L. Loesche, and T.C. O'Brien, pp. 433-64. Washington, D.C.: Information Retrieval.
124. Koulourides, T. 1962. Remineralization of enamel and dentin. *Dent. Clin. N. Amer.* July: 485-97.
125. Koulourides, T. 1966. Dynamics of tooth surface-oral fluid equilibrium. *Advances in Oral Biol.* 2:149-71.
126. Wei, S.H.Y. 1967. Remineralization of enamel and dentine—a review. *J. Dent. Child.* 34:444-51.
127. Silverstone, L.M. 1977. Remineralization phenomena. *Caries Res.* 11 (Suppl. 1):59-84.
128. Bibby, B.G. 1971. Organic enamel material and caries. *Caries Res.* 5:305-22.
129. Frank, R.M. 1965. The ultrastructure of caries resistant teeth. In *Ciba Foundation symposium: caries resistant teeth,* eds. G.E.W. Wolstenholme and M. O'Connor, pp. 169-84. Boston: Little, Brown.
130. Johansen, E. 1965. Comparison of the ultrastructure and chemical composition of sound and carious enamel from human permanent teeth. In *Tooth enamel,* eds. M.V. Stack and R.W. Fernhead, pp. 177-81. Bristol, England: John Wright & Sons.
131. Bhussry, B.R. 1958. Chemical and physical studies of enamel from human teeth. II. Specific gravity, nitrogen content, and hardness rating of discolored enamel. *J. Dent. Res.* 37:1045-53.
132. Little, M.F.; Cueto, E.S.; and Rowley, J. 1962. Chemical and physical properties of altered and sound enamel. I. Ash, Ca, P, CO_2, N, water, microradiolucency and density. *Arch. Oral Biol.* 7:173-84.
133. Bhussry, B.R. 1958. Chemical and physical studies of enamel from human teeth. III. Specific gravity, nitrogen content and histologic characteristics of opaque white enamel. *J. Dent. Res.* 37:1054-59.
134. Little, M.F.; Cooper, H.C.; and Rowley, J. 1971. Inorganic-organic interactions in human dental enamel. In *Tooth enamel II,* eds. R.W. Fernhead and M.V. Stack, pp. 100-18. Bristol, England: John Wright & Sons.
135. Turesky, S.S. 1941. Brown spots. *Tufts Dental Outlook* 2:13-17.

136. Weatherell, J.A.; Deutsch, D.; Robinson, C.; and Hallsworth, A.S. 1977. Assimilation of fluoride by enamel throughout the life of the tooth. *Caries Res.* 11(Suppl. 1):85-115.
137. Little, M.F.; Posen, J.; and Singer, L. 1962. Chemical and physical properties of altered and sound enamel. 3. Fluoride and sodium content. *J. Dent. Res.* 41:784-89.
138. Little, M.F., and Steadman, L.T. 1966. Chemical and physical properties of altered and sound enamel. IV. Trace element composition. *Arch. Oral Biol.* 11:273-78.
139. Johnson, N.W. 1967. Some aspects of the ultrastructure of early human enamel caries seen with the electron microscope. *Arch. Oral Biol.* 12:1505-21.
140. Frank, R.M., and Brendel, A. 1966. Ultrastructure of the approximal dental plaque and the underlying normal and carious enamel. *Arch. Oral Biol.* 11:883-912.
141. Pickel, F.D.; Cort, W.; Starr, N.; Bilotti, A.; and Pigman, W. 1965. Evaluation of enamel rehardening agents in saliva. *J. Dent. Res.* 44:855-59.
142. Koulourides, T.; Feagin, F.; and Pigman, W. 1965. Remineralization of dental enamel by saliva *in vitro*. *Ann. N.Y. Acad. Sci.* 131:751-57.
143. Pigman, W.; Kotwal, K.; and Koulourides, T. 1966. Calcifying ability of human body fluids. *Arch. Oral Biol.* 11:815-24.
144. Marthaler, T.M. 1978. Clinical-visual and radiographic grading of dental caries. In *Methods of caries prediction,* eds. B.G. Bibby and R.J. Shern, pp. 281-84. Washington, D.C.: Information Retrieval.
145. Kleinberg, I.; Chatterjee, R.; Domokos, A.; Castaldi, C.R.; Fain, M.; and Chebib, F. 1978. An ultraviolet photographic technique for the early detection of carious lesions. In *Methods of caries prediction,* eds. B.G. Bibby and R.J. Shern, pp. 271-79. Washington, D.C.: Information Retrieval.
146. Hyde, E.J. 1973. Caries inhibiting action of three different topically applied agents on incipient lesions in newly erupted teeth: results after 24 months. *J. Canad. Dent. Assoc.* 39:189-93.
147. Gwinnett, A.J. 1972. A comparison of proximal carious lesions as seen by clinical radiography, contact microradiography, and light microscopy. *J. Amer. Dent. Assoc.* 83:1078-80.
148. Kolehmainen, L., and Rytomaa, I. 1977. Increment of dental caries among Finnish dental students during a period of two years. *Community Dent. Oral Epidemiol.* 5:140-44.
149. Scheinin, A.; Makinen, K.K.; Tammisalo, E.; and Rekola, M. 1975. Turku sugar studies. XVIII. Incidence of dental caries in relation to 1-year consumption of xylitol chewing gum. *Acta Odontol. Scand.* 33 (Suppl. 70):307-16.
150. von der Fehr, F.R.; Löe, H.; and Theilade, E. 1970. Experimental caries in man. *Caries Res.* 4:131-48.
151. Gwinnett, A.J. 1976. The scientific basis of the sealant procedure. *J. Prev. Dent.* 3(Mar.–Apr.): 15-28.
152. Albert, M., and Grenoble, D.E. 1971. An *in vivo* study of enamel remineralization after acid etching. *J. South. Calif. State Dent. Assoc.* 39:747-51.
153. Arana, E.M. 1974. Clinical observations of enamel after acid etch procedure. *J. Amer. Dent. Assoc.* 89:1102-6.
154. Feagin, F.F., and Gonzalez, M. 1973. Fluorapatite crystal growth during remineralization of enamel surfaces. *Ala. J. Med. Sci.* 10:46-51.
155. Gonzalez, M., and Feagin, F. 1973. Electron microscopy of enamel surface after reactions of apatite accretion. *J. Oral Path.* 2:142-49.
156. Koulourides, T.; Keller, S.E.; Manson-Hing, L.; and Lilley, V. 1980. Enhancement of fluoride effectiveness by experimental cariogenic priming of human enamel. *Caries Res.* 14:32-39.

Chapter 2

Anticaries Mechanisms of Fluoride

Evidence suggests that fluoride is capable of producing a much greater cariostatic effect than is now attained with currently used preparations and procedures. This is because patients may not utilize the preparations available to them in the most effective manner. Formulations prepared for safety, patient acceptance, and convenience, as a necessity, may not have therapeutically optimal formulas, and frequently there is some question about the best method or procedure to use in the dental clinic. If the cariostatic effects of fluoride are to be maximized, the patient must be educated, improvements in formulations sought, and treatment procedures optimized. Fundamental to each of these is an understanding of how fluoride produces its anticaries effects. This is especially true since a large amount of evidence suggests that fluoride provides these effects in several ways, and that under certain conditions several mechanisms may function simultaneously.

The possibility of several anticaries mechanisms functioning simultaneously is easily seen by referring to Figure 1-1 in Chapter 1. This figure shows the three fundamental requirements for caries to develop. Two of them encompass the caries challenge (i.e., bacteria and its food supply), and the third relates to host or enamel resistance. There is considerable evidence showing that fluoride can modify or eliminate factors in each of the three areas. If one of the factors is modified or reduced in intensity, caries formation will be slowed; however, if several are modified simultaneously even greater effects should be attained.

The mechanisms by which fluoride increases caries resistance may arise from both systemic and topical applications of fluoride and can broadly be grouped as follows:

- increased enamel resistance
- increased rate of maturation
- remineralization of incipient lesions
- interference with microorganisms
- improved tooth morphology

It is the purpose of this chapter to present the evidence supporting each of these mechanisms and to discuss their relative importance as applied to the fluoride preparations currently available to dentists and patients.

Increased enamel resistance

It has been well established that dental caries is a disease involving dissolution of enamel by acids from bacterial plaque and that dissolution is inhibited by the presence of fluoride. Because fluoride forms fluorapatite, a less soluble mineral, it has long been thought that the anticaries effect of fluoride is the result of reduced solubility and that a greater amount of fluorapatite results in a greater solubility reduction. Thus, resistance to caries has been studied in the laboratory and clinic by determination of the solubility of enamel in acid and by determination of the amount of fluoride present. The following sections present a brief description of the physicochemical basis upon which fluoride reduces enamel solubility and then the evidence, both positive and negative, obtained first from solubility experiments and second from determinations of enamel fluoride levels showing their relationship to caries.

Physicochemical basis

The dissolution of dental enamel during a caries attack is a complicated and poorly understood process. This is because hydroxyapatite is a complex mineral and its solubility depends on the composition of the dissolving solution, which is also complicated and continuously changing. When enamel is exposed to a pH of about 5.5 or lower,[1] it will dissolve according to the following equation:

$$Ca_{10}(PO_4)_6(OH)_2 + 8H^+ \longrightarrow 10Ca^{++} + 6HPO_4^{=} + 2H_2O$$

Because this ordinarily occurs beneath a bacterial plaque, the concentration of calcium, phosphate, and other ions in the solution will increase. When the plaque stops producing acid (H^+), the pH rises and the amount of dissolved mineral the solution can hold will diminish. This results in the precipitation of some of the mineral. Calcium, phosphate, and other ions originally present in the plaque will add to those dissolved from the enamel and affect the pH at which precipitation begins and also the types of compounds formed. Thus, carious dissolution of enamel can be seen as a cyclic phenomenon consisting of phases of demineralization and reprecipitation that are determined by changes in the pH and ionic concentrations within the plaque and the lesion.

The presence of fluoride in the dissolution medium effectively reduces the solubility of the enamel by promoting the precipitation of hydroxyapatite and by preventing the formation of more soluble calcium phosphate minerals.[1] In addition to fluorapatite already present in the enamel, more fluorapatite may also form.

$$\underset{\text{hydroxyapatite}}{Ca_{10}(PO_4)_6(OH)_2} + 2F^- \longrightarrow \underset{\text{fluorapatite}}{Ca_{10}(PO_4)_6F_2} + 2OH^-$$

It has been shown that a small amount of fluoride in an acid solution can have a pronounced effect on hydroxyapatite (enamel) solubility.[2,3] This can be explained by the finding that when hydroxyapatite is exposed to low fluoride concentrations (about 1 ppm), a layer of fluorapatite forms on the hydroxyapatite crystals. This thin layer causes the hydroxyapatite to act as though it were all fluorapatite governing the rate of dissolution.[3,4,5]

Both of the hydroxyl groups in hydroxyapatite need not be replaced by fluoride for the hydroxyapatite to have a lower solubility. *Moreno* et al.[6] found that the lowest solubility was attained when only 58% of the hydroxyl groups were replaced by fluoride. This may be related to the hydrogen bonding that occurs between the hydroxyl (OH^-) and fluoride (F^-) ions when fluoride fills voids from missing hydroxyl groups in the apatite lattice.[7]

Another possible reason why a small amount of fluoride may have a large effect on enamel solubility is related to the dissolution pattern of the hydroxyapatite crystals. A two-site model for enamel dissolution has been proposed based on crystal morphology.[8] The model was developed after findings that enamel crystals dissolve by forming a hole along the C axis leading to a hollow shell that eventually fragments if the dissolution process is continued,[9,10] and also that acids and chelating agents (EDTA) dissolve enamel differently. Acids primarily attack the prism centers,[11,12] whereas EDTA primarily attacks the periphery of the prisms.[11,12,13] (However, variable enamel etching patterns with acid have also been reported.[14])

The two-site model states that hydroxyapatite crystals have two different sites from which dissolution can occur. One of the sites is more soluble than the other. Thus, to protect only this site, less fluoride would be required than for protection of the entire crystal.

Brown et al.[2] proposed a mechanism for the solubility-reducing effect of fluoride based on a modification of the Donnan membrane model.[16] He assumed that the plaque and outer enamel acted as a permselective membrane permitting only cations to pass through thus allowing calcium to leave the interior of the enamel and protons (H^+) to enter. From a study of phase diagrams, *Brown* concluded that the ultimate effect of fluoride on the conditions within a carious lesion is to alter the rate of diffusion of ions in a way that decreases the rate of dissolution. The diffusion rate was also affected by an artificial pellicle (i.e., salivary deposit) that slowed the formation of artificial lesions, presumably by its permselectivity.[17,18]

Caries resistance related to reduced enamel solubility

Evidence from systemically acquired fluoride

Several studies have compared caries scores to the acid solubility of teeth formed in areas with different concentrations of fluoride in the drinking water (i.e., teeth that acquired fluoride systemically—prior to the eruption of the teeth in the mouth). A positive correlation between solubility and caries was found in six studies,[19-24] but no correlation in four.[19,24-26]

A correlation between the amount of fluoride in enamel and its solubility has shown that enamel with a high fluoride level is less soluble than enamel with a low fluoride level.[27] *Isaac* et al.[28] studied different types of teeth obtained from several areas and compared the solubility of enamel to fluoride content. The findings showed a good correlation between dissolution in acid and fluoride content within a given geographic area, but also that a specific fluoride concentration was not always associated with a specific solubility (Fig. 2-1). The solubility of normal surfaces of carious teeth also was found not to differ from surfaces of noncarious teeth.[29] This suggests that there are other factors that differ between communities and that also affect solubility.

Evidence from topically acquired fluoride

Fluoride can affect the solubility of enamel not only when it is acquired during enamel formation but also when it is given as a topical application. However, because the mode of acquisition is different, the effect may be different. For example, a high level of fluoride acquired prior to eruption is more effective in slowing enamel dissolution *in vitro* than the same level acquired topically.[30]

Reduction in enamel solubility *in vivo* was shown in humans after use of fluoride dentifrices,[31-35] topical solutions,[34,36-38] and rinses.[36] A 34% reduction was found three days after a topical application of an amine fluoride solution. After using an amine fluoride dentifrice for three months, a 23% reduction was found, and after an amine fluoride mouth rinse, 22%. Daily application of 0.4% stannous fluoride gel by toothbrush gave a 25 to 30% reduction after one week.[38]

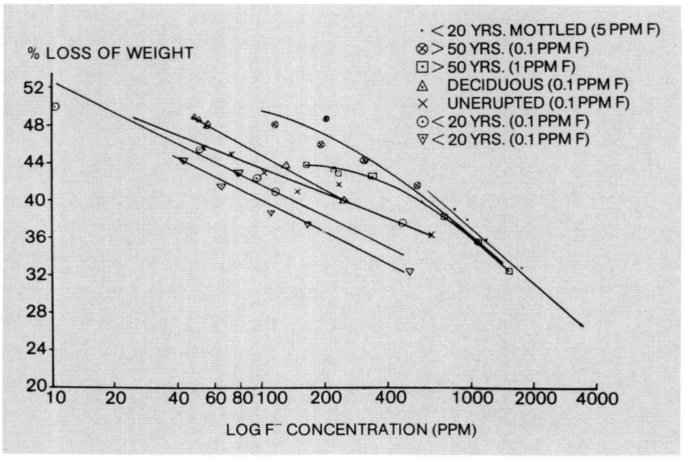

Fig. 2-1 Log F^- concentration (ppm) versus solubility rate. Successive layers of enamel exposed to acetate buffer pH 4 (1 hour).
(*Isaac* et al.[28] Reproduced with permission of the author and the *J. Dent. Res.*)

Another demonstration of the effect of fluoride on enamel solubility was obtained in studies where a gold plate was fitted over a tooth *in vivo*. This produced a stagnant area of increased caries challenge between the tooth surface and gold plate.[39] When the enamel covered by the gold plate was first treated with fluoride, the relatively sound outer layer of enamel remaining over the developing carious lesion, was thicker,[40,41] indicating greater resistance to the caries process.

Experiments with rats have also shown enamel solubility reduction after topical application of fluoride;[42,43] however, in one study it was found that the solubility reduction was not necessarily accompanied by a decrease in caries and, conversely, a diminished caries experience could occur without a reduction in enamel solubility.[44]

Caries resistance related to enamel fluoride

Evidence from systemically acquired fluoride

When teeth are formed, they acquire an amount of fluoride in the surface enamel reflecting the concentration of fluoride in the local drinking water. Thus, when teeth from different water fluoride areas are compared, it is not surprising that high enamel fluoride levels are found to be related with low caries prevalence.[21,45,46] When comparisons were made within single communities, where the range of enamel fluoride levels is less than between communities, statistically significant correlations were not found,[45,47-54] except in a study where systemic fluoride supplements were given. In this study,[55] the group that received fluoride supplements had higher enamel fluoride levels and lower caries scores.

Although all of the studies did not show a clear relationship between enamel fluoride and caries, undoubtedly because of many uncontrollable factors, it has been calculated that at least 16% of the variation in caries can be attributed to differences in enamel fluoride.[45]

A positive correlation of high enamel fluoride with caries resistance is also suggested by the caries history of subjects whose teeth were formed under the influence of fluoridated drinking water but who later moved to nonfluoridated areas. *Deatherage*[56] found that subjects who moved from fluoridated

water areas maintained some protection for as long as 20 years. Systemically administered fluoride has also been reported to provide residual protection lasting at least several years (Table 2-1).
Finally, primary enamel normally contains lower fluoride levels than permanent enamel and also appears to be less well protected by water fluoridation.[59]

Evidence from topically acquired fluoride

At least three studies have shown that fluoride acquired during *frequent* exposure to fluoride rinses or gels is not related in any simple fashion to the caries inhibition received. In Cheektowaga, New York, neutral and acidulated phosphate fluoride (APF) gels containing 0.5% fluoride were self-applied to the teeth of children each school day for two years. At the end of this time, the fluoride concentration in a thin outer layer of enamel from exfoliated deciduous teeth had increased to 4,200 ppm when the APF gel was used and 1,700 ppm when the neutral gel was used.[60] At that time, the clinical examination revealed an 80% reduction in the number of new decayed, missing, and filled teeth (DMFT) in the APF group and a 75% reduction in the neutral fluoride group.[61] The difference in caries reduction between the two groups was not statistically significant.
Similar studies were conducted with APF and neutral mouth rinses.[62,63] In these studies, enamel fluoride uptake from neutral rinses was modest (approximately 20 ppm), whereas it was significantly higher from the APF rinses (80–500 ppm). However, despite the difference in fluoride uptake, caries inhibition was similar—about 30% in all cases.[64,35] Although it appears from these studies that topically acquired enamel fluoride may not be the major reason for caries protection *during the course of the clinical trials*, when other more important mechanisms related to the frequency of fluoride exposure could have been functioning, the possibility remains that enamel fluoride may provide a future or residual benefit.
If a significant amount of topically acquired fluoride is permanently bound in the enamel and provides an anticaries effect, the effect should continue after fluoride therapy ceases. If the fluoride is not permanently bound or does not affect caries resistance, the rate of new caries formation should return to the pretreatment level. In other words, caries formation would simply be postponed. To determine residual protection, caries increments must be calculated not only during the period of fluoride application, but also for several years after treatments have ceased. Investigation of the residual anticaries effects of topical fluoride application has been carried out in only a few cases (Table 2-1).
Because the deposition of fluoride in enamel from topical fluoride treatments varies considerably with the type of fluoride and procedure, evaluation of the residual effects of those treatments expected to deposit a small amount of fluoride in enamel should be considered separately from those expected to deposit a large amount. Treatments not expected to deposit significant fluoride in sound enamel include dilute neutral fluoride, such as that used in mouth rinses, and infrequent applications of more concentrated neutral sodium fluoride. Posttreatment caries increments from several studies of this type have been reported. *Knutson* and *Armstrong*[66] reported a positive residual effect, which appeared to increase with time up to three years after a short series of 2% NaF applications. Conversely, *Sundvall-Hagland* et al.[67] found no residual effect from 2% NaF applications and, in fact, the treatment group had an increased caries rate after the first year. *Syrrist*[68] also tested 2% NaF applications and found no residual effect after the first year. *Bibby* and *Turesky*[69] applied 0.1% NaF to a very small group of subjects and reported that most of the protection was

Table 2-1 Residual anticaries effects following fluoride exposures

Study	Treatment	Caries Reduction: During treatment period	Caries Reduction: During period (years) following treatment
Deatherage[56]	F water to age 8		33% Adults (approx. 13–20 years)
Russell[57]	F water–various periods		Some (for a few years)
Way[58]	F water to age 12		21% (two years)**
Knutson and Armstrong[66]	2% NaF, 7–15 times within 8 weeks	12% (1st yr)	25% (2nd year) 33% (3rd year)
Bibby[69]	0.1% NaF, 3/year for 2 years	48%	30% (3 years)
Syrrist[68]	2% NaF, 3-4/year for 2 years	51%	1% (1st year) 38% (2nd year) 6% (3rd year) 2% (4th year) 2% (5th year)
Sundvall-Hagland et al.[67]	2% NaF 4 times within 15 days (deciduous teeth)	34% (1st yr)	+ 4% (2nd year) +60% (3rd year)
Koch[70]	0.5% NaF rinse 1/2 weeks (school) for 3 years	22%	0% (2 years)
Koch[71]	0.1% F dentifrice daily (school) for 3 years	37%	20% (2 years)
Englander et al.[72]	0.5% F gel daily (school) for 2 years	pH 4.5 gel — 81% pH 7.0 gel — 79%	63% (2 years) 55% (2 years)
Horowitz et al.[73]	APF solution 1/year for 3 years	35%	24% (2 years)
	APF solution 1/6 months for 3 years	49%	30% (2 years)
	APF gel 1/year for 3 years	26%	10% (2 years)
Houwink et al.[74]	1% SnF_2 2/year for 9 years	40%	12% (5 years)
Mellberg et al.[75]	APF gel daily 10 or 25 school days (F water)	30-35%	0% (2 years)

*42% in similar group of lifetime residents in F water area.

**Calculated on basis of 60% inhibition from F water.

maintained for three years following the applications. In more recent studies, *Koch*[70] found no residual effect from a 0.5% NaF mouth rinse given once every two weeks for three years in school, but did find residual benefits after three years of daily use of a 0.1% dentifrice.[71]

In contrast to the above studies, where the treatments were not likely to deposit much fluoride in sound enamel, several studies with acidic fluoride preparations, which deposit more fluoride in enamel, have demonstrated positive residual benefits. *Englander* et al.[72] found that most of the benefit of a daily APF gel (0.5% F) applied with custom-fitted mouth trays was maintained for at least two years. In the same study, they also used a neutral gel that was shown to deposit a relatively large amount of fluoride[60] and found a large residual benefit. *Horowitz* and *Kau*[73] used APF solution and gel (1.2% F) once or twice per year and also found significant residual benefits after two years. *Houwink* et al.[74] applied 1% fluoride as SnF_2 twice per year for nine years and found some residual effect during the following five years. In contrast to these studies, *Mellberg* et al.[75] found no residual protection after a short series of APF gel (1.2% F) applications in an area with fluoridated drinking water.

Studies of fluoride deposition in animal teeth have also suggested residual anticaries effects. In a study designed to differentiate between the possible fluoride protective mechanisms, it was found that caries formation in the rat could be inhibited by about 50% if the fluoride levels in the enamel were increased to 1,500 before instituting the cariogenic challenge[76] (Table 2-2). Lower enamel fluoride levels were less effective. A partial residual effect has also been shown in hamsters.[77]

Table 2-2 Mean caries scores in rats with different enamel fluoride levels

Water F (ppm)	Enamel F (ppm)	Caries Score
0	320	58.6
10	590	50.7 (13)*
50	1,113	33.5 (43)
100	1,492	29.7 (49)
150	1,723	26.4 (55)

*Percent caries reduction

Data from *Larson* et al.[76]

Value of Deeply Located Fluoride

In many areas on teeth the thickness of enamel may be 1,000μ (1 mm) or more, but high fluoride concentrations are found only in the outer 30 to 50μ. This is the case both when the teeth are formed in an area of optimal water fluoride or when the fluoride is acquired topically after eruption. The fact that high levels of fluoride in sound enamel normally are restricted to the outer region may be related to the extent of its protective effect. Yet it is at depths below 30 to 50μ that the major initial loss of mineral occurs during caries formation. Therefore, it should not be too surprising that an inverse correlation between caries and surface enamel fluoride is difficult to demonstrate. This is not to imply that fluoride in surface enamel has no effect on caries resistance, for it has been shown that the outer, relatively sound layer of enamel over the incipient lesion is thicker when fluoride concentrations are high.[41]

To determine the extent of the value of fluoride in deep enamel, studies will have to be conducted to compare deep enamel fluoride and caries within individual communities. It has been reported that a correlation of DMFT with the ratio of fluoride in surface enamel (3 to 5μ deep) to fluoride in deeper enamel (4 to 7μ deep) suggests that DMFT is inversely related to caries in a nonfluoridated water area.[78]

Effect of fluoride in altered enamel

Up to this point, the discussion of enamel fluoride has been concerned with sound enamel. This is primarily because every study reported in the literature where an attempt was made to relate enamel fluoride to caries has dealt with sound enamel. However, unsound enamel can acquire fluoride topically and thereby be made more resistant to acid.

There are two types of unsound enamel that fluoride can affect: developmental *hypo*mineralized and acid *de*mineralized. Developmental hypomineralized enamel refers to specific areas on the teeth that are less than fully mineralized upon eruption and therefore will acquire somewhat larger amounts of fluoride from topical exposure. They are seen as small, opaque white areas of greater caries susceptibility.[79] Developmental hypomineralized areas in rat molars[80,81] have also been found, and their increased rate of disappearance in the presence of fluoride has been well documented. Acid demineralized enamel also takes up more fluoride than sound enamel. Increased fluoride levels have been found in enamel defects,[82] caries lesions,[83] and under plaque,[84] where it is presumed that the plaque periodically provides an acid environment for the enamel.

A correlation between the amount of fluoride in altered enamel and caries would be difficult to make and interpret because of the variability in size and location of the defects and the source and time of fluoride exposure. However, there is some evidence that fluoride acquired by early lesions may increase their resistance to subsequent challenge. An example of this was shown in a study[85] with rats where the animals were exposed to fluoride and cariogenic conditions in several ways. Prior to the start of the actual experiment, the enamel fluoride was increased to varying levels by giving the rats drinking water containing different amounts of fluoride during the period in which the teeth were erupting. Subsequently, the animals were given a caries challenge with or without continuous exposure to fluoridated drinking water. Other animals were given fluoridated water but not the cariogenic challenge. At the end of the experiment, the teeth were analyzed for fluoride and examined for caries. It was found that after the initial increase in enamel fluoride produced by the early administration of fluoride, a further increase resulting from fluoridated drinking water did not occur when the dietary conditions were noncariogenic; however, significant increases occurred under cariogenic conditions (Table 2-3).

In teeth with the lowest initial fluoride levels, fluoride increased the most, resulting in similar levels for all the animals that received the cariogenic challenge and fluoridated water. When the fluoridated drinking water was not given to the animals, the higher fluoride levels initially present provided approximately 50% caries inhibition. When fluoridated drinking water also was continuously given, the caries inhibition was much greater, in the range of 80 to 94%, regardless of the enamel fluoride initially present. These results can be interpreted as follows: The acid conditions present during the cariogenic challenge produced areas of demineralization representative of an early visually nondetectable stage of caries. These early lesions acquired fluoride from the fluoridated drinking water directly in proportion to the degree of demineralization. The degree of demineralization was related to the acid resistance of the enamel, greater resistance occurring when the initial enamel fluoride levels were high. In the absence of cariogenic conditions, there was no demineralization and, therefore, no fluoride uptake. After the enamel fluoride levels were increased by the combination of the initial caries attack and fluoridated water, the teeth became more resistant to further attack and the progression of the visually nondetectable lesions to cavities was stopped. Thus, in

Table 2-3 Effect of fluoride exposure during a cariogenic challenge

	Enamel Fluoride		Percent caries reduction	
	F drinking water		Non-F water	F water
Starting levels	No cariogenic challenge	cariogenic challenge	Cariogenic challenge	Cariogenic challenge
320	296	1,634	—	80
590	1,022	1,585	13	81
1,113	1,306	2,026	43	86
1,492	1,455	1,927	49	94
1,723	1,652	1,831	55	93

Data from *Mellberg* and *Larson*[85] and Larson et al.[76]

essence, enamel resistance to caries can be increased both by high fluoride levels in sound enamel and by the presence of low fluoride concentrations in the environment.

Summary of resistance effects

It is a widely held belief that the fluoride level of sound enamel is of primary importance in determining the resistance of the tooth to dental caries and that resistance is reflected by enamel solubility measurements. There is much evidence that teeth formed in fluoridated water areas where caries prevalence is low are both higher in fluoride and lower in acid solubility than teeth formed in nonfluoridated water areas. There is also much evidence that topical application of fluoride increases fluoride levels and reduces solubility. However, the findings are equivocal when the solubilities or systemically acquired fluoride levels of teeth found in individual subjects within a particular area are compared to caries scores or when enamel fluoride levels attained after frequent topical applications are related to caries inhibition.
These equivocal or conflicting findings need not necessarily negate the assumption that enamel fluoride is of value, since they probably result partly from the inadequacy of the test methods to measure under the proper conditions or at the proper site, and partly from the likelihood that the resistance of sound enamel is only one of several mechanisms by which fluoride inhibits caries. Surface enamel fluoride has been estimated as accounting for only 16% of the total fluoride effect. Fluoride acquired by altered enamel and fluoride concentrations below the enamel surface may be other important factors that increase the resistance of enamel to caries.

Increased rate of maturation

It is common clinical experience that the resistance of teeth to caries appears to increase posteruptively with age and it is axiomatic that greater benefits are obtained by topical fluoride when it is administered shortly after eruption of the teeth. It has been thought that this is because newly erupted enamel is able to acquire more fluoride than older enamel and thus can be made more resistant to further caries attack. Although there may be some truth in this, another, possibly more valid, reason for the greater benefits of topical fluoride noted on newly erupting teeth is its effect on the rate of posteruptive enamel maturation.

The existence of posteruptive maturation as a normal process has been discussed in Chapter 1. In essence, it was stated that newly erupted enamel has areas where mineral deposition is not entirely complete. These hypomineralized areas may become fully mineralized within only a few months after eruption.

The presence of even very small amounts of fluoride in a mineralizing solution enhances the precipitation of mineral. Therefore, the greatest importance of fluoride to the maturation process probably lies in its ability to increase the *rate* of mineralization of hypomineralized areas. In addition, hypomineralized areas that mature in the presence of fluoride should contain more fluoride than enamel that was fully mineralized upon eruption. These areas will therefore be made more resistant to acid.

Evidence from water fluoridation studies

Several investigations have shown that fluoridated drinking water can prevent caries on teeth that erupt prior to the start of community water fluoridation,[79,86-89] although the benefit may not extend to highly susceptible first molars.[90] Studies of fluoridation of school drinking water at higher than normal levels have also shown benefits to previously erupted teeth.[91,92] In general, these studies show that the greatest topical benefit is obtained if exposure to fluoridated water is begun immediately after eruption. Figure 2-2 shows the effect found by *Backer-Dirks*[79] on the distal surface of first molars of children who began drinking fluoridated water at different ages. The benefits prior to age 6 could be attributed to both preeruptive and posteruptive effects. However, after age 6, the benefits were entirely posteruptive. As the tooth became older before its first exposure to fluoridated water, the protection acquired posteruptively became correspondingly less.

Evidence from topical fluoridation studies

In relatively recent years, investigators of topical fluoride applications have reported the effects on newly erupting teeth separately from those on teeth present in the mouth at the beginning of the study. In almost every case, newly erupting teeth benefited to a greater degree.[93-95] A report by *Harris*[96] stated that there is not much additional benefit when topical sodium fluoride is given each year, rather than just at ages 3, 7, 11, and 13, when most of the primary or permanent teeth erupt. Although the additional benefits attained by newly erupted teeth may be due to greater fluoride uptake by sound areas of the enamel, it is quite likely that it is due to uptake by specific (hypomineralized) areas. An increased rate of maturation, coincidental with fluoride deposition in these areas, would result in a greater percentage of them remaining sound.

Evidence from animal studies

Numerous experiments with rats and hamsters have shown that susceptibility to caries decreases rapidly with the age of the animal.[97-101] *Speirs*[101] started two groups of litter-mate rats on a cariogenic diet at either age 21 days or age 35 days. This difference of only 14 days at which the cariogenic diet was given resulted in a significant difference in the caries scores of the two groups (Fig. 2-3).

Briner and *Rosen*[102] studied the effect of fluoride on the number of detectable hypomineralized areas in rats given a cariogenic diet with or without fluoride treat-

Table 2-4 Effect of diet and fluoride treatments on number of hypomineralized areas in rat molars

Diet	Topical F*	HMA at start	HMA after 21 days
Chow	No	64.1	57.7
Cariogenic	No	64.1	119.8
Cariogenic	Yes	64.1	31.8

*0.45% F (NaF) solution twice daily for 14 days.

Data from *Briner* and *Rosen*.[102]

ments. They found that after 21 days there was a decline in the number of hypomineralized areas in animals on a noncariogenic diet, but in the animals given a cariogenic sucrose diet, the number of detectable hypomineralized areas doubled. Apparently this was the result of an increase in size or severity of initially undetectable areas. When sodium fluoride (0.45% F) applications were given to animals on the cariogenic diet, the number of detectable hypomineralized areas decreased approximately 50% (Table 2-4). This was attributed to an enhancement of maturation. The fluoride treatments promoted the deposition of calcium and phosphate from the saliva into the hypomineralized areas.[103]

Remineralization of incipient lesions

Incipient lesions of enamel, generally known as *white spots*, have long been recognized as an early clinical stage of dental caries. *G. V. Black*, the father of modern dentistry, has been credited with saying, "He who understands the white spot of enamel understands dental caries."[104] The significance of this statement has been recognized by dental researchers throughout the world who, in various ways, have undertaken the task of better defining the white spot and its changes with time.

The early years of research on the anticaries mechanism of fluoride emphasized the effect of increased acid resistance conferred by the deposition of fluoride into the enamel. Although, as discussed earlier, this mechanism was able to account for some of the effect, much remained to be explained, and the emphasis has shifted to the phenomenon of remineralization. The ever-increasing number of citations in the literature related to remineralization, as both a natural and artificially initiated mechanism for caries prevention or repair, attests to its importance in current scientific thought. Studies on remineralization were done as early as 1912 by *Head*[105] and 1921 by *Andresen*,[106] but modern research began in the 1960s with the work of *Koulourides* and *Pigman*,[107] *von der Fehr*,[108] *Backer-Dirks*,[79] and others.

The formation, appearance, histology, and fate of incipient lesions were discussed in Chapter 1. Essentially, it was stated that incipient lesions (white spots) were opaque, white areas on the enamel having a relatively sound surface but with substantial mineral loss 30 to 50μ below the surface. When the environment of the lesion was cariogenic, as under an appropriate plaque, the demineralization continued until a cavity formed. However, if the environment was changed to allow free access to saliva, the lesion often became arrested or actually disappeared because of redeposition of mineral within the lesion (remineralization). A brown color, resulting from the presence of organic material, is usually associated with an arrested lesion.

Although saliva is the natural remineralizing solution, there is evidence that fluoride and synthetic solutions are more effective. This section will present the clinical evidence supporting acceleration of remineralization by synthetic solutions and fluoride, as well as some of the methodology and findings from laboratory experiments.

Clinical acceleration of remineralization

Many attempts have been made to produce clinical remineralization of white spot lesions. In almost every case, either calcium phosphate solutions, fluoride solutions, or a combination of the two has been used. As might be expected, the composition of remineralized enamel is different from normal enamel and may vary according to the conditions employed to produce the remineralization.[109-111,143,152,153] In the case where stannous fluoride is used, tin compounds may be deposited in the lesions.

Remineralization of natural white spots

Fluoride or calcium phosphate mouthwashes were used by several investigators to arrest or remineralize white spot lesions. *McCormick* et al.[112] reported that a remineralizing mouthwash appeared to produce clinical remineralization, but the results were not statistically significant. *Koulourides* and *Axelsson*[113] followed up on the treatment of 13-year-old children once every two weeks with professional tooth cleaning using a fluoride paste. They found a yearly increment of 0.5 new lesions per child, but a reversal rate of 0.9 lesions per child. The reversals, representing a change in the clinical status of teeth from carious to sound, were believed to be due to remineralization. In much earlier work, *Andresen*[106,114] applied remineralizing powder to white spots and reported that remineralization occurred in some cases. *Wilson*[115] applied a solution of bovine enamel to teeth and reported similar findings.

Reversals of early lesions are frequently reported in clinical trials of anticaries agents, but usually have been thought to be errors in diagnosis. However, considering current knowledge of incipient lesion formation and progression, many of these may have been true reversals due to remineralization. *Muhler*[116] pointed out that a reversal rate of 2 to 3% occurred after topical application of water, but the rate was 22 to 25% after application of stannous fluoride. Since the examinations were conducted without the investigator's knowing to what group the children belonged, *Muhler* believed the reversals associated with the stannous fluoride applications were true remineralizing phenomena. *Muhler* stated that areas of teeth previously considered carious had changed from chalky white and soft to pigmented and hard, and furthermore had not increased in size. *Muhler* and co-workers published other papers showing apparent arrest of carious lesions.[117,118]

A partial remineralizing effect may theoretically be reflected in a slowing or arrestment of the growth of caries lesions. Reports of caries arrest are numerous. In 1938, *Anderson*[119] reported that white spots were arrested and rehardened under favorable conditions. *Ostrom*[120] reported that 90 to 100% of incipient lesions in a group of subjects with a mean age of 14 became arrested after semiannual application of acidulated phosphate fluoride and oral hygiene instruction. In a group with a mean age of 22 years, 100% of incipient lesions were arrested.

Hyde[121] applied either 8% stannous fluoride or acidulated phosphate fluoride (1.2% F) to

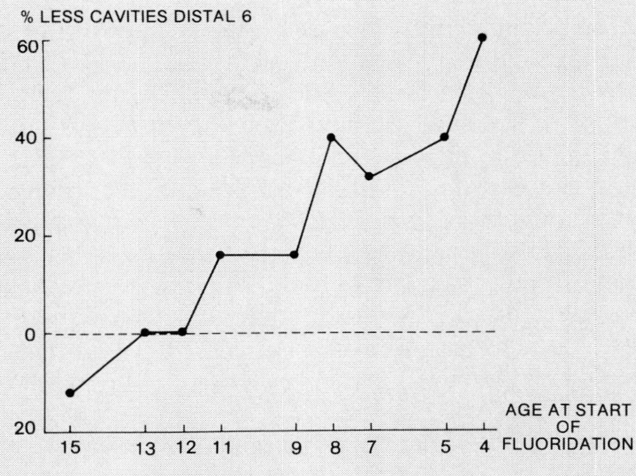

Fig. 2-2 Percentage less lesions in the distal surface of the first molar in children aged 15 years using fluoridated drinking water compared with a nonfluoridated area.
(*Backer-Dirks.*[79] Reproduced with permission of the author and the *J. Dent. Res.*)

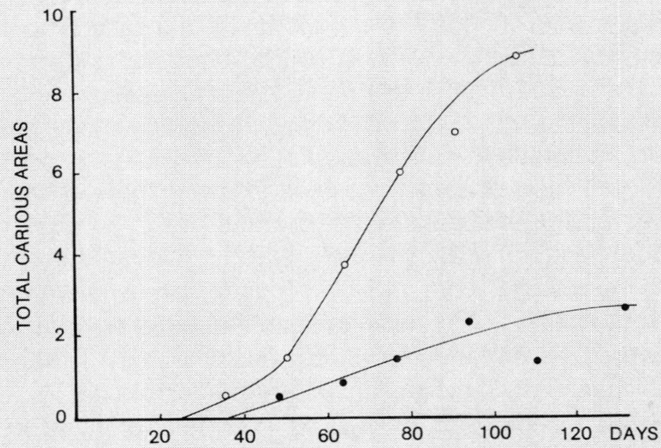

Fig. 2-3 Caries incidence, expressed as total carious areas, in two groups of litter-mates, killed at approximately three weekly intervals:

- ∘ rats maintained on high sugar diet after weaning at 21 days old.
- • rats transferred to a noncariogenic, wheat-starch diet at weaning for 14 days and then fed the cariogenic, high sugar diet from 35 days of age.

During the lactation period, the dam was fed the high sugar diet.
(*Speirs.*[101] Reproduced with permission of the author and *Caries Res.*)

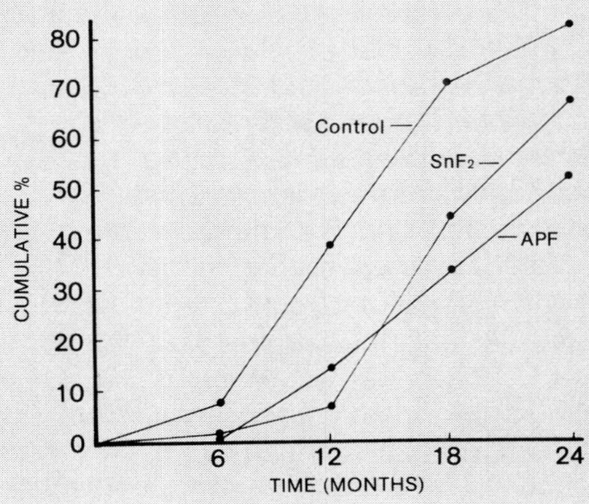

Fig. 2-4 Percent of early caries that progressed to the dentino-enamel junction during a 24-month period following treatment with fluoride.
(*Hyde.*[121] Reproduced with permission of the author and the *J. Canad. Dent. Assn.*)

incipient lesions in newly erupting first permanent molars and followed the lesions radiographically at six-month intervals for two years. Results of this study showed that although a single application was not totally effective, both agents significantly inhibited lesion growth (Fig. 2-4). Applications at more frequent intervals might have provided greater protection. Caries arrest after application of neutral sodium fluoride[122] and silver fluoride[123] has also been reported.

Remineralization of artificial white spots

Remineralization has been studied *in vivo* using artificial white spots prepared in several ways. *Nygaard-Ostby* et al.[39] developed a method to produce white spots *in vivo* by placing a gold plate over a tooth scheduled for extraction but leaving a small space between the plate and tooth where plaque could accumulate. Microscopic examination of the surface and thin sections showed the areas under the gold plate to have developed "genuine" caries. "Gold-plate" lesions were used by *von der Fehr*[108] to study remineralization. The lesions had the typical appearance of natural caries, including the X-ray dense surface layer, but when the gold plate was removed for a time, they disappeared or decreased in severity.

Koulourides[124] produced carious lesions in the mouth using an intraoral cariogenicity test. In this method, enamel slabs are mounted in partial dentures and covered with a dacron or teflon gauze, which allows plaque to accumulate beneath the gauze. Under these conditions, the enamel becomes soft (carious) and the degree of softening is related to the severity of the lesion. Removing the gauze results in a rehardening of the enamel (remineralization).

Fluoride treatment of enamel presoftened with acid or cariogenic bacteria, then carried intraorally in dentures, was found to partially remineralize the enamel.[125] Recently it has been shown[126] that incipient lesions could be formed *in vivo* by placing cups of food material on the lingual surfaces of lower incisors. Using a fluorescent dye, white spots could be detected after as little as two days of cariogenic challenge. The white spots remineralized when exposed normally to saliva.

Sognnaes[127] showed by microscopic and radiographic analysis that monkey teeth softened with acid *in vivo* had remineralized within several months. In some of his experiments he noted an increase in microdensity in as little as two days, although dye absorption indicated greater porosity than sound enamel. He also reported similar results with rats.

The development of incipient caries *in vivo* by means of frequent sucrose rinses and abstinence from oral hygiene was reported by *von der Fehr* et al.[128] These investigators found that white spot lesions developed in the gingival third of the teeth when the subjects rinsed with 50% sucrose for 23 days, but that after 30 days of meticulous oral hygiene and daily fluoride mouth rinses, the white spots remineralized and disappeared. The sucrose rinse method for incipient caries development was also applied by *Levine*.[129] He found that white spots were more rapidly remineralized by a calcium phosphate mouth rinse containing fluoride than by a 0.5% fluoride solution alone.

Remineralization in the laboratory

Formation of artificial white spots

Incipient carious lesions of enamel have been made in the laboratory for many years. Most early methods simply used an acid solution; however, this procedure tended to produce surface etching (Fig. 2-5). Nevertheless, simple acid solutions will result in a relatively sound enamel surface if the solu-

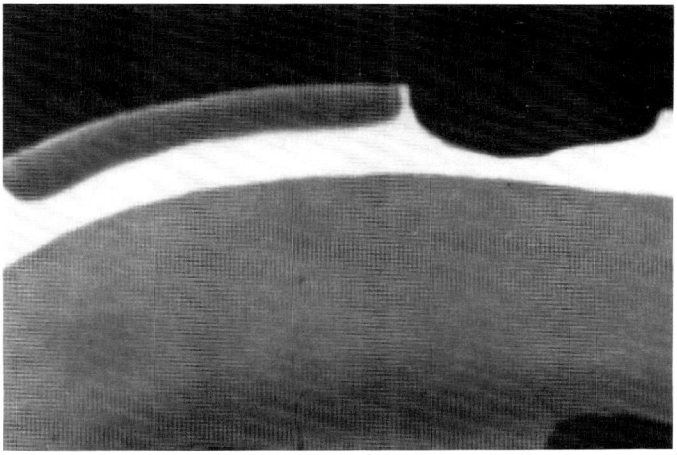

Fig. 2-5 Cross section of etched enamel surface (on right) and artificial white spot lesion. The lesion was formed in a pH 4.0, 0.1M lactic acid gel for 7 days. The etched area was treated with 0.1M lactic acid solution for 4 hours.

tions are not agitated.[130,131] A static or nonagitated system will result in slower diffusion of dissolved enamel away from the surface—a condition apparently necessary for white spot formation in acid systems. White spots closely resembling natural lesions can also be produced using acidic gels containing about 0.1 M lactic acid at pH 4 to 5.[16,132-134] The acidified gel may be regarded as a model of the plaque:enamel interface in which the transport of ions to and from the enamel is restricted by the viscosity of the gel, its calcium and phosphate concentrations, and perhaps the charge of the gel macromolecules. Lactic acid solutions containing calcium phosphate (e.g., hydroxyapatite),[17,135-137] polyphosphates, or diphosphonates[138-140] also produce white spots resembling natural lesions, as does *Streptococcus mutans* in the presence of a salivary deposit[18] or in an artificial mouth.[141]

Current investigators use either solutions or gels to produce white spots in the laboratory. Both methods appear to produce natural-appearing lesions, although with each method there are variations in the depth, thickness, and presence of the four zones described in Chapter 1. These variations are probably related to the rate at which the lesions are formed and viscosity, pH, and mineral content of the demineralizing system. Even natural lesions differ in the relative size and presence of the four zones, and both the gel and solution methods are sufficiently reproducible to be used in laboratory experiments.

The formation rate of white spot lesions *in vitro* in a gel system has been shown to be proportional to the square root of time.[142] It is more rapid at lower pH,[142-145] at lower viscosity,[145] at higher acid molarities,[146] and in enamel with a lower mineral content.[144] Figure 2-6 shows the rate of white spot formation in permanent and primary types of human and bovine teeth placed in gelatin containing lactic acid at pH 4.0. The bovine teeth formed white spots more rapidly than human teeth, and primary more rapidly than permanent.

Analysis of the mineral content of the body of the lesions has revealed the presence of dicalcium phosphate existing as brushite ($CaHPO_4{\bullet}2H_2O$),[147] monetite ($CaHPO_4$),[148] or similar material. White spots remineralized under constantly controlled conditions at pH 7.0 have shown the formation of rodlike crystals identified most likely as hydroxyapatite or fluoridated hydroxyapatite. The forma-

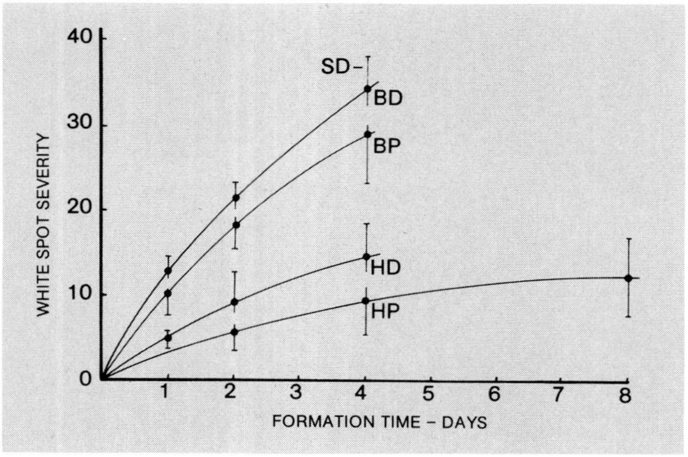

Fig. 2-6 White spot formation rate in human permanent (HP), human deciduous (HD), bovine permanent (BP), and bovine deciduous (BD) teeth in lactic acid gel at pH 4.0. (*Mellberg* and *Kellum*.[306])

tion of fluorapatite in the surface layer during white spot formation has also been reported.[149]

Fluoride treatment of sound enamel prior to exposure to an acid gel system has been reported to have no effect on the rate of white spot formation,[150,151] unless the fluoride treatment is given subsequent to a treatment with $TiCl_3$ or $ZnOCl_2$. However, when white spots are treated with fluoride and then placed in an acid gel, enlargement of the lesion is slowed.[152] Treatment of artificial white spots with a fluoride dentifrice at intervals during their formation inhibits their growth,[153] and treatment with stannous fluoride increases their hardness and radiodensity.[154,155]

Treatment of artificial white spots in bovine enamel with fluoride has resulted in fluoride concentration profiles showing greater fluoride uptake by the body of the lesion than by the surface layer[156] (Fig. 2-7).

In vitro remineralization

Much early work on remineralization was concerned with the effect of calcifying solutions on rehardening acid-softened surfaces. In this work, rehardening is assumed to be remineralization. *Koulourides* and co-workers[157] found that $CaHPO_4$ solutions could completely reharden acid-etched surfaces if the softening was not too severe. The rate of rehardening is dependent on the degree of saturation of the remineralizing solution and its pH. Although greater saturation or higher pH produce more rapid remineralization, it is less complete.[124] Rapid remineralization results in a precipitation of mineral on the enamel surface[158] or within the surface layer, restricting further ionic diffusion.[159] Complete remineralization requires optimum rather than maximum rates. Deep lesions in particular may require slow remineralization to allow diffusion into the lesion.

Silverstone[160] reported that the initial changes in mineral content during remineralization were seen in the dark zone (see Chapter 1), which was either broadened or formed in those lesions without a dark zone. However, studies with radiocalcium showed that mineral was initially deposited in the surface layer, then redissolved and deposited more deeply within the lesion.[161]

Synthetic remineralizing solutions usually contain 1 to 5mM calcium, 1 to 3mM phosphate, and have a Ca/P ratio of 1.67, the same as hydroxyapatite. They are often prepared by dissolving hydroxyapatite in acid and adjusting the pH to 6 to 7 with KOH.

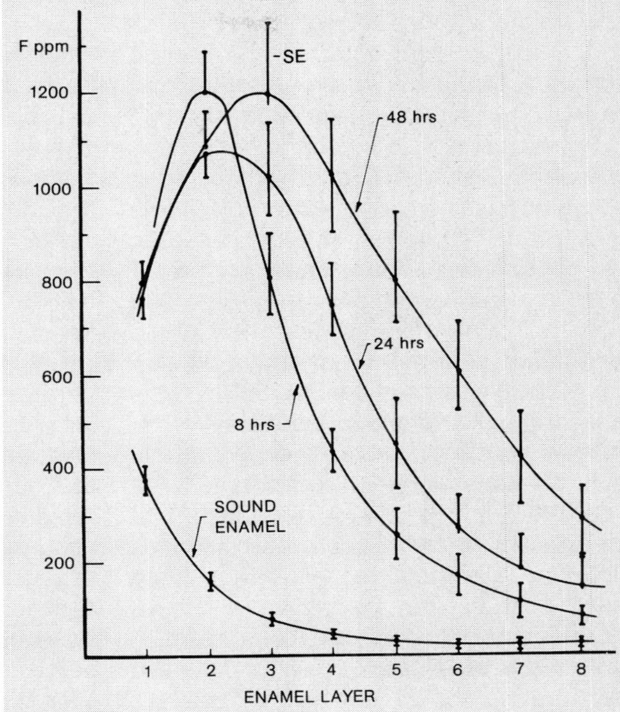

Fig. 2-7 Fluoride uptake by white spots formed in bovine enamel at pH 4.5 for 0, 8, 24, or 48 hours and then treated with 10 ppm F (as Na_2PO_3F) for 24 hours.
(*Mellberg.*[156] Reprinted with permission of *Caries Research.*)

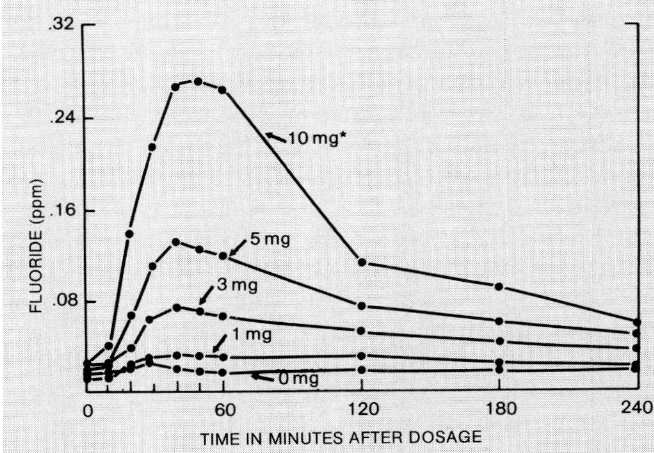

Fig. 2-8 Effect of exogenous fluoride on parotid fluid fluoride levels (N = 20). * Oral fluoride dosage.
(*Shannon.*[188] Reproduced with permission of the author and *Arch. Oral Biol.*)

Dicalcium phosphate solutions (Ca/P = 1.0) have also been used to remineralize white spots. Sodium chloride is frequently added to improve the stability and range of pH over which the solutions are active,[109] and fluoride is added to improve their effectiveness. Saliva has been found to remineralize etched enamel *in vitro*,[162,163] although it is not as good in remineralizing as are synthetic solutions.[164] The remineralizing activity of saliva has been found to vary between individuals, but is consistent in the same individual.[162] Although the concentrations of calcium and phosphate in saliva are sufficiently high to provide good remineralizing potential, salivary proteins bind as much as 50% of the calcium and 30% of the phosphate.[165] Perhaps even more important is the presence in saliva of nucleation inhibitors such as statherin.[166,167] It has also been found that remineralization of white spots by saliva is restricted to the surface, and it has been suggested that the viscosity of saliva restricts ionic diffusion into the lesion.[132] Plaque or pellicle is also likely to act as a diffusion barrier.

Effect of fluoride on remineralization

Fluoride enhances the rate of remineralization from calcium phosphate solutions. Even in minute amounts it increases the rate of precipitation of hydroxyapatite where the formation of the more soluble octacalcium phosphate would otherwise be favored.[168] Remineralization of etched surfaces is accelerated by as much as four to five times by only 1 ppm F,[124,169] and remineralization of white spots may be increased twofold. Fluoride has been shown to increase mineral deposition in sound enamel,[170] and remineralization was increased by topical fluoride applications to etched enamel prior to exposure to calcium phosphate solutions or to the oral environment.[171,172] Paradoxically, very large amounts of fluoride in calcium phosphate solutions may actually inhibit remineralization.[173] Perhaps the higher fluoride concentrations favor calcium fluoride formation, which prevents hydroxyapatite crystal growth, or rapid mineral deposition blocks diffusion pathways.

Saliva can also remineralize enamel *in vitro*, but addition of fluoride will improve the effect. However, 20 ppm F, rather than 1 ppm F, as with synthetic solutions, is required.[162]

Histological examination of microradiographs of white spot lesions has often shown a laminated appearance[132] thought to arise from transient arrest of lesion growth. *Koulourides*[174] demonstrated that laminations could be produced in artificial white spots by intermittent fluoride treatments during their formation. A study of lesions that extended into the dentin and subsequently became arrested showed the presence of a surface zone high in fluoride.[175] It was suggested that this stabilized the lesion against further demineralization.

Arrested lesions seen as brown spots have been found to be less soluble in acid.[176-178] *Little* et al.[179,180] reported that stained, but otherwise normal, enamel showed chemical and histological changes similar to those of white spots, except that they were more superficial. *Weatherell* et al.[84] found that fluoride in the gingival area of the enamel increased with age whereas in other areas there was no such increase. He suggested that this was due to acid attack followed by remineralization in areas frequently covered by fluoride-rich plaque. This finding is in agreement with *Little*'s findings since these are also the areas tending to show discoloration in older teeth. Superficial brown spots, therefore, can be considered as areas of frequent, though not severe, demineralization with almost continuous remineralization.

Remineralization has also been reported in rats. Several studies have shown that hypomineralized areas exist at the time the teeth erupt.[80,102,138,181] If the animals are maintained on a normal diet, the areas slowly mineralize. The mineralization of hypomineralized areas in rats on the normal diet is more properly termed "maturation." However, hypomineralized areas in animals on a cariogenic diet enlarge and become true incipient lesions. When these rats are given fluoride treatments, the lesions regress. This process can now properly be termed *remineralization*.

Effect of plaque on remineralization

The presence of plaque and/or pellicle obviously is important, not only in white spot formation *in vivo* but also *in vitro* and in its remineralization. Several factors can be considered. First, the plaque acts as a barrier to the treatment contacting the teeth and, second, it can act as a reservoir for acid and calcium phosphate dissolved from the enamel. It also can act as a reservoir for remineralizing agents, concentrating them near the lesion surface. Third, the plaque may inactivate the agents, for example, by complexing or reacting. In the case of fluoride, bacteria may actually take the fluoride into the cell—faster under acidic conditions, when it is needed most for countering cariogenic demineralization. As a reservoir, plaque usually contains much higher concentrations of fluoride, calcium, and phosphate than saliva.[182]

The effect of an *in vitro* produced salivary pellicle (deposit) was studied by *Zahradnik* et al.,[17] who reported that the pellicle had ionic permselective properties resulting in slower white spot formation.

Interference with microorganisms

Interference with the metabolism of microorganisms involved in caries formation has long been proposed as a possible mechanism for the topical effect of fluoride.[183] Evidence showing an effect of fluoride on plaque microorganisms has been derived from studies of single organisms, salivary sediment, and plaque itself. Although plaque obviously is the most suitable substrate for study, saliva has been utilized because of its better availability. Because saliva or salivary sediment will not entirely reflect the situation in the cariogenic plaque, evidence from salivary studies will be presented separately.

Evidence from saliva

Fluoride concentrations in saliva

Saliva can serve as a source of fluoride for the plaque and, therefore, may affect both salivary and plaque organisms. There are two major sources of salivary fluoride: (1) secretion from the salivary glands, and (2) introduction into the mouth from food, water, and fluoride preparations such as rinses or dentifrices.

Glandular Secretion: The level of fluoride secreted by the glands into the mouth depends upon many factors, but under normal conditions it is very low and in the range of 0.007 to 0.05 ppm.[184-188] Adults seem to have slightly higher levels than children. Resting saliva has slightly more fluoride than stimulated saliva,[184] but the rate or duration of flow of the stimulated saliva does not seem to affect the fluoride concentration.[188,189] Whole saliva may contain twice as much fluoride as gland saliva,[184] probably due to inclusion of nonsalivary components. Only 10% of the fluoride present in whole saliva is in a free form; the remainder is bound primarily in inorganic substances[190,191] but is released at low pH.

Ingestion of fluoride increases the concentration secreted by the glands in direct proportion to the amount ingested.[185,186,188,192,193] A 10mg does of fluoride, for example, will increase parotid fluoride levels from a normal value of 0.02 ppm F to about 0.28 ppm F (Fig. 2-8). The peak level is reached within 40 to 50 minutes followed by a rapid decline over the next hour. A slower fall follows and, if the dose is high, elevated levels may be found for several hours. The presence of ions that complex fluoride (e.g., aluminum) will reduce or delay its appearance in saliva.[194]

Extrinsic Sources: Topical application procedures increase salivary fluoride levels more than ingested fluoride. Five minutes after an application of acidulated phosphate fluoride solution (12,000 ppm F), whole saliva was found to contain approximately 100 ppm F.[187] This concentration fell rapidly, but even after ten hours was still 0.25 ppm F or roughly five to ten times the normal level in saliva, which was not reached until one week later.

Fluoride mouth rinses increase concentrations of fluoride in saliva for a shorter period, but during the rinse procedure, fluid in the mouth will contain almost as high a fluoride concentration as the rinse itself. With a 0.05% NaF solution (226 ppm F), this may be 150 ppm. After expectoration of the rinse, the fluoride concentration in the mouth falls very rapidly. Five minutes after use of a highly concentrated rinse containing 2,000 ppm F, salivary fluoride levels were only 25 ppm.[187] The level remained slightly elevated for approximately one day. Similarly, four hours after using an amine-fluoride rinse containing 10,000 ppm F, 1 ppm F was found in the saliva.[195] Although higher fluoride concentrations in the rinse and longer rinse durations increase the concentration and duration of elevated fluoride levels in saliva, use of large rinse volumes apparently does not.[196] Fluoride in the form of monofluorophosphate or amine fluoride has been reported to be retained longer than sodium fluoride.[196,197]

Brushing the teeth with 1% sodium fluoride solution (4,500 ppm F) resulted in salivary fluoride concentrations of 378 ppm F during the brushing period, but only 28 ppm F ten minutes later.[198] Immediately after brushing with a dentifrice containing 3.2% F as silicofluoride, Saxer[195] found 183 ppm F in saliva. The duration of elevated fluoride in saliva in this case was five hours. Using more conventional dentifrices (1,000 ppm F), *Birkeland*[199] found 1 ppm F in whole saliva after 30 minutes. Other investigators found elevated fluoride levels for one-half to one hour.[200,201]

The effect of chewing fluoride tablets on salivary fluoride levels has also been studied. *Parkins*[202] found that saliva contained 190 ppm F during the time a 1mg fluoride tablet was being chewed. The duration of increased salivary fluoride after tablet chewing was found to be one hour longer.[196,203]

Effect of fluoride on salivary microorganisms

Fluoride can affect microorganisms in several ways. At low fluoride concentrations it inhibits acid formation; at higher concentrations it can affect growth and metabolism; and at very high concentrations it is lethal.[204-206]

Inhibition of acid formation by salivary microorganisms has been demonstrated in numerous studies;[207-216] however, the amount required to accomplish this under actual cariogenic conditions is not known. *Jenkins*[217] found that the inhibition of bacterial acid production by microorganisms is greater at low pH. This is fortunate, since the fluoride will be most active when the conditions are most cariogenic. At pH 5, only 6 ppm F were needed to completely prevent the formation of acid from glucose. At lower fluoride concentrations, acid formation was partially inhibited; at higher concentrations (8 to 10 ppm F), the pH actually rose, probably due to the alkali-producing reactions of saliva. It has been stated[218] that sodium fluoride per se has no appreciable antibacterial power, but that undissociated molecules of HF do. At an acidic pH, the concentration of undissociated HF rises, and so then should the antibacterial effects. Support was given to this concept by *Sims,*[212] who showed that the minimum inhibitory concentration of fluoride at various pHs was more related to the undissociated HF concentration than to total F concentration. Although the sensitivity of microorganisms differed, the amount of total fluoride needed to inhibit acid formation at pH 7 was typically 100 times more than at pH 5. The amount of undissociated HF calculated to be present in the solutions, however, varies only five- to tenfold or less (Table 2-5). The amount of fluoride required for an effect on metabolism is also dependent on atmospheric conditions. For example, 200 ppm F inhibited metabolism 40% under anaerobic conditions, but had no effect under aerobic conditions.[219]

Inhibition of bacterial growth and metabolism is related, at least in part, to the effect of fluoride on enzymes. The enzyme most sensitive to fluoride during the formation of acid is enolase,[215,220] and in the formation of polysaccharides it is phosphoglucomutase.[221] It also has been suggested that the primary fluoride activity is the inhibition of glucose transfer across the cell wall.[216,222,223]

In vivo evidence for an effect of fluoride on salivary organisms has also been obtained. The formation of lactic acid from sugar was reduced for 10 to 20 minutes following rinses with 0.1 to 0.5% NaF,[208,211] and the number of viable microorganisms in whole saliva diminished for several hours after rinsing with 0.1 to 0.5% SnF_2.[224-226] Brushing with monofluorophosphate dentifrice (0.1% F) reduced the number of salivary streptococci in the mouth,[227] and topical 1% sodium fluoride applications decreased the lactobacillus count to one-sixth of pretreatment levels, an effect that persisted to some degree for as long as 24 days.[228]

Evidence from plaque studies

Fluoride concentrations in plaque

As with saliva, major factors in the effect of fluoride are its concentration in the plaque and the length of time it remains there.

Natural levels of fluoride concentration: Wide variations of fluoride concentrations in plaque have been reported;[229-235] however, most of the recent studies report concentrations in dried samples to be within the range of 25 to 50 ppm F. Assuming a wet weight to dry weight ratio of 3.5 to 7.0,[236,237] the total fluoride concentrations of plaque in its natural state would range from 3.5 to 14 ppm F, with plaque from fluoridated water areas being near the upper part of the range. This is 70 to 280 times higher than a typical 0.05 ppm F concentration of whole saliva and demonstrates that components of plaque concentrate fluoride.

State of fluoride: The concentrating effect on fluoride by plaque components results in only a small fraction of it being in the free ionic state at its natural pH.[191,230,231,238-240] It has been calculated that the concentration of free fluoride in the extracellular aqueous phase (plaque fluid) is between 0.08 and 0.8 ppm F.[241]

The actual state of the bound fluoride fraction is not entirely understood. Approximately one-half of it is released when the plaque is acidified,[240,242] and it has been thought that the released fluoride was bound to inorganic substituents, to dialyzable material,[190,231,232] or to a complex involving metal ions.[230] The remainder appears to be associated with the bacterial component of plaque, possibly within the cells[238,241] or attached to the cell walls.[243]

The distribution of fluoride in plaque apparently is not uniform since its concentration is related to the thickness of the deposit. Thick or heavy plaques usually have a lower fluo-

Table 2-5 Concentrations of fluoride and HF found to inhibit bacterial growth at various pH values

Approximate pH	S. Viridans Total F (HF)	L. Casei rhamnosos Total F (HF)	L. Plantarum Total F (HF)
7.0	210 (0.03)	1,360 (0.19)	2,100 (0.27)
6.5	145 (0.07)	1,040 (0.53)	1,770 (0.95)
6.0	90 (0.12)	740 (0.97)	1,430 (1.80)
5.5	26 (0.11)	355 (1.54)	760 (3.15)
5.0	2 (0.03)	83 (1.08)	215 (2.67)

Data from *Sims.*[212]

ride concentration than thin plaques.[244,245] This may be related to the rate of plaque growth or to a slow rate of fluoride diffusion from the surface inwards. Whatever the reason, it suggests that the concentration may be lower near the enamel surface where its presence would be most beneficial during a caries attack.

Increasing plaque fluoride: The use of fluoride-containing preparations increases the concentration of fluoride in plaque. Four hours after rinsing with 10ml of 0.2% NaF, plaque was found to contain 216 ppm F (dry weight).[245] After 24 hours, the fluoride level was still slightly elevated, but it was concluded that it did not accumulate with repeated rinses. When measured *in vivo* with an implanted electrode, a 0.2% NaF rinse raised the fluoride concentration in the interdental area to 190 ppm F immediately after rinsing and maintained an elevated level for one hour. When the electrode was covered with plaque, the length of time the fluoride remained elevated was decreased in proportion to the age of the plaque.[246] It has also been reported that plaque fluoride remains elevated longer from amine fluoride rinses than from sodium fluoride rinses.[247]

Brushing twice daily with a sodium fluoride dentifrice for four weeks resulted in an increase in plaque fluoride.[235] Before brushing, the plaque contained 24 to 45 ppm F (dry weight), but two hours after the last brushing, residual deposits contained 42 to 229 ppm F. During this time, the total amount of new plaque decreased; therefore, some of the apparent fluoride accumulation may have been the result of thinner plaque deposits. The increase in plaque fluoride associated with a sodium monofluorophosphate dentifrice was found to be related to concentrations of calcium and phosphate in the plaque.[248] *Mühlemann* et al.[234] found that partially mineralized plaque that accumulated on plastic foils attached to the teeth during a ten-day period of brushing with a sodium fluoride dentifrice (0.12% F) also had increased fluoride levels. Plaque from the dentifrice group contained 702 ppm F (dry weight), whereas plaque from the control group contained 154 ppm F.

The accumulation of fluoride by plaque growing on enamel previously given a topical fluoride application was studied by *Gron* et al.[232] They treated enamel blocks with acidulated phosphate fluoride (APF) or titanium tetrachloride ($TiCl_4$) plus APF, washed them for 1 or 24 hours, and then placed them in a plastic device that was kept in the mouth for four days. Plaque on APF-treated enamel contained 75 ppm F, and plaque on enamel treated with APF plus $TiCl_4$ contained 113 ppm F; whereas, plaque on untreated enamel contained only 15 to 20 ppm F (dry weight). The elevated fluoride levels in the plaque on the treated enamel were due to the fluoride that normally leaches off the enamel after a topical application.

Effect of fluoride on plaque quantity

Several investigators have shown that topically applied fluoride may result in less plaque accumulation. It has been reported that frequent mouth rinsing with sodium fluoride[235] or amine fluoride[249,250] solutions result in 20 to 30% less plaque on the teeth. A similar effect was found with an amine fluoride dentifrice.[251] Less plaque was also noted in subjects residing in an area with a high dental fluorosis rate, but the pattern was variable according to tooth site.[252] A trend to lower caries scores in subjects with high plaque fluoride has also been reported.[233]

Tinanoff and co-workers[253,254] found that rinsing with fluoride solutions reduced the bacterial colonization on enamel implants. Stannous fluoride was more effective than other agents and appeared to reduce the adhesion of bacteria to bacteria and bacteria to enamel. Although *Tinanoff* found that stannous chloride was not nearly as effective as stannous fluoride,[253] some evidence[255] suggests that much of the effect is due to the stannous ion. *Svatum* found that a stannous fluoride dentifrice, when held on the teeth in a cap splint, also reduced plaque accumulation[256] and acidogenesis.[257]

The accumulation of plaque during a three-day period following an APF gel application to clean teeth was significantly less than on untreated teeth,[258] and a series of five to ten daily APF gel applications (1.2% F) in mouthpieces also significantly reduced plaque scores for at least six days.[259,260] Furthermore, the amount of *Streptococcus mutans* in the plaque of these subjects was reduced by 75% and lower *S. mutans* levels persisted for at least 12 weeks. It is possible that the duration of this effect was related to the duration of loss of fluoride from the treated enamel. Enamel fluoride loss after two similar series of five and ten APF gel applications was found to persist for approximately 90 to 150 days respectively.[261]

After use of APF, SnF_2, or sequential application of both agents, *Woods*[262] also found less *S. mutans* seven days later. *Woods*[263] also determined the effect of a stannous fluoride prophylaxis paste applied for two and one-half minutes with a toothbrush. One week after application, he found 57% less *S. mutans* in the plaque. Elimination of *S. mutans* in proximal sites with stannous fluoride on dental floss was accomplished by *Keene* et al.,[264] who noted that many of the sites remained free of *S. mutans* for as long as two months. Less plaque was also found on teeth in animals after fluoride applications,[265,266] and on amalgams containing stannous fluoride.[267]

Effect of fluoride on plaque metabolism

The effect of fluoride on plaque metabolism may be reflected in a change in the relative numbers of organisms, the amount of intracellular and extracellular polysaccharide present, or in its acid-forming ability.

Differences in the relative numbers of polysaccharide-producing organisms were noted by a number of investigators. *Loesche* and co-workers[259,260] found that a series of APF gel (1.2% F) applications reduced *S. mutans*, the most cariogenic organism, but did not effect *Streptococcus sanguis.* They reasoned that since *S. sanguis* is able to colonize soft tissues in the mouth, whereas *S. mutans* colonizes only hard tissues, recolonization of the teeth would more easily occur with *S. sanguis.* However, the amount of *S. sanguis* in plaque was found in another study to be inversely related to the concentration of fluoride in the drinking water.[270] A fluoride gel containing 0.5% fluoride did not affect the composition of dental plaque according to *Myers* and *Handleman*[271] and

Jordan et al.,[272] although *Jordan* et al. did not take their plaque sample until 11 months after fluoride application.

Plaque in contact with even low fluoride concentrations in drinking water is different from plaque originating in nonfluoridated water areas, according to several investigators. *DeStoppelaar* et al.,[268] *Broukal* and *Zajicek*[273] and *Van Houte* et al.[274] reported that fewer polysaccharide-producing streptococci were present in human plaque from fluoridated water areas, and *Bowen*[269] reported a similar finding in monkeys receiving 2 ppm F water.

Sodium fluoride, stannous fluoride, and sodium monofluorophosphate rinses and dentifrices were all effective in reducing the amount of intracellular polysaccharide content of human plaque.[275] Intracellular polysaccharide is important since it can be utilized by the organism for acid production during periods between eating. The polysaccharide reducing effect of fluoride did not persist for long with any of these agents, but of those tested, the effect of monofluorophosphate remained longer, and in addition was also found to reduce extracellular polysaccharide, the material providing much of the plaque matrix. The formation of the water insoluble fraction may be affected more than the soluble fraction.[276] Extracellular polysaccharide formation *in vitro* by four strains of *S. mutans* can be inhibited by 70 ppm F according to *Bowen* and *Hewitt*.[277]

Norman et al.[278] found that plaque overlying silicate restorations had a different composition and suggested that the difference might have been due to the effect of fluoride leached from the silicate.

Acid formation by human plaque *in vitro* is inhibited by fluoride. Addition of sucrose to plaque collected from children living in areas having fluoridated and nonfluoridated water resulted in a lessened pH drop in plaque from the fluoridated areas.[238] Although the differences were very small, the experiment showed that naturally occurring fluoride can affect plaque. Further evidence was provided by plaque collected from the same subjects before and after water fluoridation where an inhibition of acid production was found after water fluoridation.[279] Similarly, less acid formation was found in the plaque of monkeys on 2 ppm F water.[269] The magnitude of the effect of plaque fluoride during these *in vitro* experiments would be expected to depend upon the magnitude of the artificial caries challenge and lack of oral environment. Since the challenge can be considered great in these experiments, some of the natural inhibitory effect of fluoride could have been overcome. However, *in vivo* experiments were also conducted where fluoride in sugar solutions was applied to plaque *in vivo* and shown to reduce the amount of acid formed in humans[280,281] and monkeys.[282,283] A drop of 2% sodium fluoride solution applied to plaque prior to a 10% glucose rinse also resulted in a smaller pH drop.[284] Fluoride rinses were found to reduce the acidogenic potential of plaque for 15 minutes.[211,285]

Effect of enamel fluoride

It sometimes has been thought that the fluoride in plaque arises from the enamel, and in some cases this is true, although only for relatively short periods. *Zwemer*[286] treated enamel of isolated mandibular central incisors *in vivo* with 4% sodium fluoride for 20 minutes. At intervals after the application, bacterial suspensions were applied to the teeth and the amount of lactic acid produced by the suspension was determined. It was found that acid production was inhibited 56% immediately following the application, but only 14% 24 hours later. No inhibition could be detected after one week. Similarly, *Wooley* and *Rickles*[287] measured the pH drop caused by applications of 2% sodium fluoride. They also found an effect that persisted for approximately three to four days, but was absent after one week. *Bergman*[284] found no effect several months after three topical applications of 2% sodium fluoride. Several days after use of 10 to 50 ppm F water or repeated 0.5% fluoride gel applications to hamsters, their plaque was found not to be different from plaque of control animals as measured by the amount of pH drop upon application of sucrose solutions.[266,268] The duration of bacterial inhibition produced by these treatments is undoubtedly related to the length of time that fluoride is lost from the topically treated teeth.

The duration of loss will depend upon the type of treatment given and may range from less than one day after rinses[187] to as long as eight months after a series of APF gel applications.[261] When the period of fluoride loss from the enamel is over and only permanently bound fluoride remains, fluoride levels undoubtedly will return to normal. This is suggested by the finding that plaque grown on shark enamel, which has 33,000 ppm F and is almost entirely fluorapatite,[289] does not contain higher fluoride concentrations than plaque grown on untreated human enamel.[232] Although it has been found[290] that enamel under plaque with a high fluoride concentration may also have high fluoride, it was suggested that the increased enamel fluoride originated from the plaque. This agrees with the suggestion made by *Weatherell* et al.[84,291] that enamel undergoing periodic demineralization and remineralization will concentrate fluoride from the overlying plaque. In an *in vitro* experiment, it was shown that more fluoride was taken up by enamel under fermenting plaque.[292] *Briner* and *Francis*[293] questioned the validity of pH measurement as a reflection of inhibition of acid formation. In one experiment, they showed that lactic acid formation could be reduced 45% without a significant change in pH. They reasoned that this was due to the consumption of hydrogen ions by the enamel dissolution process and the buffering effect of lactate and phosphate ions released. Both of these effects tend to raise the pH when enamel is dissolved, whereas in the absence of dissolution the pH remains low. Untreated but naturally fluoridated mottled enamel (with its firmly bound fluoride) had 32% less lactic acid formation.

Fluoride in enamel has also been thought to have an effect on pellicle or plaque accumulation and composition.[294] It has been found that less salivary material is retained on fluorapatite than on hydroxyapatite;[295] that fluoride and monofluorophosphate are able to desorb protein and bacteria from hydroxyapatite;[296] and that adsorption of a tyrosine-rich salivary peptide (statherin) and proline-rich peptide is greater on fluorapatite.[297] This suggests that the composition of pellicle may be different on enamel with a high fluoride composition.

Bacterial resistance to fluoride

When certain microorganisms were grown under conditions of ever-increasing fluoride concentrations, they developed a resistance to fluoride up to concentrations of 1,900 ppm.[298-300] However, when the organisms were then transferred to a nonfluoride medium, they lost their resistance to fluoride. During the time when they were resistant to fluoride, they were less cariogenic than non-resistant strains.[301] No reports have appeared in the literature describing fluoride-resistant strains *in vivo*.

Summary of effects on Microorganisms

Plaque contains higher levels of fluoride than saliva, showing that it is capable of concentrating and retaining it by means of combination with inorganic or organic materials. Although only a small amount of fluoride in the aqueous phase of plaque is in a free ionic state (0.1 to 1.0 ppm), much more is released (1 to 5 ppm) when the pH is

Table 2-6 Effects of fluoride supplements on enamel fluoride, fluorosis, fissure morphology, and dental caries

Group	Enamel F (ppm)	Fluorosis (Percent very mild to moderate)	Shallow fissures (Percent)	Caries (DFS)
I. F. Supplements	3,060	67	47	1.57
II. No Supplements	1,700	4	4	7.93
III. F Water	2,320	33	24	3.16

Data from *Aasenden* and *Peebles*.[305]

lowered to levels found during caries formation.

The concentration of fluoride in plaque from communities with fluoridated drinking water is about twice as high as in nonfluoridated communities. After use of fluoride mouth rinses or dentifrices, it can reach 100 ppm for periods of minutes, although it may remain elevated for several hours or more.

The natural low concentrations of fluoride in plaque at acid pH (1 to 5 ppm) have been found to reduce the amount of acid formation, while the higher concentrations (e.g., 70 ppm) achieved after the use of fluoride rinses or dentifrices are able to reduce the formation of polysaccharides. Much higher concentrations (10,000 ppm) are lethal to bacteria and a reduction *in vivo* of *Streptococcus mutans* was shown after repeated use of APF gel in mouthpieces. Fluoride that is firmly bound to enamel will not have an effect unless it is released during caries dissolution, whereupon it may attenuate further acid formation.

Taken as a whole, these findings indicate that the concentration of fluoride in plaque is not sufficient to render it totally nonpathogenic, but that it may contribute to the anticaries activity of the agent. Because of the nature of antibacterial effects, fluoride will be more effective as its concentration and frequency of use are increased.

Improved tooth morphology

The areas of the teeth most susceptible to dental caries are the occlusal surfaces, and those with deep fissures are considered to be the most prone to caries. Studies of the effect of water fluoridation on tooth size and shape have suggested that fluoride tended to make the teeth slightly smaller[302] and, more important, to give them shallower fissures.[302-304] The reduction in fissure size associated with water fluoridation is modest; consequently, the effect on dental caries by this mechanism is questionable. However, a study of the use of systemic fluoride supplements indicated an anticaries effect due to altered tooth morphology, although the assessment of the fissures was subjective. *Aasenden* and *Peebles*[305] studied three groups of children. Group I consisted of children from an area with nonfluoridated drinking water who received fluoride supplements from shortly after birth. The daily dose was 0.5mg F until age 3 and 1.0mg F thereafter. Group II consisted of children from the same community but who did not receive fluoride supplements. Group III consisted of children from an area with fluoridated water. The morphology of the pits and fissures was recorded as "typical" or "atypically shallow." Atypical fissure angles appeared wide, the explorer did not catch in either pits or fissures, and the finding was general throughout the mouth, with both deciduous and permanent teeth having the favorable morphology. Table 2-6 shows the results of this study. The fluoride supplements produced teeth with more fluoride, more fluorosis, more shallow fissures, and significantly lower caries scores. The degree of fluorosis found was not considered to be an esthetic problem, but indicated that the amount of supplement given during the early stages of enamel formation was at the borderline of the tolerable limit.

Relationship of fluoride treatment to possible anticaries mechanisms

The previous sections in this chapter described some of the evidence in support of different mechanisms for the anticaries effects of fluoride. It was shown that some mechanisms require that fluoride be present in enamel but that for some others it was not necessary; some effects persist for long periods, whereas others are transient. From these findings, it is obvious that fluoride may function by one or more mechanisms, depending upon how it is used.

Systemic fluoride treatments

The use of fluoride supplements will increase the concentration of fluoride in sound enamel prior to its exposure to the cariogenic conditions of the oral cavity. Supplements have also been shown to result in shallower fissures that appear to be less susceptible to caries. These effects depend on the supplements being given during formation of the tooth. Once the tooth has erupted it can no longer be expected to benefit systemically, except for a transient slight elevation of salivary fluoride. An increase in enamel fluoride level may occur when fluoride is made available shortly before tooth eruption, but an effect on fissure morphology probably requires fluoride exposure during an earlier stage of crown formation.

Topical fluoride treatments

Effects of treatment formulation and use

Several factors will determine how effective a topical agent can be and how well it will function by each mechanism. The concentration of fluoride in the treatment preparation is significant. All else being equal, the higher the concentration, the greater the anticaries effect. A small difference in concentration will not be important, but a 25 or 50% increase will produce greater fluoride deposition in sound enamel and incipient lesions, greater penetration of fluoride into deeper enamel, and will have a greater inhibiting effect on bacteria. It must be cautioned that the concentrations of fluoride listed on the label of topical preparations cannot always be taken as the amount of useful fluoride present. This is particularly true in the case of prophylaxis pastes where thickening agents, abrasives, humectants, and other materials are present (see Chapter 6), which may reduce the availability of fluoride to the tooth.

The second factor of importance in determining the effectiveness of an infrequently used topical fluoride agent is the quantity of fluoride actually deposited and retained in the enamel and plaque. While this is dependent to a large degree upon the concentration of fluoride in the preparation, many other factors are also involved. Generally, available evidence suggests that the more fluoride that is taken up by enamel and plaque, the better is the anticaries effect.

Penetration of fluoride into enamel is another factor to consider in evaluating a topical fluoride agent. While it is true that the early carious lesion begins at the outer enamel surface, the major demineralization really takes place below the surface. It seems probable that greater penetration of fluoride into subsurface enamel will result in greater resistance of the tooth to decay. Penetration of fluoride will be greater from preparations having a higher fluoride concentration and a lower pH, and after a greater number of applications.

Although fluoride uptake from various topical agents by incipient lesions and other defects may be much more important than uptake by sound enamel, most of the data available, particularly from *in vivo* sources, are related to sound enamel. This is unfortunate; it is difficult to compare treatments in respect to this factor because some treatment modes (e.g., frequently used low fluoride concentrations) increase the fluoride concentration of incipient lesions much more than suggested by experiments with sound enamel. Likewise, comparison of the amounts of fluoride deposited in plaque from various preparations is helpful in evaluating the potential anticaries efficacy of a treatment.

Finally, and perhaps most important, the efficacy of a topical fluoride preparation is related to its frequency of use. The benefit of frequency is probably related to a maintenance of fluoride in the plaque, which may serve as a reservoir to provide fluoride for remineralization and antibacterial effects. The availability of fluoride during a caries attack may be the single most important factor in minimizing the effect of the acid exposure. Frequent application of potent preparations (e.g., 0.5% F) will increase plaque fluoride to higher levels and also increase enamel fluoride more than infrequent applications.

Mechanisms of topical agents

Based upon the preceding discussion, the possible mechanisms functioning during or after the use of commonly used fluoride preparations can be considered.

A common dental office procedure is the annual or semiannual application of concentrated fluoride solutions or gels. Since these treatments are given only once or twice per year, the mechanism of action will primarily depend upon increasing the resistance of sound or altered enamel to acid and, therefore, a measure of fluoride uptake may provide a good prediction of the relative effect of different agents. In addition, remineralization may be enhanced through the formation of a reservoir of fluoride in incipient lesions. The annual or semiannual treatment cannot be expected to have a long-lasting effect on plaque bacteria or to have an effect on enamel defects that form after the treatment is given.

Fluoride prophylaxis pastes should work in the same manner as the annual or semiannual applications, except that since pastes are usually less potent in depositing fluoride in enamel, they can be expected to be less effective than solutions. Prophylaxis pastes have been used in both self-brushing and professional application techniques. The greater thoroughness of professional applications could be expected to result in greater benefits.

Mouth rinses, when used very frequently, appear to be more effective than prophylaxis pastes, even though they may not always be particularly effective in depositing fluoride in sound enamel. The two most important factors in determining the efficacy of the mouth rinse are the concentration of fluoride in the rinse and its frequency of use. Since fluoride uptake from rinses by sound enamel is low,

Table 2-7 Possible anticaries mechanisms of fluoride therapy forms

Mechanism	Supplement	Dentifrice	Rinse	Frequent topical	Annual topical	Prophylaxis paste
Increased enamel resistance	+	O	O	+	+	+
Remineralization	+*	+	+	+	O	O
Antibacterial	+*	+	+	+		
Improved morphology	+					

+ Significant effect possible. O Effect possible on incipient lesions. * From F tablets if chewed and swished.

it is likely that uptake by incipient lesions or other enamel defects, an effect on plaque bacteria, and the promotion of remineralization produce the caries inhibitions found.

Fluoride tablets, in addition to providing the intended systemic effect on unerupted teeth, are also able to provide a topical effect if chewed prior to swallowing. If done on a daily basis, thoroughly chewed and swished tablets could be expected to function similarly to mouth rinse solutions.

Fluoride-containing dentifrices that do not deposit very much fluoride in sound enamel probably function in much the same manner as fluoride mouth rinses.

Finally, repeated application of a relatively high concentration of fluoride in a gel by mouthpiece appears to be the most effective technique available today. Since applications are usually intended to be given very frequently, are of moderately high fluoride concentration, and provide very good fluoride uptake, this procedure can call into play all three of the major anticaries mechanisms. The high enamel fluoride concentration obtained by repetitive mouthpiece applications should ensure some degree of caries inhibitions long after fluoride applications are stopped.

A summary of the anticaries mechanisms provided by the different treatment forms is given in Table 2-7. The indication that several treatment forms function by the same mechanism does not mean that they function with equal intensity by each mechanism or that the effect of each mechanism is directly additive. Although each effect is probably partially additive, evidence is not available to quantitate the degree to which this occurs. However, in general, use of higher fluoride concentrations and greater frequency will favor a more pronounced anticaries effect.

References

1. McCann, H.G., and Brudevold, F. 1966. The mechanism of the caries inhibiting effect of fluoride. In *Environmental variables in oral disease*, eds. S.J. Kreshover and F.J. McClure, pp. 103-28. Washington, D.C.: AAAS, Pub. No. 81.
2. Brown, W.E.; Gregory, T.M.; and Chow, L.C. 1977. Effects of fluoride on enamel solubility and cariostasis. *Caries Res.* 11 (Suppl. 1):118-41.
3. Brudevold, F., and McCann, H.G. 1968. Enamel solubility tests and their significance in regard to dental caries. *Ann. N.Y. Acad. Sci.* 153:20-51.
4. Mir, N.A.; Higuchi, W.I.; and Hefferren, J.J. 1969. The mechanism of action of solution fluoride upon the demineralization rate of human enamel. *Arch. Oral Biol.* 14:901-20.
5. Wier, D.R.; Chien, S.H.; and Block, C.A. 1972. Transformation of hydroxyapatite to fluorapatite. *Soil Sci. Am. Proc.* 36:285-88.
6. Moreno, E.C.; Kresak, M.; and Zahradnik, R.T.

1974. Fluoridated hydroxyapatite solubility and caries formation. *Nature (Lond.)* 247:64-65.
7. Young, R.A.; van der Lugt, W.; and Elliott, J.C. 1969. Mechanism for fluorine inhibition of diffusion in hydroxyapatite. *Nature (Lond.)* 223:729-30.
8. Fox, J.L.; Higuchi, W.I.; Awzi, M.B.; and Maw-Sheng Wu. 1978. A new two-site model for hydroxyapatite dissolution in acidic media. *J. Coll. Interface Sci.* 67:312-30.
9. Scott, D.B.; Simmelink, J.W.; and Nygaard, V. 1971. Mineralization of dental enamel. In: *Chemistry and physiology of enamel,* pp. 6-24. Ann Arbor: University of Michigan Press.
10. Swancar, J.R.; Scott, D.B.; Simmelink, J.W.; and Smith, T.J. 1971. The morphology of enamel crystals. In *Tooth Enamel II,* eds. R. W. Fernhead and M. V. Stack, pp 233-39. Bristol, England: John Wright & Sons.
11. Johnson, N.W., Poole, D.F.G.; and Tyler, J.E. 1971. Factors affecting the differential dissolution of human enamel in acid and EDTA. A scanning electron microscope study. *Arch. Oral Biol.* 16:385-96.
12. Nichol, T.; Judd, G.; and Ansell, G.S. 1973. Two stage model for human enamel demineralization as determined by scanning electron microscope analysis. *J. Dent. Res.* 52:487-93.
13. Hoffman, S.; McEwan, W.S.; and Drew, C.M. 1969. Scanning electron microscope studies of EDTA-treated enamel. *J. Dent. Res.* 48: 1234-42.
14. Silverstone, L.M.; Saxton, C.A.; Dogon, I.L.; and Fejerskov, O. 1975. Variations in the pattern of acid etching of human dental enamel examined by scanning electron microscopy. *Caries Res.* 9:373-87.
15. Arends, J. 1973. Dislocations and dissolution of enamel. Theoretical considerations. *Caries Res.* 7:261-68.
16. von Bartheld, F. 1961. Membrane phenomena in carious dissolution of the teeth. *Arch. Oral Biol.* 6:284-303.
17. Zahradnik, R.T.; Moreno, E.C.; and Burke, E.J. 1976. Effect of salivary pellicle on enamel subsurface demineralization *in vitro*. *J. Dent. Res.* 55:664-70.
18. Zahradnik, R.T., and Moreno, E.C. 1977. *In vitro* enamel demineralization by streptococcus mutans in the presence of salivary pellicles. *J. Dent. Res.* 56:1107-10.
19. Jenkins, G.N.; Armstrong, P.A.; and Speirs, R.L. 1952. Laboratory investigations on the relation of fluorine to dental caries on Tyneside and District. *Proc. Royal Soc. Med.* 45:517-25.
20. Healy, W.B., and Ludwig, T.G. 1966. Enamel solubility studies on New Zealand teeth. *N. Zealand Dent. J.* 62: 276-78.
21. Charlton, G., and Shamshula, R. 1970. Fluoride, enamel solubility and dental caries. *J. Dent. Res.* 49:650.
22. Cutress, T.W., and Malthus, R.S. 1970. The fluoride concentrations and acid solubility of teeth from fluoridated (1 ppm) and low fluoride areas. *N. Zealand Dent. J.* 66:229-34.
23. Little, M.F.; Losee, F.; and Barret, K. 1974. Fluoride and acid resistance vs DMFT in outer enamel from low and high F areas. *J. Dent. Res.* 53: IADR abstr. #434.
24. Finn, S.B., and De Marco, C. 1956. The effect of artificial water fluoridation on the solubility of tooth enamel. *J. Dent. Res.* 35:185-88.
25. Lamberts, B.M.; Keene, H.J.; and Levin, S. 1976. Enamel solubility rate measurements in vivo on Naval recruits. *J. Dent. Res.* 55:797-804.
26. Kraske, L.M., and Zahran, M. 1965. Relationship of enamel solubility to caries experience. *J. Dent. Res.* 44:1413.
27. Cutress, T.W. 1972. The inorganic composition and solubility of dental enamel from several specified population groups. *Arch. Oral Biol.* 17: 93-109.
28. Isaac, S.; Brudevold, F.; Smith, F.A.; and Gardner, D.E. 1958. Solubility rate and natural fluoride content of surface and subsurface enamel. *J. Dent. Res.* 37:254-63.
29. Brudevold, F. 1948. A study of the phosphate solubility of the human enamel surface. *J. Dent. Res.* 27:320-29.
30. Nicholson, C.R., and Mellberg, J.R. 1969. Effect of natural fluoride concentration of human tooth enamel on fluoride uptake *in vitro*. *J. Dent. Res.* 48:302-6.
31. Eigen, E.; Volpe, A.R.; Lapeyroleries, F.M.; Weiss, S.; and King, W.J. 1963. An *in vivo* technique for determining the effect of agents on enamel solubility in human subjects. *Arch. Oral Biol.* 8:459-60.
32. Herd, J.K., and Overell, B.G. 1964. Effect of toothpaste containing sodium monofluorophosphate on enamel solubility *in vivo*. *Brit. Dent. J.* 117:286-91.
33. Morley, C.W. and Holmes, A.W. 1965. *In vivo* assessment of tooth enamel solubility in acid. *Brit. Dent. J.* 118: 71-76.
34. King, W.J.; Weiss, S.; Volpe, A.R.; and Eigen, E. 1965. *In vivo* tooth surface solubility studies. *Ann. N. Y. Acad. Sci.* 131:713-26.
35. Kawasaki, T.; Takeuchi, M.; and Amano, F. 1974. Effect of pre-test food uptake and the use of stannous fluoride dentifrice on the biopsy

method for the acid resistance of surface enamel. *J. Dent. Health (Jap.)* 24:120-23.

36. Gulzow, H.J., and Jellinghous, M. 1973. Caries prophylaxis by local application of fluorides as solution, jelly or lacquer. *Deutsch Zahnaerztl Z.* 28:592-97.
37. von der Fehr, F.R.; Møller, I.J.; Steinnes, E.; and Poulsen, S. 1971. The effect of topical fluoride treatments on the *in vivo* solubility of young incisors. *Caries Res.* 5:22.
38. Feller, R.P. 1974. Reduction of enamel solubility by daily use of a 0.4% stannous fluoride gel. *J. Dent. Res.* 53:1280-83.
39. Nygaard-Ostby, B.; Morch, T.; and Hals, E. 1957. A method for caries production on selected tooth surfaces *in vivo. Acta Odont. Scand.* 15:357-63.
40. von der Fehr, F.R. 1961. The effect of fluorides on the caries resistance of enamel. *Acta Odont. Scand.* 19: 431-42.
41. von der Fehr, F.R. 1967. A study of carious lesions produced *in vivo* in unabraded, abraded, exposed and F-treated human enamel surfaces, with emphasis on the x-ray dense outer layer. *Arch. Oral Biol.* 12:797-814.
42. Konig, C.G.; Marthaler, T.M.; and Mühlemann, H.R. 1958. Inter-relation between enamel solubility reduction and caries inhibition. *Helv. Odont. Acta* 2:34-39.
43. Regolati, B.; Schait, A.; Schmid, R.; and Mühlemann, H. R. 1975. Effect of enamel solubility reducing agents on erosion in the rat. *Helva Odont. Acta* 19:31-36.
44. Greer, R.M., and Hartles, R.L. 1968. A study of the effects of the topical application of solutions and dentifrices containing fluorides on the incidence of caries and the surface solubility of the molar teeth of the albino rat. *Arch. Oral Biol.* 13:115-24.
45. De Paola, P.F.; Brudevold, F.; Aasenden, R.; Moreno, E.C.; Englander, H.R.; Bakhos, Y.; Bookstein, F.; and Warram, J. 1975. A pilot study of the relationship between caries experience and surface enamel fluoride in man. *Arch. Oral Biol.* 20: 859-64.
46. Keene, H.J.; Mellberg, J.R.; and Nicholson, C.R. 1973. History of fluoride, dental fluorosis, and concentrations of fluoride in surface layer of enamel of caries-free Naval recruits. *J. Pub. Health Dent.* 33:142-48.
47. Candeli, A.; Scavizzi, F.; and Marci, F. 1970. The relationship between fluoride concentration and the caries frequency of different tooth surfaces in a high fluoride area. *Caries Res.* 4: 69-77.
48. Gedalia, I.; Rosenweig, K.A.; and Sadeh, A. 1961. Fluoride content of superficial enamel layer and its correlation with F content of saliva, tooth age and DMFT count. *J. Dent. Res.* 40:865-69.
49. Englander, H.R., and Mellberg, J.R. 1976. Failure to demonstrate an association between enamel fluoride concentration and dental caries in the deciduous dentition. *J. Dent. Res.* 55: 707.
50. Poulsen, S., and Larsen, M.J. 1975. Dental caries in relation to fluoride content of enamel in the primary dentition. *Caries Res.* 9:59-65.
51. Bischoff, J.I.; van der Merwe, E.H.M.; Retief, D.H.; Barbakow, F.N.; and Cleaton-Jones, P.E. 1976. Relationship between fluoride concentrations in enamel, DMFT index, and degree of fluorosis in a community residing in an area with a high level of fluoride. *J. Dent. Res.* 55:37-42.
52. Keene, H.J.; Grossman, F.D.; Pederson, E.D.; Mellberg, J.R.; and Nicholson, C.R. 1975. Caries experience and fluoride concentration of surface enamel in dental fluorosis patients. *Caries Res. 9:247-50.*
53. van der Merwe, E.H.M.; Bischoff, J.I.; Fatti, L.P.; Retief, D.H.; Barbakow, F.H.; and Friedman, M. 1977. Relationship between fluoride in enamel, DMFT index and fluorosis in high — and low — fluoride areas in South Africa. *Community Dent. Oral Epidemiol.* 5:61-64.
54. Richards, A.; Larsen, M.J.; Fejerskov, O.; and Thylstrup, A. 1977. Fluoride content of buccal surface enamel and its relation to dental caries in children. *Arch. Oral Biol.* 22:425-28.
55. Aasenden, R., and Peebles, T.C. 1974. Effects of fluoride supplementation from birth on deciduous and permanent teeth. *Arch. Oral Biol.* 19:321-26.
56. Deatherage, C.F. 1943. Fluoride domestic waters and dental caries experience in 2,026 white Illinois Selective Service men. *J. Dent. Res.* 22:129-37.
57. Russell, A.L. 1949. Dental effects of exposure to fluoride bearing Dakota sandstone waters at various ages and for various lengths of time. *J. Dent. Res.* 28:600-12.
58. Way, R.M. 1964. The effect on dental caries of a change from a naturally fluoridated to a fluoride-free communal water. *J. Dent. Child.* 31 (No. 2):151-57.
59. Backer-Dirks, O. 1974. The benefits of water fluoridation. *Caries Res.* 8 (Suppl. No. 1.):2-15.
60. Mellberg, J.R.; Englander, H.R.; and Nicholson, C.R. 1967. Acquisition of fluoride *in vivo* by deciduous enamel from daily topical sodium fluoride applications over 21 months. *Arch. Oral Biol.* 12:1139-48.

61. Englander, H.R.; Keyes, P.H.; Gestwicki, M.; and Sultz, H.A. 1967. Clinical anticaries effect of repeated topical sodium fluoride applications by mouthpieces. *J. Amer. Dent. Assoc.* 75:638-44.
62. Mellberg, J.R., and Nicholson, C.R. 1974. Weekly mouthrinsing with 3000 ppm of fluoride; the effect of concentration of fluoride in the enamel. *J. Pub. Health Dent.* 34:2-7.
63. Mellberg, J.R., and Nicholson, C.R. 1974. Fluoride uptake in vivo by deciduous enamel of children from neutral fluoride and APF mouthrinses. *Caries Res.* 8:148-54.
64. Aasenden, R.; De Paola, P.F.; and Brudevold, F. 1972. Effects of daily rinsing and ingestion of fluoride solutions upon dental caries and enamel fluoride. *Arch. Oral Biol.* 17: 1705-14.
65. Heifetz, S.B.; Driscoll, W.S.; and Creighton, W.E. 1973. The effect on dental caries of weekly rinsing with a neutral sodium fluoride or an acidulted phosphate-fluoride mouthwash. *J. Amer. Dent. Assoc.* 87:364-68.
66. Knutson, J.W., and Armstrong, W.D. 1946. Effect of topically applied sodium fluoride on dental caries experience III. Report of findings for the third study year. *Pub. Health Rept.* 61:1683-89.
67. Sundvall-Hagland, I.; Brudevold, F.; Armstrong, W.D.; Gardner, D.E.; and Smith, F.A. 1959. A comparison of the increment of fluoride in enamel and the reduction in dental caries resulting from topical fluoride applications. *Arch. Oral Biol.* 1: 74-79.
68. Syrrist, A. 1956. A 7-year report on the effect of topical applications of sodium fluoride on dental caries. *Odont. Rev.* 7:386-96.
69. Bibby, B.G., and Turesky, S.S. 1947. A note on the duration of caries inhibition produced by fluoride applications. *J. Dent. Res.* 26:105-8.
70. Koch, G. 1969. Caries increment in school children during and two years after the end of supervised rinsing of the mouth with sodium fluoride solution. *Odont. Rev.* 20:323-30.
71. Koch, G. 1970. Long term study of effect of supervised toothbrushing with a sodium fluoride dentifrice. *Caries Res.* 149-57.
72. Englander, H.R.; Carlos, J.P.; Senning, R.S.; and Mellberg, J.R. 1969. Residual anticaries effect of repeated topical sodium fluoride applications by mouthpieces. *J. Amer. Dent. Assoc.* 78:783-87.
73. Horowitz, H.S., and Kau, M.C.W. 1974. Retained anti-caries protection from topically applied acidulated phosphate-fluoride: 30 and 36 mouth post-treatment effects. *J. Prev. Dent.* 1: 22-27.
74. Houwink, B.; Backer-Dirks, O.; and Kwant, G.W. 1974. A nine year study of topical application with stannous fluoride in identical twins and the caries experience five years after ending the applications. *Caries Res.* 8:27-38.
75. Mellberg, J.R.; Franchi, G.J.; Englander, H.R.; Mosely, G.W.; and Nicholson, C.R. 1978. Short intensive topical APF applications and dental caries in a fluoridated area. *Community Dent. Oral Epidemiol.* 6:117-20.
76. Larson, R.H.; Mellberg, J.R.; Englander, H.R.; and Senning, R.S. 1976. Caries inhibition in the rat by water-borne and enamel-bound fluoride. *Caries Res.* 10:321-31.
77. Englander, H.R., and Keyes, P.H. 1967. Residual anticaries effect of topical sodium fluoride applications in the Syrian hamster. *J. Dent. Res.* 46:264-67.
78. Charleton, G.; Schamschula, R.G.; and Blainey, B.L. 1975. Analysis of the relationship of enamel fluoride to caries incidence. *J. Dent. Res.* 54:665.
79. Backer-Dirks, O. 1966. Post-eruptive changes in dental enamel. *J. Dent. Res.* 45:503-11.
80. Francis, M.D., and Briner, W.W. 1966. The development and regression of hypomineralized areas of rat molars. *Arch. Oral Biol.* 11:349-54.
81. Fitzgerald, R.J., and Konig, K.G. 1968. Maturation of dental enamel in germ-free and monoinfected Sprague-Dawley rats. *Helv. Odont. Acta* 12:55-61.
82. Little, M.F.; Casciani, F.S.; and Rowley, J. 1967. Site of fluoride accumulation in intact erupted human enamel. *Arch. Oral Biol.* 12:839-47.
83. Levine, R.S. 1972. Distribution of fluoride in active and arrested carious lesions in dentin. *J. Dent. Res.* 51: 1025-29.
84. Weatherell, J.A.; Robinson, C.; and Hallsworth, A.S. 1972. Changes in the fluoride concentration of the labial enamel surface with age. *Caries Res.* 6:312-24.
85. Mellberg, J.R., and Larson, R.H. 1978. Effect of a cariogenic challenge on fluoride uptake by enamel of rats receiving fluoridated drinking water. *Caries Res.* 12:137-41.
86. Klein, H. 1945. Dental caries experience in relocated children exposed to water containing fluoride. I. Incidence of new caries after two years of exposure among previously caries-free permanent teeth. *Pub. Health Rept.* 60:1462-67.
87. Klein, H. 1946. Dental caries (DMF) experience in relocated children exposed to water containing fluorine. II. *J. Amer. Dent. Assoc.* 33:1136-41.
88. Hayes, R.L.; Littleton, N.W.; and White, C.L. 1957. Post-eruptive effects of fluoridation on first permanent molars of children in Grand

Rapids, Michigan. *Am. J. Pub. Health* 47:192-99.
89. Backer-Dirks, O.; Houwink, B.; and Kwant, G.W. 1961. Some special features of the caries preventive effect of water fluoridation. *Arch. Oral Biol.* 4:187-92.
90. Russell, A. L., and White, C. L. 1961. Dental caries in Maryland children after seven years of fluoridation. *Pub. Health Rept.* 76:1087-93.
91. Horowitz, H. S.; Heifetz, S. B.; and Law, F. E. 1972. Effect of school water fluoridation on dental caries: final results in Elk Lake, Pa., after 12 years. *J. Amer. Dent. Assoc.* 84:832-38.
92. Heifetz, S.B., and Horowitz, H.S. 1974. Effect of school water fluoridation on dental caries: interim results in Seagrove, N.C., after four years. *J. Amer. Dent. Assoc.* 88:352-55.
93. Muhler, J.C. 1960. The anticariogenic effectiveness of a single application of stannous fluoride in children residing in an optimal communal fluoride area. II. Results at the end of 30 months. *J. Amer. Dent. Assoc.* 61:431-38.
94. Wellock, W. D.; Maitland, A.; and Brudevold, F. 1965. Caries increments, tooth discoloration, and state of oral hygiene in children given single annual applications of acid phosphate fluoride and stannous fluoride. *Arch. Oral Biol.* 10:453-60.
95. De Paola, P.F., and Mellberg, J.R. 1973. Caries experience and fluoride uptake in children receiving semi-annual prophylaxes with an acidulated phosphate fluoride paste. *J. Amer. Dent. Assoc.* 87:155-59.
96. Harris, R. 1959. Observations on the effect of topical sodium fluoride on caries incidence in children. *Aust. Dent. J.* 4:257-60.
97. Volker, J.F., and Klapper, C.E. 1954. Some observations on dental caries in Syrian hamsters. *Oral Surg.* 7:207-12.
98. Konig, K.G.; Mühlemann, H.R.; Schait, A.; and Schmid, R. 1965. The effect of post-eruptive fluoride uptake and enamel maturation on dental caries in Osborne-Mendel rats. *Helv. Odont. Acta* 9:135-40.
99. Konig, K.G. 1965. Caries resistance in experimental animals. In *Caries resistant teeth*, eds. G.E.W. Wolstenholme and M. O'Connor, pp. 87-106. Ciba Foundation Symposium, (Churchill, London).
100. Larson, R.H., and Fitzgerald, R.J. 1964. Caries development in rats of different ages with controlled flora. *Arch. Oral Biol.* 9:705-12.
101. Speirs, R.L. 1967. Factors influencing "maturation" of developmental hypomineralized areas in the enamel of rat molars. *Caries Res.* 1:15-31.
102. Briner, W.W., and Rosen, S. 1967. Effect of fluoride on hypomineralized areas in the molars of rats fed a cariogenic diet. *Arch. Oral Biol.* 12:1077-84.
103. Fanning, R.J.; Shaw, J.H.; and Sognnaes, R.F. 1954. Salivary contribution to enamel maturation and caries resistance. *J. Amer. Dent. Assoc.* 49:668-71.
104. Rowe, N.H. 1977. *Introduction to symposium on: incipient caries of enamel.* Ann Arbor: University of Mich. Nov. 11-12.
105. Head, J. 1912. A study of saliva and its action on tooth enamel in reference to its hardening and softening. *J.A.M.A.* 59:2118-22.
106. Andresen, V. 1921. Uber mineralization und remineralization des Zahnschmelzes. *Dtsch. Mschr. Zahnheilk.* 39:97.
107. Koulourides, T., and Pigman, W. 1960. Studies on rehardening of artificially softened enamel. *J. Dent. Res.* 39:198.
108. von der Fehr, F.R. 1965. Maturation and remineralization. *Adv. Fluor. Res.* 3:83-95.
109. Poole, D.F.G., and Silverstone, L. M. 1973. Remineralization of enamel. In *Hard tissue growth, repair and remineralization.* Ciba Foundation Symposium II.
110. Mühlemann, H.R.; Lenz, H.; and Rossinsky, K. 1964. Electron microscopic appearance of rehardened enamel. *Helv. Odont. Acta* 8:108-11.
111. Wei, S.H.Y. 1970. Electron microprobe analysis of the remineralization of enamel. *J. Dent. Res.* 49:612-25.
112. McCormick, J.; Manson-Hing, L.; Wolff, A.E.; and Koulourides, T. 1970. Remineralizing mouthwash rationale and a pilot clinical study. *Ala. J. Med. Sci.* 7:92-97.
113. Koulourides, T., and Axelsson, P. 1977. Experimental and clinical studies of caries arrestment. *Caries Res.* 11:130.
114. Andresen, V. 1922. Mineralisationszemente zur behandlung der Caries incipiens. *Dtsch. Mschr. Zahnheilk.* 40:707.
115. Wilson, L.A. 1928. Is the artificial calcification and recalcification of dental enamel possible? *Dent. Digest* 34:689.
116. Muhler, J.C. 1960. Stannous fluoride enamel pigmentation—evidence of caries arrestment. *J. Dent. Child.* 27:157-61.
117. Muhler, J.C.; Spear, L.B.; Bixler, D.; and Stookey, G. K. 1967. The arrestment of incipient dental caries in adults after the use of three different forms of SnF_2 therapy: results after 30 months. *J. Amer. Dent. Assoc.* 75:1402-06.
118. Mercer, V.H., and Muhler, J.C. 1965. The clinical demonstration of caries arrestment following topical stannous fluoride treatments. *J.*

Dent. Child. 32:65-72.
119. Anderson, B.G. 1938. Clinical study of arresting dental caries. *J. Dent. Res.* 17:443-52.
120. Ostrom, C.A. 1978. Effectiveness of a preventive dentistry delivery system. *J. Amer. Dent. Assoc.* 97:29-36.
121. Hyde, E.J. 1973. Caries inhibiting action of three different topically applied agents on incipient lesion in newly erupted teeth: results after 24 months. *J. Canad. Dent. Assoc.* 39:189-93.
122. Hollender, L., and Koch, G. 1969. Influence of topical application of fluoride on rate of progress of carious lesions in children. *Odont. Revy.* 20:37-41.
123. Nishino, M. 1969. Studies on the topical applications of ammoniacal silver fluoride for the arrestment of dental caries. *J. Osaka Univ. Dent. Soc.* 14:1-14.
124. Koulourides, T. 1968. Experimental changes of enamel mineral density. In *Art and science of dental caries research* ed. R. S. Harris. New York: Academic Press.
125. Koulourides, T.; Phantumvanit, P.; Munksgaard, E.C.; and Hausch, T. 1974. An intraoral model used for studies of fluoride incorporation in enamel. *J. Oral Path.* 3:185-96.
126. Bibby, B.G.; Zero, D.; and Deeney, M. 1978. Experimental white spot development in vital teeth. *Ann. Mtg. Int. Assoc. Dent. Res.* Abstr. No. 1102.
127. Sognnaes, R.F. 1963. Dental hard tissue destruction with special reference to idiopathic erosions. In *Mechanisms of hard tissue destruction,* ed. R.F. Sognnaes. Washington, D.C.: AAAS, Publ. No. 75.
128. von der Fehr, F.R.; Loe, N.; and Theilade, E. 1970. Experimental caries in man. *Caries Res.* 4:131-48.
129. Levine, R.S. 1975. An initial clinical assessment of a mineralizing mouthrinse. *Brit. Dent. J.* 138:249-53.
130. Sperber, G.H., and Buonocore, M.G. 1963. Effect of different acids on character of demineralization of enamel surfaces. *J. Dent. Res.* 42:707-23.
131. Sperber, G.H., and Buonocore, M.G. 1963. Enamel surface in white spot formation. *J. Dent. Res.* 42:724-31.
132. Silverstone, L.M. 1977. Structural alterations of human dental enamel during the incipient lesion development. In *Proc. symp. on incipient caries of enamel.* ed. N. H. Rowe, pp. 3-50. Ann Arbor: Univ. of Mich. Press.
133. Gray, J.A., and Francis, M.D. 1963. Physical chemistry of enamel dissolution. In *Mechanisms of hard tissue destruction.* ed. R.F. Sognnaes, pp. 213-60. Washington, D.C.: AAAS, Publ. No. 75.
134. Grieve, A.R. 1978. The production of secondary caries-like lesions *in vitro*. *Caries Res.* 12:35-42.
135. Besic, F.C. 1953. Caries-like enamel changes by chemical means. *J. Dent. Res.* 32:830-39.
136. Wei, S.H.Y., and Koulourides, T. 1972. Electron microprobe and microhardness studies of enamel remineralization. *J. Dent. Res.* 51:648-51.
137. Manson-hing, L.R.; Keller, S.E.; Feagin, F.F.; and Koulourides, T. 1972. Microradiographic comparison of artificial caries systems. *J. Dent. Res.* 51:923-28.
138. Francis, M.D.; Briner, W.W.; and Gray, J.A. 1973. Chemical agents in the control of calcification processes in biological systems. In *Hard tissue growth, repair and remineralization.* Ciba Foundation Symposium II.
139. Featherstone, J.D.B. 1977. Diffusion phenomena during artificial carious lesion formation. *J. Dent. Res.* 56: D48-D52.
140. Woltgens, J.H.M. 1975. Influence of diphosphonates and sodium fluoride on the development of artificial lesions. *Caries Res.* 9:438-44.
141. Levine, R.S., and Coulter, W.A. 1976. A preliminary report on human enamel demineralization in an artificial mouth. *Arch. Oral Biol.* 21:137-39.
142. Davidson, C.L.; Boom, G.; and Arends, J. 1973. Calcium distribution in human and bovine surface enamel. *Caries Res.* 7:349-59.
143. Groeneveld, A., and Arends, J. 1975. Influence of pH and demineralization time on mineral content, thickness of surface layer and depth of artificial caries lesions. *Caries Res.* 9:36-44.
144. Groeneveld, A.; Purdell-Lewis, D.J.; and Arends, J. 1975. Influence of the mineral content of enamel on caries-like lesions produced in hydroxyethyl cellulose buffer solutions. *Caries Res.* 9:127-38.
145. Manson-Hing, L.R.; Keller, S.W.; Feagin, F.F.; and Koulourides, T. 1972. Microradiographic comparison of artificial caries systems. *J. Dent. Res.* 51:923-28.
146. Groeneveld, A.; Theuns, H.H.; and Kalter, P.G.E. 1978. Microradiography of developing artificial dental caries-like lesions in man. *Arch. Oral Biol.* 23:75-83.
147. Davidson, C.L.; Arends, J.; and Hoekstra, I. 1976. Density changes in enamel after decalcification. *J. Biomechanics* 9:81-85.
148. Featherstone, J.D.B.; Duncan, J.F.; and Cutress, T.W. 1978. Crystallographic changes in human tooth enamel during *in vitro* caries

simulation. *Arch. Oral Biol.* 23:405-13.

149. Larsen, M.J. 1974. Demineralization of human enamel. *Scand. J. Dent. Res.* 82:491-95.

150. Clarkson, B.H., and Silverstone, L.M. 1974. The effects on enamel of several different topical fluoride agents *in vitro*. *J. Int. Assoc. Dent. Child.* 5:27-32.

151. Clarkson, B.H. 1978. The effect of metal/fluoride complexes on fluoride uptake and caries-like lesion formation in enamel. *J. Dent. Res.* 57:784-89.

152. Purdell-Lewis, D.J.; Groeneveld, A.; and Arends, J. 1978. The effect of demineralization of SnF_2-treated white spot enamel lesions. *Caries Res.* 12:52-59.

153. Buonocore, M.G., and Gwinnett, A.J. 1967. Chemical, polarized light, and microradiographic study of the effects of various toothpastes on "white spot" formation *in vitro*. *J. Oral Ther. Pharm.* 3:321-29.

154. Purdell-Lewis, D.J.; Arends, J.; and Groeneveld, A. 1978. The effect of differing concentrations of SnF_2 on demineralized enamel. *Caries Res.* 12:43-51.

155. Purdell-Lewis, D.J.; Groeneveld, A.; and Arends, J. 1976. Microhardness and densitometric measurements of the effect of 4% SnF_2 solution on artificial white spot lesions. *Caries Res.* 10:216-26.

156. Mellberg, J.R. 1980. Penetration of fluorine from sodium monofluorophosphate into artificially produced incipient enamel lesions. *Caries Res.* 14:115-20.

157. Koulourides, T.; Cueto, H.; and Pigman, W. 1961. Rehardening of softened enamel surfaces of human teeth by solutions of calcium phosphate. *Nature (Lond.)* 189:226-27.

158. Wei, S.H.Y., and Wefel, J.S. 1976. In vitro interactions between the surfaces of enamel white spots and calcifying solutions. *J. Dent. Res.* 55:135-41.

159. Johansson, B. 1965. Remineralization of slightly etched enamel. *J. Dent. Res.* 44:64-70.

160. Silverstone, L.M. 1972. Remineralization of human enamel *in vitro*. *Proc. Royal Soc. Med.* 65:906-8.

161. ten Cate, J.M.; Flim, G.J.; and Arends, J. 1977. Site of enamel-lesion-remineralization. *J. Dent. Res.* 56:D146.

162. Koulourides, T.; Feagin, F.; and Pigman, W. 1965. Remineralization of dental enamel by saliva *in vitro*. *Ann. N.Y. Acad. Sci.* 131:751-57.

163. Pigman, W.; Kotwal, K.; and Koulourides, T. 1966. Calcifying ability of human body fluids. *Arch. Oral Biol.* 11:815-24.

164. Silverstone, L.M., and Poole, D.F.G. 1969. Histologic and ultrastructural features of remineralized enamel. *J. Dent. Res.* 48:766-70.

165. Gron, P. 1973. Remineralization of enamel lesions *in vivo*. *Oral Sci. Rev.* 3:84-99.

166. Gron, P., and Hay, D.I. 1976. Inhibition of calcium phosphate precipitation by human salivary secretions. *Arch. Oral Biol.* 21:201-5.

167. Schlesinger, D.H., and Hay, D.I. 1977. Complete covalent structure of Statherin, a tyrosine rich acidic peptide which inhibits calcium phosphate precipitation from human parotid saliva. *J. Biological Chem.* 252:1689-95.

168. Brown, W.E.; Smith, J.P.; Lehr, J.R.; and Frazier, A. W. 1962. Crystallographic and chemical relations between octacalcium phosphate and hydroxyapatite. *Nature (Lond.)* 196:1050-55.

169. Pigman, W.; Cueto, H; and Baugh, D. 1964. Conditions affecting the rehardening of softened enamel. *J. Dent. Res.* 43:1187-95.

170. Silverstone, L.M., and Johnson, N.W. 1971. The effect on sound enamel of exposures to calcifying fluids *in vitro*. *Caries Res.* 5:323-42.

171. Gron, P., and Amdur, B.H. 1975. The effect of topically applied fluoride on enamel remineralization *in vitro*. *Arch. Oral Biol.* 20:223-24.

172. Koulourides, T.; Keller, S.; Manson-Hing, L; and Boddan, R. 1971. Fluoride topicals tested intraorally on sample enamel in humans. *Ann. Mtg. Int. Assoc. Dent. Res.* Abstr. No. 363.

173. Levine, R.S., and Rowles, S.L. 1973 Further studies on the remineralization of human carious dentin *in vitro*. *Arch. Oral Biol.* 18:1351-56.

174. Koulourides, T. 1978. Tooth surface adaptation to the cariogenic challenge. *Ann. Mtg. Int. Assoc. Dent. Res.* Abstr. No. 430.

175. Levine, R.S. 1972. Distribution of fluoride in active and arrested carious lesions of dentin. *J. Dent. Res.* 51:1025-29.

176. Miller, W.D. 1905. A study of certain questions relating to the pathology of the teeth. *Dent. Cosmos* 47:18-39.

177. Beust, T.B. 1930. Microorganisms and caries. *J. Amer. Dent. Assoc.* 17:1536-44.

178. Enright, J.J., and Friesell, H.E. 1933. Studies of the cause and nature of dental caries. *J. Amer. Dent. Assoc.* 20:897-910.

179. Little, M.F.; Cueto, E.S.; and Rowley, J. 1962. Chemical and physical properties of altered and sound enamel. I. Ash, Ca, P, CO_2, N, water, microradiolucency and density. *Arch. Oral Biol.* 7:173-84.

180. Little, M.F.; Posen, J.; and Singer, L. 1962. Chemical and physical properties of altered and sound enamel. III. Fluoride and sodium content. *J. Dent. Res.* 41:784-89.

181. Francis, M.D. 1966. The effectiveness of antica-

ries agents in rats using an incipient lesion method. *Arch. Oral Biol.* 11:349-54.

182. Gron, P. 1977. Can incipient lesions be arrested? *Proceedings of symposium on incipient caries of enamel,* ed. N. H. Rowe, pp. 145-69. Ann Arbor: Univ. of Michigan.
183. Jenkins, G.N. 1963. Theories on the mode of action of fluoride in reducing dental decay. *J. Dent. Res.* 42: 444-52.
184. Yao, K., and Gron, P. 1970. Fluoride concentrations in duct saliva and in whole saliva. *Caries Res.* 4:321-31.
185. Gron, P.; McCann, H.G.; and Brudevold, F. 1968. The direct determination of fluoride in human saliva by a fluoride electrode. *Arch. Oral Biol.* 13:203-13.
186. Ericsson, Y. 1969. Fluoride excretion in human saliva and milk. *Caries Res.* 3:159-66.
187. Aasenden, R.; Brudevold, F.; and Richardson, B. 1968. Clearance of fluoride from the mouth after topical treatment or the use of a fluoride mouthrinse. *Arch. Oral Biol.* 13: 625-36.
188. Shannon, I.L., and Edmonds, E.J. 1972. Effect of fluoride dosage on human parotid saliva fluoride levels. *Arch. Oral Biol.* 17:1303-9.
189. Shannon, I.L.; Suddick, R.P.; and Edmonds, E.J. 1973. Effect of rate of gland function on parotid saliva fluoride concentration. *Caries Res.* 7:1-10.
190. Birkeland, J.M., and Rolla, G. 1972. *In vitro* affinity of fluoride to proteins, dextrans, bacteria and salivary components. *Arch. Oral Biol.* 17:455-63.
191. Birkeland, J.M. 1973. The effect of pH on the interaction of fluoride and salivary ions. *Caries Res.* 7:1-8.
192. Carlson, C.N.; Armstrong, W.D.; and Singer, L. 1960. Distribution and excretion of radio-fluoride in the human. *Proc. Soc. Exp. Biol. Med.* 104:235-39.
193. Ahrens, G. 1965. Investigations into the salivary excretion of fluoride after oral ingestion of sodium fluoride and tablets containing fluoride *J. Dent. Res.* 44 (Abstr.):1144.
194. Brudevold, F.; Bakhos, Y.; and Gron, P. 1973. Fluoride in human saliva after ingestion of aluminum chloride and sodium fluoride or sodium monofluorophosphate. *Arch. Oral Biol.* 18:699-706.
195. Saxer, U.P. 1970. Oral fluoride clearance after application of fluoride containing dentifrices or rinsing fluids. *Schweiz. Mschr. Zahnheilk* 80:237-42.
196. DeBoever, J., and Mühlemann, H.R. 1970. Radiotelemetric determination of oral fluoride clearance after local application of fluoride. *Schweiz. Mschr. Zahnheilk.* 80:225-36.
197. Silvera, R.S.; Gabathuler, H.; and Mühlemann, H.R. 1974. Salivary fluoride levels after mouthrinsing with inorganic fluoride and amine fluoride. *Helv. Odont. Acta* 18 (Suppl. VIII):79-81.
198. Marthaler, T.M., and Schait, A. 1968. Fluoride concentrations in saliva during and after supervised toothbrushing with 1 percent sodium fluoride solution. *Helv. Odont. Acta* 12:33-38.
199. Birkeland, J.M. 1971. Fluoride ion activity *in vitro* and *in vivo* of two sodium fluoride dentifrices. *Caries Res.* 5:193-201.
200. Graf, H., and Mühlemann, H.R. 1969. Oral telemetry of fluoride ion activity. *Arch. Oral Biol.* 14:259-63.
201. Duckworth, R., and Joyston-Bechal, S. 1966. The distribution of dentifrice fluoride during and after toothbrushing. *Adv. F Res. Dent. Caries Prev.* 4:113-19.
202. Parkins, F.M. 1971. Fluoride concentrations in saliva after chewing fluoride tablets. *J. Dent. Res.* 50:515.
203. Shields, W.F., and Mühlemann, H.R. 1975. Simultaneous pH and fluoride telemetry from the oral cavity. *Helv. Odont. Acta* 19:18-26.
204. Bibby, B.G., and van Kesteren, M. 1940. The effect of fluorine on mouth bacteria. *J. Dent. Res.* 19:391-402.
205. Simonson, L.G., and Shklair, I.L. 1972. The in vitro inhibitory effect of fluoride ion on streptococcus mutans. Ann. Mtgs. Int. Assoc. Dent. Res. Abstr. No. 77.
206. Shiota, T. 1956. Effect of sodium fluoride on oral lactobacilli isolated from the rat. *J. Dent. Res.* 35: 939-46.
207. Clapper, W.E. 1947. The effect of sodium fluoride on the metabolism of oral lactobacilli. *Proc. Soc. Exp. Biol. Med.* 65:333-36.
208. Ericsson, Y., and Hellstrom, I. 1952. The lactic acid content of the saliva after carbohydrate ingestion II. Source of the salivary lactic acid and inhibition of its formation. *Acta Odont. Scand.* 10:118-33.
209. Wright, D.N., and Jenkins, G.N. 1954. The effect of fluoride in the acid production of saliva glucose mixture. *Brit. Dent. J.* 96:30-33.
210. Lilienthal, B. 1956. The effect of fluoride on acid formation by salivary sediment. *J. Dent. Res.* 35:197-204.
211. Hellstom, I. 1960. Fluorine retention following sodium fluoride mouthwashing. *Acta Odont. Scand.* 18:263-78.
212. Sims, W. 1966. The effect of sodium fluoride on the rate of acid production of surface aggregates of streptococci and lactobacilli. *J. Dent.*

Res. 45:915-20.

213. Jenkins, G.N.; Ferguson, D.B.; and Edgar, W.M. 1967. Fluoride and the metabolism of salivary bacteria. *Acta Odont. Helv.* 11:2-10.

214. Kleinberg, I. 1967. Effect of varying sediment and glucose concentrations on the pH and acid production in human salivary sediment mixtures. *Arch. Oral Biol.* 12:1457-73.

215. Capozzi, L.; Brunetti, P.; Negri, P.L.; and Migliorini, E. 1967. Enzymatic mechanism of action of some fluorine compounds. *Caries Res.* 1:69-77.

216. Sandham, H.J., and Kleinberg, I. 1973. Effect of fluoride on carbon dioxide and acid formation in salivary sediment mixtures incubated with glucose. *Arch. Oral Biol.* 18:211-25.

217. Jenkins, G. N. 1959. The effect of pH on the fluoride inhibition of salivary acid production. *Arch. Oral Biol.* 1:33-41.

218. Roberts, M.H., and Rahn, O. 1946. Antisepsis and ionization of sodium fluoride. *J. Bact.* 52:612-13.

219. Molan, P.C., and Hartles, R.L. 1966. The differential effect of NaF on the aerobic and anaerobic metabolism of the human oral flora. *Arch. Oral Biol.* 11:1163-70.

220. Cimasoni, G. 1970. Fluoride and enzymes. In *Fluoride in medicine,* ed. T.L. Vischer. Bern: Huber.

221. Najjar, V.A. 1955. *Methods in enzymology,* ed. S.P. Colowick and O.K. Kaplan, pp. 298-99. New York: Academic Press.

222. Sandham, H.J., and Kleinberg, I. 1969. The effect of fluoride on the interrelation between glucose utilization, pH and carbohydrate storage in a salivary sediment system. *Arch. Oral Biol.* 14:619-28.

223. Weiss, S.; King, W.J.; Kestenbaum, R.C.; and Donohue, J.J. 1965. Influence of various factors on polysaccharide synthesis in *Streptococcus mitis. Ann. N.Y. Acad. Sci.* 131:839-50.

224. Segreto, V.A., and Jerman, A.C. 1970. Effect of 0.1% and 0.5% SnF_2 mouthwashes on whole saliva. *Ann. Mtg. Int. Assoc. Dent. Res.* Abstr. No. 301.

225. Plies, S.M. 1972. The in vivo effect of a 0.1% stannous fluoride mouthwash on various oral microorganisms. *Tex. Rep. Biol. Med.* 30:163-80.

226. Andres, C.J.; Schaeffer, J.C.; and Windeler, A.S., Jr. 1974. Comparison of antibacterial properties of stannous fluoride and sodium fluoride mouthwashes. *J. Dent. Res.* 53:457-60.

227. Woods, R. 1969. The effect of Na_2FPO_3 on salivary bacteria. *J. Dent. Res.* 48:1085-86.

228. Kozouskova, J.; Kubaniova, Z.; Psenak, M.; and Maternov, M. 1967. Vliv NaF lokalni aplikaci Na ustni laktobacily. *Dent. Abstr.* 12:345.

229. Dawes, C.; Jenkins, G.N.; Hardwick, J.L.; and Leach, S. 1965. The relation between the fluoride concentrations in the dental plaque and in drinking water. *Brit. Dent. J.* 119:164-67.

230. Edgar, W.M., and Jenkins, G.N. 1972. The ionizable F of plaque. *Ann. Mtg. Int. Assoc. Dent. Res.* Abstr. No. 173.

231. Singer, L.; Jarvey, B.A.; Venkateswarlu, P.; and Armstrong, W.D. 1970. Fluoride in plaque. *J. Dent. Res.* 49:455.

232. Gron, P.; Yao, K.; and Spinelli, M. 1969. A study of inorganic constituents in dental plaque. *J. Dent. Res.* 48: 799-805.

233. Agus, H.M.; Schamshula, R.G.; Barmes, D.E.; and Bunzel, M. 1976. Associations between the total fluoride content of dental plaque and individual caries experience in Australian children. *Community Dent. Oral Epidemiol.* 4:210-14.

234. Mühlemann, H.R.; Schait, A.; and Schroeder, H.E. 1964. Salivary origin of fluorine in calcified dental plaques. *Helv. Odont. Acta* 8:128-29.

235. Birkeland, J.M. 1972. Fluoride content of dental plaque after brushing with a fluoride dentifrice. *Scand. J. Dent. Res.* 80:80-81.

236. Edgar, W.M., and Tatevossian, A. 1971. The aqueous phase of plaque. In *Tooth Enamel II,* pp. 229-32. Bristol: Wright.

237. Birkeland, J.M. 1970. Direct potentiometric determination of fluoride in soft tooth deposits. *Caries Res.* 4:243-55.

238. Jenkins, G.N.; Edgar, W. M.; and Ferguson, D.B. 1969. The distribution and metabolic effects of human plaque fluorine. *Arch. Oral Biol.* 14:105-19.

239. Tatevossian, A., and Gould, C.T. 1976. The composition of the aqueous phase in human dental plaque. *Arch. Oral Biol.* 21:319-26.

240. Birkeland, J.M., and Charleton, G. 1976. Effect of pH on the fluoride ion activity of plaque. *Caries Res.* 10:72-80.

241. Jenkins, G.N., and Edgar, W.M. 1977. Distribution and forms of F in saliva and plaque. *Caries Res.* 11 (Suppl. 1):226-42.

242. Ferguson, D.B., and Jenkins, G.N. 1965. Some observations on the fluoride of dental plaque. *J. Dent. Res.* 44:1173.

243. Kasket, S., and Rodriguez, V.M. 1976. Fluoride accumulation by a strain of human oral *Streptococcous sanguis. Arch. Oral Biol.* 21:459-64.

244. Hardwick, J.L., and Leach, S.A. 1963. The fluoride content of the dental plaque. *Adv. F. Res. Dent. Caries Prev.* 2:151-58.

245. Birkeland, J.M.; Jorkjend, L.; and von der Fehr,

F.R. 1971. The influence of fluoride rinses on the fluoride content of dental plaques in children. *Caries Res.* 5:169-79.

246. Hassell, T.M.; Gabathuler, H.; and Mühlemann, H.R. 1971. Telemetric recording of fluorine in the interdental area. *Helv. Odont. Acta* 15:36-41.

247. Flessa, H.J., and Gulzow, H.J. 1970. The duration of presence of sodium fluoride and amine-fluoride in plaque. *Deutsch Zahnaerztl Z.* 25:252-59; *Oral Res.* Abstr. 5:6206.

248. Mainwaring, P.J. 1976. Fluoride, calcium and phosphorus concentrations in plaque following the use of a sodium monofluorophosphate toothpaste (NaMFP) containing calcium glycerophosphate (CaGP). Part II. *J. Dent. Res.* 55:D142.

249. Shern, R.J.; Rundell, B.B.; and DeFerver, C.J. 1974. Effects of an amine fluoride mouth rinse on the formation and microbial content of plaque. *Helv. Odont. Acta* 18 (Suppl. VIII): 57-62.

250. Mühlemann, H.R., and Strub, J.R. 1975. Inhibition of plaque growth with taurolin, vantocil and amine fluoride. *Helv. Odont. Acta* 19:57-60.

251. Lobene, R.R., and Soparkar, P.M. 1974. The effects of amine fluorides on human plaque and gingivitis. *Ann. Mtg. Int. Assoc. Dent. Res.* Abstr. No. 369.

252. Poulsen, S., and Møller, I. J. 1974. Dental plaque and gingivitis in relation to dental fluorosis in Khouribga, Morocco. *J. Dent. Res.* 53(Abstr.):1108.

253. Tinanoff, N.; Brady, J.M.; and Gross, A. 1976. The effect of NaF and SnF_2 mouthrinses on bacterial colonization of tooth enamel: TEM and SEM studies. *Caries Res.* 10: 415-26.

254. Gross, A., and Tinanoff, N. 1977. Effect of SnF_2 mouthrinse on initial bacterial colonization of tooth enamel. *J. Dent. Res.* 56:1179-83.

255. Lilienthal, B. 1956. The effect of a stannous fluoride mouthwash on acid formation in the mouth and some observations on the mechanism of inhibition. *Aust. Dent. J.* 1:221-27.

256. Svatun, B. 1978. Plaque-inhibiting effect of dentifrices containing stannous fluoride. *Acta Odont. Scand.* 36:205-10.

257. Svatun, B., and Attramadal, A. 1978. The effect of stannous fluoride on human plaque acidogenicity in situ (Stephen curve). *Acta Odont. Scand.* 36:211-12.

258. Pearlman, B.A., and Joyston-Bechal, S. 1973. Pilot study of the use of fluoride as a plaque preventive agent. *J. Dent. Res.* 52 (Abstr.):953.

259. Loesche, W.J.; Murray, R.J.; and Mellberg, J.R. 1973. The effect of topical acidulated fluoride on percentage of *Streptococcus mutans* and *Streptococcus sanguis* in interproximal plaque sample. *Caries Res.* 7:283-96.

260. Loesche, W.J.; Syed, S.A.; Murray, R.J.; and Mellberg, J.R. 1975. Effect of topical acidulated phosphate fluoride on percentage of *Streptococcus mutans* and *Streptococcus sanguis* in plaque. II. Pooled occlusal and pooled approximal samples. *Caries Res.* 9:139-55.

261. Mellberg, J.R.; Nicholson, C.R.; Franchi, G.J.; Englander, H.R.; and Mosley, G.W. 1977. Enamel fluoride uptake from intensive APF gel applications *in vivo*. *J. Dent. Res.* 56:716-21.

262. Woods, R. 1971. The short term effect of topical fluoride applications on the concentration of streptococcus in dental plaque. *Aust. Dent. J.* 16:152-55.

263. Woods, R.G. 1971. Toothbrush applied prophylactic paste and *Streptococcus mutans* in plaque. *J. Dent. Res.* 50:747-48.

264. Keene, H.J.; Shklair, I.L.; and Mickel, G.J. 1977. Effect of multiple dental floss—SnF_2 treatment on *Streptococcus mutans* in interproximal plaque. *J. Dent. Res.* 56: 21-27.

265. Keyes, P.H.; Rowberry, S.A.; Englander, H.R.; and Fitzgerald, R.J. 1966. Bio-assays of medicaments for the control of dentobacterial plaque, dental caries, and periodontal lesions in Syrian hamsters. *J. Oral Ther. Pharm.* 3:157-73.

266. Englander, H.R., and Keyes, P.H. 1968. Acid production in the dental plaque of hamsters protected from dental caries with sodium fluoride. *J. Oral Ther. Pharm.* 4:382-87.

267. Winkworth, R.J., and Jerman, A.C. 1973. *Plaque formation compared on surfaces of stannous fluoride containing and conventional amalgams.* U. S. Air Force Department: SAM-TR-73-25.

268. DeStoppelaar, J.D.; van Houte, J.; and Backer-Dirks, O. 1969. The relationship between extracellular polysaccharide producing streptococci and smooth surface caries in 13 year old children. *Caries Res.* 3:190-9.

269. Bowen, W. H. 1972. The effect of fluoride and molybdate on caries activity and the composition of plaque in monkeys. *Caries Res.* 6:254-55.

270. Kilian, M.; Thylstrup, A.; and Fejerskov, O. 1977. Microbial composition of dental plaque of Tanzanian children as related to water fluoride concentration and degree of dental fluorosis. *Caries Res.* 11:115.

271. Myers, M., and Handleman, S.L. 1971. Effect of daily application of fluoride in a custom fitted mouthpiece on plaque flora associated with dental decay. *J. Dent. Res.* 50: 597-603.

272. Jordan, H.V.; Englander, H.R.; and Lim, S. 1969. Potentially cariogenic streptococci in selected population groups in the western hemisphere. *J. Amer. Dent. Assoc.* 78:1331-35.

273. Broukal, Z., and Zajicek, O. 1974. Amount and distribution of extracellular polysaccharides in dental microbial plaque. *Caries Res.* 8:97-104.

274. van Houte, J.; Backer-Dirks, O.; DeStoppelaar, J.D.; and Jansen, H.M. 1969. Iodophilic polysaccharide producing bacteria and dental caries in children consuming fluoridated and non-fluoridated drinking water. *Caries Res.* 3:178-89.

275. Saxton, C.A., and Critchley, P. 1972. The effect of fluoride and monofluorophosphate on polysaccharide synthesis in human plaque *in vivo*. *Caries Res.* 6:254.

276. Shimura, N., and Onisi, M. 1978. The effect of sodium fluoride on the bacterial production of polysaccharide and subsequent adsorption on hydroxyapatite. *J. Dent. Res.* 57:928-31.

277. Bowen, W.H., and Hewitt, M.J. 1974. Effect of fluoride on extracellular polysaccharide production by *Streptococcus mutans*. *J. Dent. Res.* 53:627-629.

278. Norman, R.D.; Mehra, R.V.; Swartz, M.L.; and Phillips, R.W. 1972. Effects of restorative materials on plaque composition. *J. Dent. Res.* 51:1596-01.

279. Edgar, W.M.; Jenkins, G.N.; and Tatevossian, A. 1970. The inhibitory action of fluoride on plaque bacteria—further evidence. *Brit. Dent. J.* 128:129-32.

280. Stralfors, A. 1950. The bacterial chemistry of dental plaques. *Odont. Tidskr.* 58:155-341.

281. Neff, D. 1967. Acid production from different carbohydrate sources in human plaque in situ. *Caries Res.* 1:78-87.

282. Bowen, W.H., and Eastoe, J.E. 1967. The effect of sugar solutions containing fluoride and molybdate ions on the pH of plaque in monkeys. *Caries Res.* 1:130-36.

283. Cornick, D.E.R. 1968. Effect of fluorine and magnesium on acid production in plaque deposited on indwelling glass electrodes in monkeys *(Macaca Irus)*. *J. Dent. Res.* 47:974.

284. Bergman, G. 1952. Plaque test on teeth topically treated with sodium fluoride. *Acta Odont. Scand.* 10:111-17.

285. Stephen, K.W., and Jenkins, G.N. 1971. Studies on some factors affecting plaque pH. *Caries Res.* 5 (Abstr.): 28.

286. Zwemer, J.D. 1957. Lactic acid formation by lactobacilli exposed to fluoridized enamel. *J. Dent. Res.* 36:182-91.

287. Wooley, L.H., and Rickles, N.H. 1971. Inhibition of acidogenesis in human dental plaque in situ following the use of topical sodium fluoride. *Arch. Oral Biol.* 16:1187-94.

288. Fitzgerald, D.B., and Fitzgerald, R.J. 1973. Plaque acid production in hamsters pre-treated with fluoride. *J. Dent. Res.* 52:111-15.

289. Glas, J.E. 1962. Studies on the ultrastructure of dental enamel. VI. Crystal chemistry of shark's teeth. *Odont. Revy.* 13:315-26.

290. Charleton, G.; Blainey, B.; and Shamshula, R.G. 1974. Associations between dental plaque and fluoride in human surface enamel. *Arch. Oral Biol.* 19:139-43.

291. Weatherell, J.A.; Hallsworth, A.S.; and Robinson, C. 1973. The effect of tooth wear on the distribution of fluoride in the enamel surface of human teeth. *Arch. Oral Biol.* 18:1175-89.

292. Turtola, L.O. 1977. Enamel microhardness and fluoride uptake underneath fermenting and non-fermenting artificial plaque. *Scand. J. Dent. Res.* 85:373-79.

293. Briner, W.W., and Francis, M.D. 1962. The effect of enamel fluoride on acid production by *Lactobacillus casei*. *Arch. Oral Biol.* 7:541-50.

294. Rolla, G. 1977. Effects of fluoride on plaque formation. *Caries Res.* 11 (Suppl. 1):243-61.

295. Ericson, T., and Ericsson, Y. 1967. Effect of partial fluorine substitution on the phosphate exchange and protein adsorption of hydroxyapatite. *Helv. Odont. Acta* 11:10-14.

296. Rolla, G., and Melsen, B. 1975. Descrption of protein and bacteria from hydroxyapatite by fluoride and monofluorophosphate. *Caries Res.* 9:66-73.

297. Moreno, E.C.; Kresac, M.; and Hay, D.I. 1978. Adsorption of two human parotid salivary macromolecules on hydroxy-, fluorhydroxy- and fluroapatites. *Arch. Oral Biol.* 23:525-33.

298. Williams, R.A.D. 1967. The growth of Lancefield Group D streptococci in the presence of sodium fluoride. *Arch. Oral Biol.* 12:109-17.

299. Hamilton, I.R. 1969. Studies with fluoride-sensitive and fluoride-resistant strains of *Streptococcus salivarius*. II. Fluoride inhibition of glucose metabolism. *Canad. J. Microbiol.* 15:1021-27.

300. Kruger, W.W.; Frea, J.I.; and Rosen, S. 1973. Characterization of fluoride resistant mutants of *Streptococcus mutans*. *Ann. Mtg. Int. Assoc. Dent. Res.* Abstr. No. 115.

301. Rosen, S.; Frea, J.I.; and Hsu, S.M. 1978. Effect of fluoride resistant microorganisms on dental caries. *J. Dent. Res.* 57:180.

302. Cooper, V.K., and Ludwig, T.G. 1965. Effect of fluoride and of soil trace elements on the morphology of the permanent molars in man. *N. Z. Dent. J.* 61:33-40.

303. Simpson, W.J., and Castaldi, C.R. 1969. A study of crown morphology of newly-erupted first permanent molars in Wetaskium, Alberta, (optimum fluoridated) and Camrose, Alberta (low fluoride). *Odont. Revy* 20:1-14.
304. Lovius, B.B.J., and Goose, D.H. 1969. The effect of fluoridation of water on tooth morphology. *Brit. Dent. J.* 127:322-24.
305. Aasenden, R., and Peebles, T.C. 1974. Effects of fluoride supplementation from birth on human deciduous and permanent teeth. *Arch. Oral Biol.* 19:321-26.
306. Mellberg, J.R., and Kellum, W.R. 1979. Comparison of enamel white spot formation rate in human, bovine, deciduous and permanent teeth. *Ann. Mtg. Int. Assoc. Dent. Res.* Abstr. No. 291.

Chapter 3

Fluoride Metabolism

In 1972, *Schwarz* and *Wilne*[1] reported that diets containing less than 2.5 ppm F resulted in poor growth in the rat and concluded that fluoride is an essential trace element for normal growth in this animal. The importance of this finding to human nutrition can only be surmised, yet it would appear that the need of fluoride in the rat reflects a need in other mammals. The size of this need for general human health is not known, but at the very least, it is clearly demonstrated by its effect on dental caries.

Source of human fluoride

The principal source of fluoride ingested by humans is water, but some is also derived from certain plants, marine animals, and even dust particles. Although rain may pick up fluoride from the spray of sea water, coal smoke, or volcanic emissions, most of the fluoride in water is due to its solvent action on rocks and minerals. The concentration of fluoride in ground water depends on the amount of fluoride-containing mineral present, the temperature and pH of the water, and its flow rate. The major fluoride-containing mineral is fluorite or fluorspar (CaF_2), which is 49% fluoride, but many other minerals also contain significant amounts.[2] Usually the concentration is low, (less than 1 ppm), but it can also be several times higher. When fluoride is dissolved in water from mineral sources it is present in ionic form (F^-), which is the same as when it is added through water fluoridation systems. In other words, there is no difference between natural and controlled water fluoridation.

The amount of fluoride ingested by drinking and from food depends on the concentration of fluoride in the water, the size and age of the person, and on personal and dietary habits. The mean consumption of drinking water and total fluids by children according to age is given in Table 3-1. Total fluids include milk, carbonated beverage, soup, etc. Milk, which is very low in fluoride, may account for one-third to one-half of total daily fluid. Adults in thirst-producing occupations may consume several liters of water per day.

The amount of drinking water consumed is influenced by the temperature of the area. *Galagan* and *Vermillion*[3] calculated that water intake within areas where the mean maximum temperature is between 50°F and 80°F varied according to the following equation:

$$\text{oz. } H_2O/\text{lb.} = -0.038 + 0.0062F^\circ$$

Thus a 100 lb. person living in an area with a mean maximum temperature of 80°F (e.g., southern U.S.) would consume an average of 1,354 ml. Where the mean maximum tem-

Table 3-1 Mean daily drinking water and total fluid consumption according to age

Age (years)	Drinking water	Total fluid
0 — 0.5	298	743
0.5 — 1	140	774
1 — 2	238	768
2 — 3	298	901
3 — 5	349	926
5 — 8	389	1,102
8 — 12	493	1,290
> 12	301	1,247

Data from *Walker* et al.[94]

perature is 60°F (e.g., northern U.S.), water consumption would average 988 ml.

Food materials per se are relatively poor as fluoride sources, with some exceptions. Salt water fish, particularly when the bones are included,[4] are high in fluoride. Tea also contains much fluoride and may supply 0.3 to 0.8 mg. F per day.[5] Of course, food prepared in areas with fluoridated water will contain more fluoride than food prepared in areas without fluoridated water. The diets from 16 hospitals throughout the United States were analyzed for fluoride by *Kramer* et al.[6] (Table 3-2) Since the analyses included the water used in the food preparation, hospitals in fluoridated areas had higher fluoride contents than those in nonfluoridated areas. However, there was no correlation between the water fluoride and dietary fluoride within the fluoridated areas, thus showing the difficulty of giving precise values for dietary fluoride.

Estimates of total daily fluoride ingestion in the adult have varied between 0.4 mg and 5.0 mg per day,[7-9] but most fall within the 1.0–3.0 mg range.[10] Total fluoride intake by infants has been estimated from analysis of commercial infant food to be 0.32 mg/day at age 1–4 weeks rising to 1.23 mg at age 4–6 months.[11] These values would be higher if fluoridated water were used for diluting the food and lower if whole human or cow's milk constituted a large part of the diet.[11,12] According to *Forsman*,[13] infant diets prepared with water containing 0.2 ppm F supply 0.23 mg fluoride at age 2 weeks and 0.3 mg at age 10 weeks. When the water contains 1.2 ppm fluoride, the values are 0.83 mg and 1.10 mg respectively. Based on body weight, the young child usually ingests several times more fluoride than the adult. Adult ingestion is in the range 0.02–0.05 mg/kg, whereas infants ingest 0.1–0.2 mg/kg body weight.[11,13]

In addition to food and water, fluoride may also be ingested intentionally as fluoride supplements (F-vitamins, F-drops, etc.) or unintentionally from topical fluoride applications (fluoride dentifrices, rinses, annual topical applications, etc.). Ingestion from these sources will be discussed in subsequent chapters dealing with the appropriate form of fluoride therapy. In general, however, it can be said that infrequently applied topical fluoride, or even the frequent application of low fluoride therapy, will not increase fluoride intake to an excessive level.

Table 3-2 Fluoride ingested in food

City	F in drinking water (ppm)	Total F in food (mg)
Nonfluoridated areas		
Birmingham, Ala.	0.08	0.78
Iron Mountain, Mich.	0.08	1.03
Chicago, Ill.*	0.33	0.86
Houston, Tex.	0.44	0.95
Fluoridated Areas		
Durham, N.C.	0.53	2.62
Corvallis, Ore.	0.60	3.44
Tuscaloosa, Ala.	0.76	2.94
Martiney, Calif.	0.81	1.73
Milwaukee, Wis.	0.85	3.41
New York, N.Y.	0.88	2.55
St. Louis, Mo.	0.91	2.10
Chicago, Ill.	0.95	1.97
Madison, Wis.	1.11	2.88
Louisville, Ky.	1.14	1.98
Lexington, Ky.	1.15	2.84
Cleveland, Ohio	1.27	3.05

*Prior to fluoridation.

Data from *Kramer* et al.[6]

Fluoride absorption

Once ingested, inorganic ionic fluoride is normally rapidly and nearly completely absorbed by the stomach and intestines. Absorption appears to be passive in nature and no active transport is involved in the process.[14] Apparently, simple diffusion determines the rate. Because fluoride appears in the blood very rapidly, the stomach is probably the major site of absorption, at least for soluble or dissolved fluoride. However, diffusion of fluoride through the intestine is more rapid than through the stomach and absorption at this site will also occur.[14] A small amount may also be absorbed through the oral tissue.[15]

The solubility of the fluoride compound has a great effect on the amount and rate of fluoride absorbed. Very soluble compounds are absorbed rapidly and nearly completely. Insoluble or partly soluble compounds are absorbed according to the degree of solubility (Table 3-3). Thus, approximately 97% of fluoride from a 6 mg dose of sodium fluoride is absorbed, whereas comparable figures for solid calcium fluoride and bone meal are 62% and 37% respectively. When calcium fluoride is put into solution prior to ingestion, it is absorbed approximately in the same way as sodium fluoride.

The presence of large amounts of elements such as calcium and aluminum, which form insoluble fluoride compounds or fluoride

Table 3-3 Typical fluoride absorption, excretion and storage of various fluoride materials in the adult after ingestion

Fluoride source	Fluoride dose (mg)	Percentage in feces	Percentage absorbed	Percentage in urine	Percentage stored*
NaF solution	6.47	2.9	97.1	37.4	61.3
CaF_2 solution	6.25	4.3	95.7	34.7	63.7
CaF_2 solid	6.43	37.9	62.1	27.7	55.4
Bone meal	6.31	63.2	36.8	17.1	53.4

*Percentage of absorbed fluoride.

Data from *Largent.*[22]

complexes, will inhibit or prevent fluoride absorption.[16,17] However, the effect on fluoride absorption of calcium in a high calcium human diet has been found to be negligible.[18] Studies of the absorption of fluoride from prenatal vitamin-mineral tablets containing large amounts of calcium revealed that the fluoride in most of the tablets was either not absorbed or absorbed only to a limited degree. If the fluoride was put into the tablet coating where it was dissolved and absorbed prior to release of the calcium compounds, very good absorption was obtained.[19] Fluoride in sodium monofluorophosphate is covalently bonded and, therefore, much less affected by calcium. Although it is slowly hydrolyzed to ionic fluoride by enzymes or acid, it may be absorbed intact.[20]

Fluorides that occur naturally in water or are added to communal water supplies in order to increase the fluoride content are essentially absorbed completely. Organic fluoride compounds having covalent fluorine bonds rather than ionic bonds may also readily be absorbed, but they are not applicable to this discussion since they are not generally reactive with minerals and therefore are not used in the treatment of dental caries. In addition to sodium monofluorophosphate, a few other inorganic compounds also exist in which fluoride is bonded covalently. These compounds (e.g., KPF_6 and KBF_4) are physiologically inert, although they are readily absorbed.[21]

Fluoride inhaled in vapors and dust can also contribute to body fluoride levels. While fluoride in this form is readily absorbed through the lungs,[22] it is considered primarily an occupational health hazard in certain industries and is not a widespread or normal occurrence.

Physiological distribution

Fluoride in blood

The rapidity of fluoride absorption can be seen from the appearance of fluoride in the blood. The maximum plasma fluoride concentration is found 30-60 minutes after ingestion of a dose of soluble fluoride.[23,24] Figure 3-1 shows plasma fluoride concentrations from one subject after ingestion of single oral doses of 1.5 to 10 mg F as sodium fluoride. After the initial rapid increase, the fluoride concentrations declined for the next several hours reaching a normal level about 24 hours after the 10 mg F dose. The calculated half-life of fluoride in plasma after ingestion of a dose of fluoride has been found to vary with the particular subject and the size of the dose, but it is within the range of 2-9 hours.[24]

When fluoride doses were repeatedly ingested by a subject at 12-hour intervals, plasma fluoride levels were as shown in Figure 3-2. There was no additive effect of the repeated doses except that the plasma half-life tended to be slightly longer.[24] In addition, slightly higher maxima were consistently found when the dose was given in the morning after a 12-hour fast than when given in the evening.

Fluoride exists in both ionic and bound forms in the plasma,[25,26] with the bound form being present in larger quantity. The unbound or ionic form varies according to the concentration of fluoride in the drinking water.[26,27] When the water contains 0.25 ppm F, plasma may contain 0.01 ppm ionic F, but when the water contains 1.2 ppm F, ionic fluoride in plasma increases to 0.025 ppm. In an area with 9.6 ppm F water, ionic plasma fluoride levels varied between 0.02 ppm and 0.10 ppm F[27] with the higher levels being found in older individuals (probably because of slower skeletal growth).

Fluoride in saliva

Fluoride concentrations in human saliva are slightly less than those found in plasma,[23,28] ranging from less than 0.01 ppm to 0.05 ppm.[29,30] *Ekstrand* et al.[24] found a saliva/plasma fluoride ratio of 0.64 after single oral fluoride doses. The rapid rate of fluoride absorption is reflected in its appearance in saliva. *Shannon* and *Edmonds*[32] measured fluoride in saliva at intervals following ingestion of several different fluoride doses (see Fig. 2-8) and found the peak concentration within one hour. In other studies, *Shannon* and co-workers[31] found that unstimulated saliva contains more fluoride than stimulated, but that the rate of stimulation does not effect the concentration.

The type of fluoride compound ingested also alters the extent of salivary response.[32] (Fig. 3-3) Sodium fluoride, stannous fluoride, and sodium monofluorophosphate all increase salivary fluoride levels more than aluminum fluoride or calcium fluoride, probably because of complexation or low solubility of the aluminum and calcium salts. A similar effect of aluminum was reported by *Brudevold* et al.[33]

Fluoride in milk

Fluoride levels in human milk are in the range of 0.02 to 0.05 ppm[28,34] and are not significantly changed by moderate changes in fluoride ingestion. *Ericsson*[28] found no change 2 hours after ingestion of 300 ml of 5.5 ppm F water and *Backer-Dirks* et al.[34] found similar levels of 0.05 ppm in milk from subjects living in areas having 0.1 and 1.0 ppm F in the drinking water.

Fluoride in cow's milk was found to be higher than in human milk[34,35] and also was found to rise when the animals were on a high fluoride diet. These findings were attributed to the higher total fluoride intake by the cow.

Fluoride in hard tissues

Bone

The major site of fluoride accumulation in the body is the hard tissues, for which it has a special affinity. Approximately one-half of a dose of fluoride ingested in excess of normal is deposited and retained in the mineral fraction of the bones.[22] The exact amount retained is dependent upon the amount ingested and absorbed, the duration of fluoride exposure, and the metabolic activity of

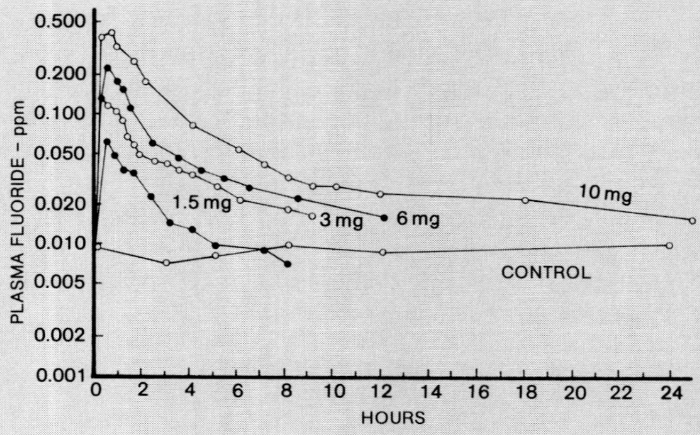

Fig. 3-1 Plasma ionic fluoride concentrations in a single subject following four different doses of fluorides, and the plasma fluoride concentration during a control day on a standardized low F diet.
(*Ekstrand* et al.[24] Reproduced with permission of the author and the *Europ. J. Clin. Pharm.*)

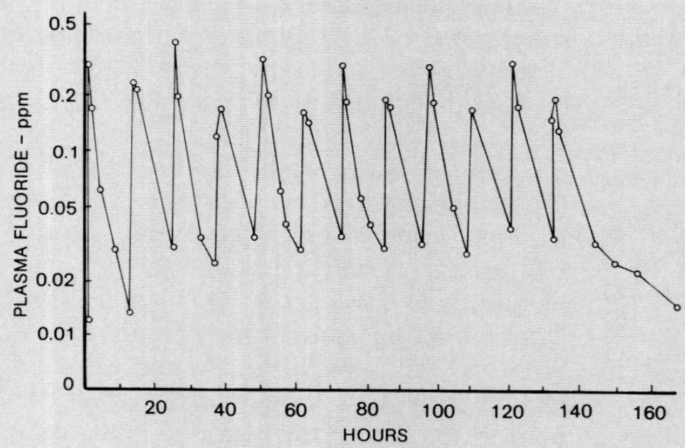

Fig. 3-2 Plasma ionic fluoride concentration in a single subject after multiple dosing of 4.5 mg F every 12 hours. The dose was taken at 8 A.M. and 8 P.M. for 6 days.
(*Ekstrand* et al.[24] Reproduced with permission of the author and the *Europ. J. Clin. Pharm.*)

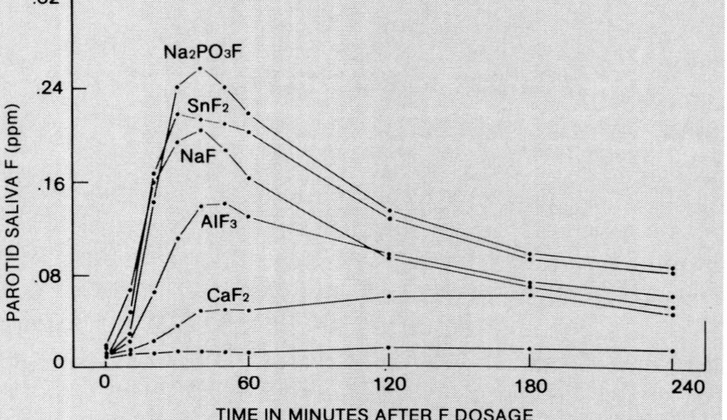

Fig. 3-3 Ionic fluoride concentrations in parotid saliva after ingestion of different fluoride salts.
(*Shannon* and *Edmonds*.[32] Reproduced with permission of the authors and the *J. Dent. Res.*)

Table 3-4 Fluoride concentrations at 5μ in enamel from primary teeth formed in fluoridated and nonfluoridated water areas

City	Reference	Number of teeth	Fluoride concentration (ppm ± SD)
Nonfluoridated water			
Cambridge, Mass.	95	51	492 ± 187
Norwood, Mass.	96	58	595 ± 170
Sunbury, Pa.	97	102	675 ± 240
Cheektowaga, N.Y.	98	39	680 ± 450
Knoxville, Tenn.	99	86	733 ± 329
Portland, Ore.	100	39	809 ± 465
North Dakota*	101	52	702 ± 240
Mississippi*	102	70	695 ± 254
Fluoridated water			
Charlotte, N.C.	103	106	892 ± 309
Governor's Island, N.Y.	104	163	918 ± 323
Lexington, Ky.	99	75	946 ± 346
Stickney, Ill.	105	161	1,071 ± 380

*Several cities.

the tissue involved. Younger or more rapidly growing bones acquire fluoride at a more rapid rate.[36] The quantity of fluoride accumulated by the skeleton is closely related to the concentration of fluoride in the drinking water, although it would be influenced by large deviations from normal levels of fluoride in the diet. *Zipkin* et al.[37] showed a linear relationship between fluoride in drinking water and fluoride in bones (Fig. 3-4). Bone continues to take up fluoride throughout the lifetime of the subject and increases in concentration with age.[37] Numerous studies have established that fluoride is bound within the bone by replacing hydroxyl or bicarbonate groups normally associated with hydroxyapatite structures and that it increases the crystallinity or crystal size of the apatite.[38] The accumulation of large amounts of fluoride by bone also results in a decrease of citrate[39] and an increase in magnesium content.[40]

Dental tissues

Fluoride is deposited in dental tissues in several fashions during the life of the tooth. Initial deposition occurs while the organic and mineral phases are being laid down. Next, fluoride is deposited from the tissue fluids during the preeruptive maturation phase prior to eruption, and finally, fluoride is acquired topically by enamel during the posteruptive maturation and aging period. This latter period includes deposition in hypomineralized areas, demineralized areas, and other defects in enamel.

Preeruptive fluoride acquisition—Studies with the rat, cow[41,42] and pig[43] have shown that during the initial stages of enamel formation the fluoride concentration is much higher than it is upon completion. Figure 3-5 shows the fluoride concentrations in developing pig enamel as mineral accumulates to a final density of about 2.9. After an initial rise in

Table 3-5 Fluoride concentrations in an outer layer of enamel of permanent teeth formed in different water fluoride areas

Water F (ppm)	Number of teeth	Enamel F (ppm)	Layer thickness (μ)
0.07	20	555 ± 260*	16.3 ± 2.6*
0.1	25	516 ± 289	16.6 ± 1.9
0.7	15	1,106 ± 255	16.8 ± 3.2
1.3	20	1,732 ± 391	13.6 ± 0.8
1.7	20	2,358 ± 679	14.4 ± 1.9
2.2	25	2,783 ± 652	13.6 ± 1.7
2.5	21	2,535 ± 825	12.8 ± 2.8
3-5	20	2,648 ± 763	12.9 ± 2.5

*Mean ± standard deviation.

Data from *Shannon* and *Trodahl*.[44]

fluoride concentration (to about 240 ppm in this case), it rapidly declines as the mineral density and degree of enamel formation increases. This phase of enamel formation is then followed by a preeruptive maturation phase where significant additional fluoride is acquired from the tissue fluids.

As the unerupted enamel becomes more fully mineralized during the preeruptive maturation phase, fluoride is less able to penetrate and fluoride deposition becomes increasingly restricted to the surface. As a result, the surface acquires much higher concentrations than the interior. Although enamel thickness may total 1,000μ, high fluoride concentrations are normally found only in the outer 30-50μ. Figure 3-6 shows typical fluoride concentrations acquired systemically by enamel of permanent and primary teeth from optimally and suboptimally fluoridated water areas. Because the amount of fluoride acquired by the outer enamel depends on the concentration of fluoride in the tissue fluids bathing the teeth and the length of time between mineralization and eruption, the longer preeruptive stage of permanent teeth produces higher enamel fluoride levels than in primary teeth.

Most of the fluoride contained in sound enamel is acquired preeruptively and, as stated earlier, is dependent on the supply of fluoride to the tissue. Because tissue fluoride is related to fluoride intake, fluoride concentrations in enamel can be related to fluoride in drinking water. Table 3-4 lists fluoride concentrations at a depth of 5μ in enamel of primary teeth from several optimally and suboptionally or nonfluoridated communities. The difference in mean enamel fluoride concentration between the two groups is 200 to 300 ppm or approximately 25 to 35% higher in the fluoridated areas. Differences of 200 ppm may even be found between areas considered nonfluoridated because some of these areas do have fluoride in their drinking water, but at less than the optimal level.

Fluoride concentrations in layers of enamel from permanent teeth formed in areas having water fluoride ranging from 5 ppm to less than 0.1 ppm[44] are shown in Table 3-5. The layers range in thickness from 12 to 16μ with midpoints of 6 to 8μ—slightly greater than the 5μ depth given for the fluoride concentrations of primary teeth in Table 3-4. Correcting for this difference will slightly increase the fluoride concentrations shown for the permanent teeth.

Table 3-6 lists the enamel fluoride concentrations found in very superficial layers of permanent enamel.[45] As in the other tables,

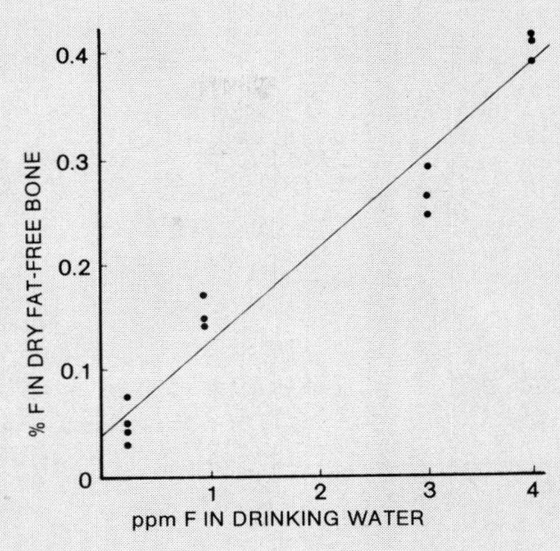

Fig. 3-4 Relation of fluoride concentration in human bones to fluoride concentration in drinking water.
(Adapted from *Zipkin* et al.[37])

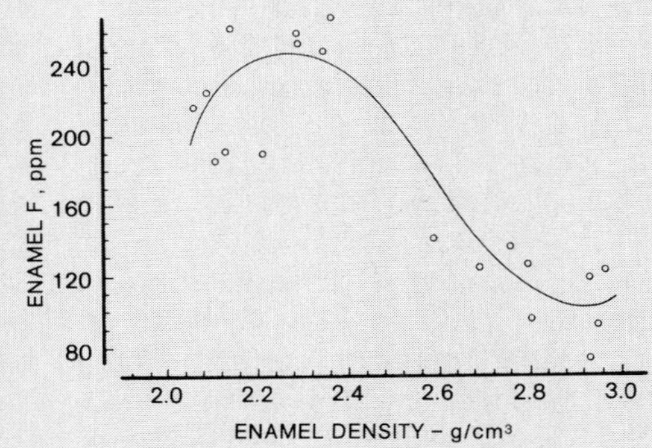

Fig. 3-5 Fluoride concentrations at different stages of density in developing pig enamel.
(*Speirs.*[43] Reproduced with permission of the author and *Arch. Oral Biol.*)

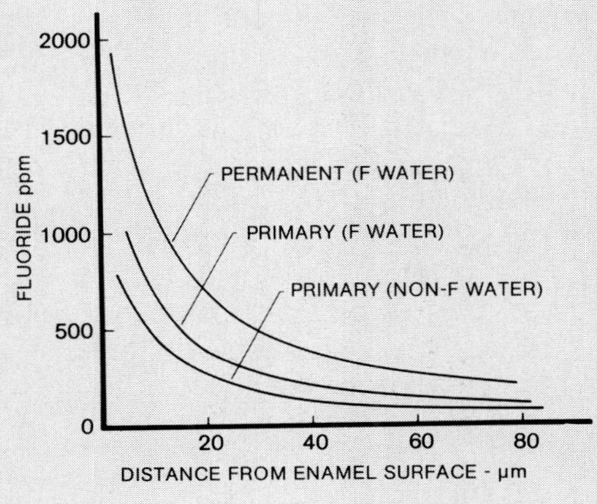

Fig. 3-6 Fluoride concentrations in human enamel according to depth.
(*Mellberg.*[107] Reproduced with permission of the *J. Prev. Dent.*)

Table 3-6 Fluoride concentrations in an outer thin layer of enamel from permanent central incisors

Location	Water	Sampling depth (μ)	Mean F Concentration (ppm)
Boston, Mass.	0.1 ppm	2.2	1,711
Danvers, Mass.	fluoridated	2.0	2,217
Kalamazoo, Mich.	fluoridated	1.6	2,577
Charlotte, N.C.	fluoridated	1.4	2,687
Stickney, Ill.	fluoridated	1.7	3,191
Midland, Tex.	5–7 ppm*	2.0	4,867

*Until 10 months prior to study.

Data from *Aasenden.*[45]

the positive correlation between water fluoride and enamel fluoride is clearly evident. It was also observed in this study that enamel from males contained approximately 10% more fluoride than enamel from females. It was suggested that this was the result of a longer preeruptive maturation time in males.

Even though teeth from different subjects may be formed in the same area, they can vary considerably in fluoride content. Figure 3-7 shows the frequency of primary teeth with various F concentrations at depths of 5μ from areas with optimally and suboptimally fluoridated drinking water. A coefficient of variation (percent standard deviation) of approximately 30% in the fluoride concentration within a group of teeth from a defined area is the usual finding. The fluoride concentration of different teeth in the same mouth as well as different areas of the same tooth also varies,[46-48] but this is mainly the result of caries activity and enamel attrition (wear) rather than from developmental causes.[49] However, newly erupted teeth have been found to contain more fluoride near the incisal edge,[47] possibly because the incisal enamel has a longer preeruptive stage.

Fluoride concentrations in dentin and cementum are higher than in enamel,[50-52] probably because of greater porosity and the longer time during which they can acquire fluoride from tissue fluids. A cross-sectional representation of fluoride concentration in root tissue is given in Figure 3-8.[50] Where the tissue is in contact with circulating fluids (i.e., at pulp and cementum surfaces), the fluoride concentration is high, but where diffusion is hindered, the concentration is low. A generalized cross-sectional representation of a tooth crown showing enamel and dentin is given in Figure 3-9.

Post-eruptive fluoride acquisition—Although mineralization of enamel is essentially complete upon eruption of the tooth, areas still remain where mineral may be deposited. Many of these areas, seen as opaque white spots, disappear with time[53] and it is assumed that they have acquired calcium, phosphate and fluoride from saliva. Solid evidence for *posteruptive fluoride acquisition* by this mechanism in the human is lacking, however studies of newly erupted teeth in the rat clearly show that hypomineralized areas acquire fluoride and are mineralized more rapidly in the presence of fluoride.[54] The normal increase in total enamel fluoride in a human tooth by this mechanism probably is not great, although it may be quite important for the inhibition of caries.

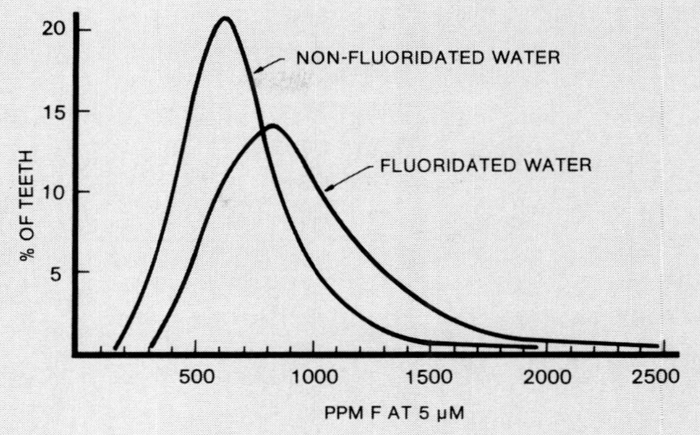

Fig. 3-7 Frequency distribution of primary teeth containing various concentrations of fluoride at 5 μ depth. (*Mellberg.*[107] Reproduced with permission of the *J. Prev. Dent.*)

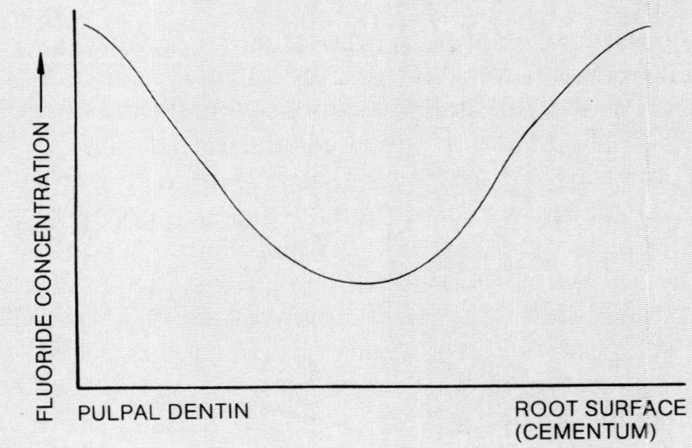

Fig. 3-8 Generalized fluoride distribution profile in roots of human teeth. (Adapted from *Yoon* et al.[50])

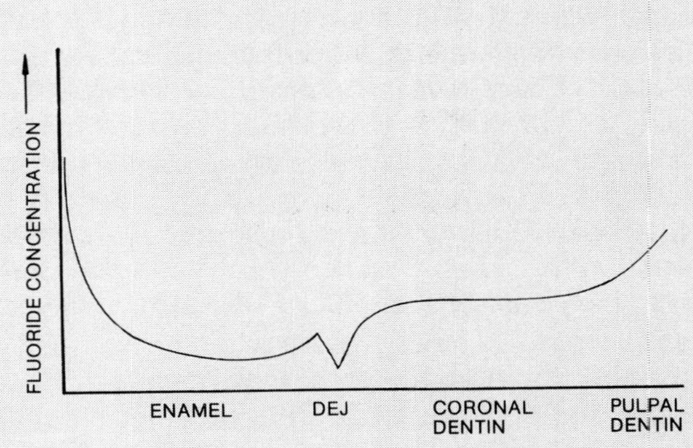

Fig. 3-9 Generalized fluoride distribution profile in enamel and dentin of the crowns of human teeth.
(Adapted from *Yoon* et al.[50])

Table 3-7 Fluoride in sound and defective human permanent enamel

Type of enamel	Fluoride concentration (ppm)* Age groups (years) 20	40–49
Sound	250	430
White spot	873	1,100
Diffusely discolored	808	3,043
Brown	1,075	2,035

*Enamel layer approximately 50 μ thick.
Data from *Little* et al.[106]

The greatest posteruptive deposition of fluoride probably arises from deposition in defects that form as the enamel is attacked by its environment. In the presence of fluoride, any change that increases the enamel porosity or allows deposition of mineral will result in an increase in enamel fluoride. Areas of enamel with obvious defects, for example, white spots (incipient lesions), brown spots (arrested lesions), or carious cavities, are found to contain more fluoride than sound enamel (Table 3-7). The apparent association of fluoride with enamel color probably results from a simultaneous deposition of proteinaceous material,[55] which increases with age. The active incipient carious lesion is white due to subsurface mineral loss, but if it becomes arrested, it will turn dark as it accumulates precipitated protein and mineral. Enamel may also accumulate fluoride at the margins of silicate fillings as a result of leaching from the fluoride-rich silicate.[49]

Not all aging factors produce an accumulation of enamel fluoride. *Weatherell* and coworkers[47–49] reported analyses showing that wear or other abrasive forces remove some of the original surface, exposing enamel with a lower fluoride concentration. Fluoride concentrations in labial and buccal enamel surfaces of incisors, canines and premolars are higher near the biting edge when young, but become lower with increasing age. Simultaneously, fluoride concentrations of the gingival area increase with age. This latter finding probably reflects the fact that the gingival area is often covered by plaque that contains fluoride. The regular formation of acid by the plaque dissolves small amounts of enamel, much of which is reprecipitated in the presence of fluoride as fluoride-containing apatites. Examples of extreme changes of fluoride concentration in young and old enamel are shown in Figure 3-10. Because not all teeth exhibit such uniform patterns, simple statements regarding the pattern of fluoride over the enamel surface cannot be made accurately.

Fluoride excretion

Although fluoride is excreted in feces and sweat and is lost by way of hair, skin, and saliva, the principal route of elimination of soluble fluoride is by way of the urine. In fact, urinary fluoride has been widely regarded as one of the best indicators of fluoride ingestion. *Hodge* et al.[56] differentiated fluoride excretion in individuals according to whether they are in "steady-state," (i.e., have been ingesting the same amount of fluoride for a long period) or whether they have received elevated quantities for short periods. The elimination of fluoride under these two circumstances will differ.

Individuals who are in steady-state excrete approximately 80–90% of the total ingested soluble fluoride in urine and approximately 10% in feces. In most cases, part of the fluoride is retained (positive balance) and accumulates throughout the individual's lifetime. If the individual changes to a lower fluoride intake, a negative balance occurs

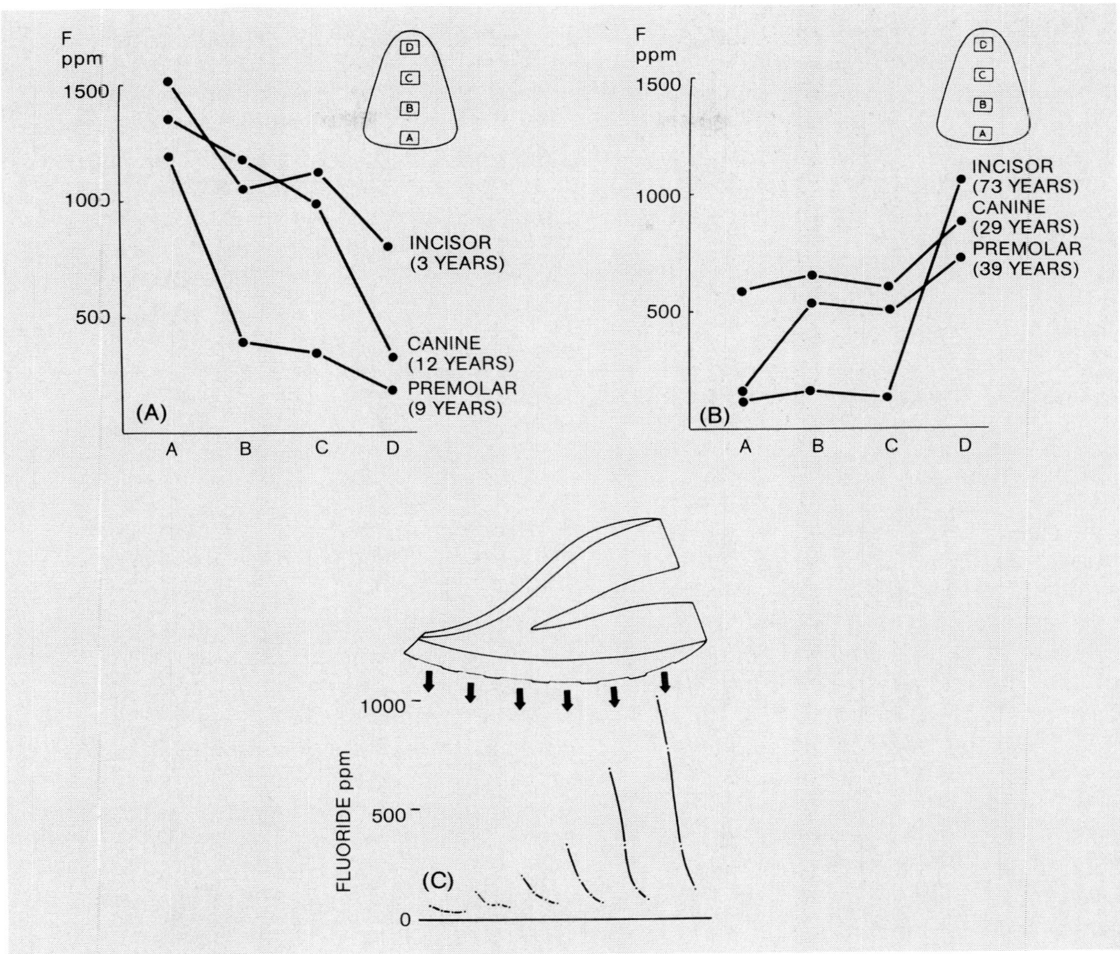

Fig. 3-10 Fluoride distribution in surface enamel.
A) Fluoride distribution in the labial or buccal surfaces of three young anterior teeth.
B) Fluoride distribution in the labial or buccal surfaces of older anterior teeth.
C) Variations in the gradient of fluoride concentration from surface to interior of enamel at six different sites in the labial surface of an incisor of unknown age.
(*Weatherell* et al.[47] Reproduced with permission of the authors and *Caries Res.*)

where bone fluoride slowly mobilizes until the body reaches a new steady-state. The process is slow but is evident from slowly changing urine fluoride levels. It required more than two years for adults to reach a steady urine fluoride output after a change from drinking water containing 8.0 ppm F to water containing 1.0 ppm F.[57] The amount of ingested fluoride retained by individuals on a steady-state intake has been a matter of debate. *Hodge* et al.[56] believed that only a small amount is retained and quote data from a number of investigators. Findings from one study reviewed by *Hodge* are given in Table 3-8. *Spencer* et al.,[9,58] on the other hand, in carefully controlled studies in a hospital met-

Table 3-8 Fluoride balance in humans*

F in water supply (ppm)	Age (years)	Length of residence (years)	Time of observation (days)	F ingested daily (mg)			F excreted daily (mg)			Balance (mg/day)
				Fluid	Food	Total	Feces	Urine	Total	
2.0	35	10	96	2.4	1.2	3.6	0.4	2.9	3.3	+ 0.3
5.5	55	29	60	3.8	1.3	5.1	0.6	4.5	6.1	0.0
6.1	57	34	133	6.7	1.0	7.7	0.4	8.1	8.5	− 0.8
8.0	57	19	140	11.3	2.5	13.8	1.4	10.4	11.8	+ 2.0
20.0	30	8	45	20.8	1.5	22.3	1.4	12.3	13.7	+ 8.6

*Selected data from *Largent*.[22]

abolic ward, found that roughly 50% of ingested fluoride is retained, even by individuals on a steady-state intake.

Spencer et al.[59] studied the fluoride balance of subjects who received 9.1 mg fluoride per day for 32 days in addition to the 4.4 mg that they normally consumed in their food and water. They found that 40% of the fluoride supplement was consistently retained during the 32-day test period and that urine fluoride levels returned to normal 6 to 12 days later. Only about 10% of the fluoride retained during the test period was excreted after discontinuation of fluoride. Similarly, after a test period of 3 months, during which 45 mg of additional fluoride per day was ingested, only 2% of the retained fluoride was excreted.[60]

An explanation for the difference between the findings of *Hodge* and *Spencer* may be that the skeletons of *Spencer*'s subjects were not saturated with fluoride and therefore retained most of what they acquired during the relatively short steady-state periods of increased fluoride ingestion. It has been reported that fluoride in bone reaches a plateau with age, which suggests an equilibrium between bone fluoride and tissue fluoride.[61]

Excretion of fluoride from a single dose has been found by most investigators to be roughly 50%. Individuals in an active state of bone growth will excrete less fluoride than older individuals and will take longer to reach a steady-state. *Gedalia*[62] found that young children had lower urinary fluoride and greater fluoride storage. Another example was shown in a community where urinary fluoride levels in adults went from 0.3 ppm F prior to fluoridation to 1.0 ppm F within 1 month after fluoridation. In children, however, urinary fluoride levels took 3 years to go from 0.3 ppm F to 0.9 ppm F.[63] The pre- and postfluoridation urine fluoride levels were similar to the water fluoride concentrations, thus supporting the frequent assumption that urine fluoride reflects the water fluoride level. This was not found to be valid when the water contained a very low fluoride level (0.02 ppm), but urine contained 0.42 ppm.[64] It is likely that the urine fluoride in this case is reflecting fluoride ingestion from food material, which likely contained water from different communities having higher water fluoride levels.

Excretion of a single dose of ingested fluoride is very rapid with approximately 30% being found in the urine within four hours.[65]

Essentially all remaining fluoride not retained in the bone is excreted within 24 hours.
The rate of fluoride excretion and the amount of fluoride retained from an administered dose is markedly influenced by the acid-base state of the individual.[66] Because undissociated HF permeates kidney tubules much more rapidly than ionic F^-, an acid urine results in the reabsorption of urinary fluoride. In an alkaline urine, less fluoride is reabsorbed and therefore remains in the tubules and is excreted. Analysis of tissue after administration of fluoride to rats given ammonium chloride in their drinking water to produce an acid urine showed much higher fluoride levels than in rats given water with sodium bicarbonate.[66] Urine fluoride excretion was twice as high in the alkalotic (bicarbonate) animals, and they were able to tolerate a toxic dose 90% greater than the acidotic animals.

Fluoride toxicity

Accumulated evidence from numerous studies shows that the prolonged use of fluoride at recommended levels does not produce harmful physiological effects in the human. Except for dental fluorosis, this has been found true even when individuals consume drinking water containing up to 8.0 ppm F—about 8 times the recommended amount. However, like every chemical, there are safe limits for fluoride ingestion beyond which harmful effects occur. These effects can be classified as acute, due to a single ingestion of a large amount of fluoride, or chronic, due to long-term ingestion of smaller amounts. A summary list of the toxic effects of various levels of fluoride is given in Table 3-9.

Acute toxicity

Ingestion of an acute fatal dose of fluoride is very rare. The amount of soluble fluoride considered lethal when taken orally is 35-70 mg F per kg body weight.[67] This is equivalent to 5 to 10 g sodium fluoride for a 70 kg adult or about 1.0 to 2.0 g sodium fluoride for a 15 kg child. Amounts less than this, however, may cause nausea and vomiting.
Symptoms of acute toxicity occur rapidly. There is diffuse abdominal pain, diarrhea, vomiting, excess salivation, and thirst. Rapid measures to reduce fluoride absorption should be started by inducing vomiting and then large volumes of calcium, as in lime water or milk, should be given. Administration of aluminum hydroxide gels should be exceptionally good for binding fluoride.[67] Because an alkaline urine prevents fluoride reabsorption, it has been suggested that expeditious manipulation of urinary pH by diuresis with an alkalinizing agent might favorably affect the clinical outcome in cases of acute fluoride poisoning.[66] Because of rapid elimination of fluoride in the urine, a subject surviving the first 24 hours has a good prognosis.[68]

Chronic toxicity

Soft tissue

Chronic health problems of the soft tissues related to prolonged ingestion of fluoride in moderate excess have not been encountered, although numerous studies have been conducted.[69] This is undoubtedly related to the very low levels of fluoride (less than 1 ppm) present in soft tissues as a result of rapid and efficient urinary excretion and sequestration by bone.

Bone

When excessive fluoride (e.g., in drinking water containing more than 8 ppm F) is ingested daily for many years, symptoms of

Table 3-9 Toxic effects of fluoride in the human

Concentration or dose of F	Medium	Effects
2 ppm or more	Water	Mottled enamel
5 ppm	Water	No osteosclerosis
8 ppm	Water	10% osteosclerosis
20–80 mg/day or more	Water or air	Crippling fluorosis
50 ppm	Food or water	Thyroid changes
100 ppm	Food or water	Growth retardation
More than 125 ppm	Food or water	Kidney changes
2.5–5.0 g	Acute dose	Death

Data from *Smith* and *Hodge*.[107]

skeletal fluorosis may occur. Severe cases are normally found only in warm climates where the drinking water contains very high levels of fluoride or where industrial workers are unnecessarily exposed to materials, such as cryolite, containing large amounts of fluoride. When this occurs, bone density slowly increases, the joints stiffen and become painful, and movement becomes restricted.[70] Modern health practices have essentially eliminated this problem.

The ingestion of slightly elevated doses of fluoride for many years, however, has also been associated with beneficial effects. In an epidemiological study by *Bernstein* et al.,[71] it was found that ingestion of drinking water containing 3–6 ppm F might have been beneficial in the prevention of osteoporosis and possibly aortic calcification. Increased density and thickened cortical bone and periosteum were found in subjects residing in an area with 8 ppm F in the drinking water by *Leone* et al.,[72] who considered these changes beneficial since they counteracted the osteoporotic changes of aging.

Dental fluorosis

Dental fluorosis is an abnormal development of the teeth that occurs primarily in the enamel and appears in a mild form as white opacities over the enamel surface. Because the disruption will most likely occur during the early stages of enamel formation, and certainly prior to eruption, excess fluoride in any amount cannot produce opacities in an erupted tooth. However, it must be emphasized that not all opacities that may be present are due to fluoride. *Small* and *Murray*[73] found 97 other causes of enamel opacities, and *Murray* and *Shaw*[74] found that over 80% of the subjects examined in a low fluoride area had some kind of enamel opacity. Some investigators have actually reported that there are fewer opacities in fluoridated areas than non-fluoridated areas.[75,76] The discovery that one type of enamel opacity is due to fluoride is closely associated with the history of water fluoridation. In the search for the cause of mottled enamel (dental fluorosis) it was found that drinking water with excess natural fluoride produced fluorosis, but that when the water contained amounts near 1 ppm, caries formation was inhibited.

As described by *Fejerskov* et al.,[77] the first signs of dental fluorosis are fine striae of accentuated perikymata appearing as horizontal white lines evenly distributed over the enamel surface. In more affected teeth, the lines become broader and more pronounced, occasionally merging to form irregularly scattered, cloudy or paper-white areas. With increasing severity, the irregular opaque areas merge until extensive areas appear chalky white. Pitting can occur, either as minute depressions or as single or multiple circular holes indicating a loss of the outermost surface enamel. Horizontal bands of pits are often observed, which in very severe cases tend to merge into large "corroded" areas. In the most severe cases, the entire enamel surface appears corroded. Discoloration may occur to varying degrees due to the posteruptive environment. In general, increased levels of fluorosis are associated with a reduced resistance to abrasion. The general morphology of fluorosed teeth is not different from normal. Several examples of fluorotic teeth are shown in Chapter 4 (see Fig. 4-2).

Fluorosis occurs symetrically within the dental arches; the premolar is usually the tooth most affected, followed by the second molar, maxillary incisor, canine, first molar, and mandibular incisor. Fluorosis is usually limited to the permanent dentition, but the primary teeth may also be affected.[13,78] The reason for this may be related to a modifying effect of the placenta on fluoride transfer to the fetus[79] or to a shorter period of enamel formation.

Histologically, fluorosed enamel consists of areas of diffuse hypomineralization or porosity below a well-mineralized surface layer. In severe cases, hypomineralization below the surface may reach 25% or more.[80] Although the severest porosity occurs in the outer third of the enamel, it also extends more deeply; the entire enamel and even the dentin may be affected to some degree.[77] Because of the high degree of porosity in severe fluorosis and the brittleness of the outer layer, it is thought that the pits or "corrosion" of the surface is due to loss of enamel and not the result of a failure of enamel production. *Thylstrup* and *Fejerskov*[81] suggest that a pore volume of greater than 10-15% is conducive to mechanical damage and loss of surface.

The prevalence of dental fluorosis is directly related to the concentration of fluoride in the drinking water or other excess ingestion of fluoride. Given the same level of water fluoride, it is more prevalent in warmer climates or where fluoride-rich diets occur in conjunction with high fluoride water. Malnutrition or low dietary calcium may be a contributing factor.[82-84] Protein deficiency in animals reduces bone fluoride uptake[85-86] and enhances the formation of dental fluorosis.[87] Since the skeleton normally takes up fluoride rapidly from an ingested dose, it may be expected that a normally growing skeleton will modify the fluoride exposure to the rest of the body and thereby reduce fluorosis.

Fejerskov et al.[77] listed three possible ways in which fluoride might cause fluorosis:

—effect on ameloblasts
—effect on nucleation and crystal growth
—effect on calcium homeostasis

After assessing the available literature, they concluded that experimental data indicate that fluoride might interact with the cellular processes during enamel matrix secretion and that there is evidence to suggest that impairment of the processes of matrix maturation could occur. Because crystal formation and growth are greatly affected by fluoride, its presence in excess might disrupt these processes. Finally, they suggested that a significant lowering of serum calcium leading to an increased concentration of parathyroid hormone (which, in turn, results in mobilization of calcium) might be a causative factor.

A problem with understanding the effect of fluoride on enamel formation is the fact that serum fluoride levels are very low. However, it has been shown that peak levels of fluoride occur in the serum after fluoride ingestion,[24] and it has been found that a peak level of approximately 10μM (0.2 ppm) or more is associated with development of fluorosis.[88,89] As shown in Figure 3-2, a dose of 4.5 mg F taken by a 49 kg individual was sufficient to produce a peak level of 0.2 ppm F (200μg/ml). A dose of 4.5 mg/49 kg is near the 0.1 mg/kg body weight found to be borderline for producing fluorosis in the rat.[13,90] Based on normal fluoride ingestion, Toth[91] calculated that a "dangerous" dose for children age 7 to 9 years is 0.1 mg/kg and that younger children could tolerate slightly more fluoride and older individuals slightly less.

Another explanation for the effect of low serum fluoride was offered by *Weatherell* et al.[92] They noted that a fraction of the fluoride in developing enamel is released at a certain stage of development (see Fig. 3-5), and that this labile fluoride may provide a sufficiently high concentration to affect the ameloblast.

Brudevold et al.[93] found that, in general, the concentration of fluoride in fluorosed rat enamel is higher than in normal rat enamel, but that many nonfluorosed teeth had more fluoride than some fluorosed teeth. They suggested that this was because fluorosis was caused by a disruption of the enamel matrix and that most of the fluoride incorporation occurs after the matrix is formed. They further suggested that this situation may be used to safely produce very high enamel fluoride concentrations by administering low fluoride during the period of matrix formation and a higher dose later. Since the matrix of esthetically important teeth is formed during the first four years of life, daily doses of more than 1 mg may be beneficial after this age.

Summary

The principal source of fluoride ingested by humans is drinking water, but food is also an important contributor. The amount of fluoride ingested by an individual varies considerably, but for an adult is usually in the range of 1 to 3 mg per day. Based on body weight, a child usually ingests several times more fluoride than an adult.

Ingested soluble fluoride is rapidly absorbed from the stomach and intestines and distributed throughout the body. Fluoride in an insoluble or complexed form is absorbed more slowly. The peak level of fluoride in blood is found 30 to 60 minutes after ingestion. Normal blood fluoride levels are very low (near 0.03 ppm F), but may increase to 0.50 ppm or more after large doses. Fluoride levels in saliva are about 65% of the blood levels.

Bone is the major site of fluoride accumulation in the body, but a small amount is also acquired by the dental tissues. Most enamel fluoride is acquired before the tooth erupts, unless the patient is on intensive topical fluoride treatment and the highest concentrations are found in the outer 30 to 50 μ (0.03 to 0.05 mm). Permanent teeth have higher fluoride levels than primary teeth because of a longer preeruptive maturation period. Enamel fluoride concentrations depend on the amount of fluoride ingested prior to eruption and are related to the concentration of fluoride in the drinking water, but vary widely even within a single geographic area. Fluoride is acquired by the enamel of erupted teeth mostly in defects and enamel exposed to caries activity.

Elimination of ingested fluoride is rapid and primarily by way of the urine. Approximately 30% is eliminated within 4 hours after ingestion, and the remainder within 24 hours. The half-life of fluoride in the blood varies between 2 to 9 hours. An individual who has ingested the same amount of fluoride for a long period is considered to be in steady-state. Under these conditions, approximately 80 to 90% of ingested fluoride is eliminated in the urine and 10% in the feces. If the individual changes to a lower intake, fluoride will slowly mobilize from the bones and be eliminated in the urine until a new steady-state is reached. When a single dose of fluoride, in excess of normal, is ingested, approximately 50% is retained by the bones. There is evidence that the rate of fluoride elimination is more rapid from an alkaline urine.

While recommended fluoride concentrations cause no harm, excessive amounts can be toxic. Acute lethal toxicity occurs from 35 to 70 mg/kg body weight, equivalent to 5 to 10 g sodium fluoride for an adult or 1 to 2 g sodium fluoride for a small child. Lower doses cause nausea and vomiting. Chronic ingestion of excess fluoride in lower doses (e.g., 8 ppm F in the drinking water) may cause bone fluorosis, but the initial effects are seen in the dentition. Dental fluorosis is caused by a disruption of early enamel formation and in mild forms is noted as white opacities over the surface. Not all white areas on enamel, however, are caused by fluoride. Because fluorosis is caused during the early stage of enamel formation and most fluoride is acquired during the maturation period, fluorosis and enamel fluoride levels need not be related. It also follows that fluorosis cannot be caused after the enamel has been formed.

References

1. Schwarz, K., and Wilne, D.B. 1972. Fluorine requirements for growth in the rat. *Bio-Inorganic Chem.* 1:331-38.
2. Bell, M.E., and Ludwig, T.G. 1970. Ingestion from water. In *Fluorides and human health*, pp. 18-32. World Health Organization.
3. Galagan, D.J., and Vermillion, J.R. 1957. Determining the optimum fluoride concentrations *Public Health, Rep., Wash.* 72:491-93.
4. Hodge, H.C., and Smith, F.A. 1970. Minerals: fluorine and dental caries. In *Dietary chemicals vs dental caries.* Am. Chem. Soc. Pub. No. 94.
5. Duckworth, S.C., and Duckworth, R. 1978. The ingestion of fluoride in tea. *Brit. Dent. J.* 145:368-70.
6. Kramer, L.; Osis, D.; Wiatrowski, E.; and Spencer, H. 1974. Dietary fluoride in different areas in the U.S. *Am. J. Clin. Nutr.* 27:590-94.
7. Machle, W.; Scott, E.W.; and Largent, E.J. 1942. The absorption and excretion of fluorides. I. The normal fluoride balance. *J. Ind. Hyg. Toxicol.* 24:199-204.
8. Auermann, E., and Borris, W. 1971. Fluoride intake in individuals in various age groups and under special conditions. *Caries Res.* 5:11.
9. Spencer, H.; Osis, D.; Wiatrowski, E.; and Samachson, J. 1970. Availability of fluoride from fish protein concentrate and from sodium fluoride in man. *J. Nutr.* 100:1415-24.
10. Myers, H.M. 1978. *Fluorides and dental fluorosis.* Basel: Karger.
11. Wiatrowski, E.; Kramer, L.; Osis, D.; and Spencer, H. Dietary fluoride intake of infants. *Pediatrics* 55:517-22.
12. Ericsson, Y., and Ribelius, U. 1971. Wide variations of fluoride supply to infants and their effect. *Caries Res.* 5:78-88.
13. Forsman, B. 1977. Early supply of fluoride and enamel fluorosis. *Scand. J. Dent. Res.* 85:22-30.
14. Stookey, G.K.; Crane, D.B.; and Muhler, J.C. 1964. *In vitro* studies concerning fluoride absorption. *Proc. Soc. Exp. Biol. Med.* 115:298-301.
15. Patten, J.R.; Whitford, G.M.; Stringer, G.I.; and Pashley, D.H. 1978. Oral absorption of radioactive fluoride and iodide in rats. *Arch. Oral Biol.* 23:215-17.
16. Weedle, D.A., and Muhler, J.C. 1954. The effects of inorganic salts on fluorine storage in the rat. *J. Nutr.* 54:437-44.
17. Mellberg, J.R. 1965. Stabilization of fluoride solutions in glass containers. *J. Pharm. Sci.* 54:615-16.
18. Spencer, H.; Lewin, I.; Fowler, J.; and Samachson, J. 1969. Effect of NaF on calcium absorption and balance in man. *Am. J. Clin. Nutr.* 22:381-90.
19. Grodberg, M.G., and Mellberg, J.R. 1967. *Multiple layer tablet with calcium salt central core separated from soluble fluoride outer coating.* U.S. Pat. 3,345,265.
20. Ericsson, Y. 1967. Biologic splitting of PO_3F^- ions. *Caries Res.* 1:144-52.
21. Zipkin, I., and Likins, R.C. 1957. Absorption of various fluorine compounds from the gastrointestinal tract of the rat. *Am. J. Physiol.* 191:549-50.
22. Largent, E.J. 1961. *Fluorosis: the health aspects of fluorine compounds.* Columbus: Ohio State Univ. Press.

23. Carlson, C.H.; Armstrong, W.D.; and Singer, L. 1960. Distribution and excretion of radiofluoride in the human. *Proc. Soc. Exp. Biol. Med.* 104:235-39.
24. Ekstrand, J.; Alvan, G.; Boreus, L.O.; and Norlin, A. 1977. Pharmacokinetics of fluoride in man after single and multiple oral doses. *Europ. J. Clin. Pharm.* 12:311-17.
25. Taves, D.R. 1968. Evidence that there are two forms of fluoride in human serum. *Nature* 217:1050-51.
26. Venkateswarlu, P. 1975. Determination of total fluorine in serum and other biological materials by oxygen bomb and reverse extraction techniques. *Analyt. Biochem.* 68:512-21.
27. Ekstrand, J. 1978. Relationship between fluoride in the drinking water and the plasma fluoride concentration in man. *Caries Res.* 12:123-27.
28. Ericsson, Y. 1969. Fluoride excretion in human saliva and milk. *Caries Res.* 3:159-66.
29. Yao, K., and Gron, P. 1970. Fluoride concentrations in duct saliva and in whole saliva. *Caries Res.* 4:321-31.
30. Shannon, I.L. 1977. Biochemistry of fluoride in saliva. *Caries Res.* 11 (Suppl. 1):206-25.
31. Shannon, I.L.; Suddick, R.P.; and Edmonds, E. J. 1973. Effect of rate of gland function on parotid saliva fluoride concentration. *Caries Res.* 7:1-10.
32. Shannon, I.L., and Edmonds, E.J. 1978. Fluoride levels in human parotid saliva following ingestion of fluoride compounds of varying solubility. *J. Dent. Res.* 56:1521-25.
33. Brudevold, F.; Bakhos, Y.; and Gron, P. 1973. Fluoride in human saliva after ingestion of aluminum chloride and sodium fluoride or sodium monofluorophosphate. *Arch. Oral Biol.* 18:699-706.
34. Backer-Dirks, O.; Jongeling-Eijndhoven, J.M.P.A.; Flissebaalje, T. D.; and Gedalia, I. 1974. Total and free ionic fluoride in human and cow's milk as determined by gas-liquid chromatography and the fluoride electrode. *Caries Res.* 8:181-86.
35. Adair, S.M., and Wei, S.H.Y. 1978. Supplemental fluoride recommendations for infants based on dietary fluoride intake. *Caries Res.* 12:76-82.
36. Zipkin, I., and McClure, F.J. 1952. Fluorine in the bones and teeth of the growing rat. *J. Nutr.* 47:611-20.
37. Zipkin, I.; McClure, F.J.; Leone, N.C.; and Lee, W.A. 1958. Fluoride deposition in human bones after prolonged ingestion of fluoride in drinking water. *Publ. Hlth. Rep.* 73:732-40.
38. Eanes, E.D.; Zipkin, I.; Harper, R.A.; and Posner, A.S. 1965. Small angle x-ray diffraction analysis of the effect of fluoride on human bone apatite. *Arch. Oral Biol.* 10:161-73.
39. Zipkin, I.; Schraer, R.; Schraer, H.; and Lee, W.A. 1963. The effect of fluoride on the citrate content of bones of the growing rat. *Arch. Oral Biol.* 8:119-26.
40. Zipkin, I.; McClure, F.J.; and Lee, W.A. 1960. Relation of the fluoride content of human bone to its chemical composition. *Arch. Oral Biol.* 2:190-95.
41. Weatherell, J.A.; Deutsch, D.; Robinson, C.; and Hallsworth, A.S. 1975. Fluoride concentrations in developing enamel. *Nature (Lond.)* 256:230-32.
42. Crenshaw, M.A.; Wennberg, A.; and Bauden, J.W. 1978. Fluoride-binding by organic matrix of developing bovine enamel. *Arch. Oral Biol.* 23:285-87.
43. Speirs, R.L. 1978. Incorporation of a dietary fluoride supplement into bone and developing teeth of the domestic pig. *Arch. Oral Biol.* 23:1013-17.
44. Shannon, I.L., and Trodahl, J.N. 1977. Effect of waterborne fluoride on fluoride concentration and solubility of dental enamel. *Aust. Dent. J.* 22:428-31.
45. Aasenden, R. 1974. Fluoride concentrations in the surface tooth enamel of young men and women. *Arch. Oral Biol.* 19:697-701.
46. Gedalia, I., and Kalderon, S. 1964. Fluoride in the surface enamel of teeth from the same mouth. *J. Dent. Res.* 43:44-49.
47. Weatherell, J.A.; Robinson, C.; and Hallsworth, A.S. 1972. Changes in the fluoride concentration of the labial enamel surface with age. *Caries Res.* 6:312-24.
48. Weatherell, J.A.; Hallsworth, A.S.; and Robinson, C. 1973. The effect of tooth wear on the distribution of fluoride in the enamel surface of human teeth. *Arch. Oral Biol.* 18:1175-89.
49. Hallsworth, A.S., and Weatherell, J.A. 1969. The microdistribution, uptake and loss of fluoride in human enamel. *Caries Res.* 3:109-18.
50. Yoon, S.H.; Brudevold, F.; Gardner, D.E.; and Smith, F.A. 1960. Distribution of fluoride in teeth from areas with different levels of fluoride in the water supply. *J. Dent. Res.* 39:845-56.
51. Yardeni, J.; Gedalia, I.; and Kohn, M. 1963. Fluoride concentrations of dental calculus, surface enamel and cementum. *Arch. Oral Biol.* 8:697-701.
52. Stepnick, R.J.; Nakata, T.M.; and Zipkin, I. 1975. The effects of age and fluoride exposure on fluoride, citrate and carbonate content of

human cementum. J. Periodontal. 46:45-50.
53. Backer Dirks, O. 1966. Post-eruptive changes in dental enamel. *J. Dent. Res.* 45:503-11.
54. Briner, W.W., and Rosen, S. 1967. Effect of fluoride on hypomineralized areas in the molars of rats fed a cariogenic diet. *Arch. Oral Biol.* 12:1077-84.
55. Bibby, B.G. 1971. Organic enamel material and caries. *Caries Res.* 5:305-22.
56. Hodge, H.C.; Smith, F.A.; and Gedalia, I. 1970. Excretion of fluorides. In *Fluorides and Human Health.* Geneva: World Health Organization Monograph #59.
57. Likins, R.C.; McClure, F.J.; and Steere, A.C. 1956. Urinary excretion of fluoride following defluoridation of a water supply. *Publ. Hlth. Rep.* 71:217-20.
58. Spencer, H.; Lewin, I.; Wiatrowski, E.; and Samachson, J. 1970. Fluoride metabolism in man. *Am. J. Med.* 49:807-13.
59. Spencer, H.; Kramer, L; Osis, D.; and Wiatrowski, E. 1975. Excretion of retained fluoride in man. *J. Appl. Physiol.* 38:282-87.
60. Spencer, H.; Osis, D.; and Wiatrowski, E. 1974. Studies of fluoride metabolism in man. In *Trace substances in environmental health-VII,* ed. D.D. Hemphill, pp. 289-294. Columbia: Univ. Missouri Press.
61. Jackson, D., and Weidman, S.M. 1958. Fluorine in human bone related to age and water supply of different regions. *J. Pathol. Bacteriol.* 76:451-59.
62. Gedalia, I. 1958. Urinary fluoride levels of children and adults. *J. Dent. Res.* 37:601-4.
63. Zipkin, I.; Likins, R.C.; and McClure, F.J. 1956. Urinary fluoride levels associated with use of fluoridated waters. *Publ. Health Rep.* 71:767-72.
64. Shannon, I.L., and Sanders, D.M. 1979. Urinary fluoride concentrations in 6- to 9-year old children's drinking water with a very low fluoride level. *Caries Res.* 13:18-22.
65. Zipkin, I.; Lee, W.A.; and Leone, N.C. 1957. Rate of urinary fluoride output in normal adults. *Am. J. Pub. Health* 47:848-51.
66. Whitford, G.M., and Pashley, D.H. 1979. The effect of body fluid pH on fluoride distribution, toxicity, and renal clearance. In *Continuing evaluation of the use of fluorides, AAAS selected symposium II.* eds. E. Johansen, D.R. Taves, and T.O. Olsen.
67. Gosselin, R.E.; Hodge, H.C.; Smith, R.P.; and Gleason, M. N. 1976. *Clinical toxicology of commercial products.* 4th ed. Section III, pp. 159-63. Baltimore: Williams & Wilkins.
68. Hodge, H.C., and Smith, F.A. 1965. Biologic effects of inorganic fluorides. In *Fluorine chemistry.* Vol. 4. ed. J.H. Simons. New York: Academic Press.
69. *Fluorides and human health.* 1970. Geneva: World Health Organization Monograph #59.
70. Singh, A., and Jolly, S.S. 1970. Chronic toxic effects on the skeletal system. *Fluorides and human health,* pp. 238-49. Geneva: World Health Organization Monograph #59.
71. Bernstein, D.S.; Sodowsky, N.; Hegsted, D.M.; Guri, C.D.; and Stare, F.J. 1966. Prevalence of osteoporosis in high- and low-fluoride areas in North Dakota. *J. Amer. Dent. Assoc. 198:499-504.*
72. Leone, N.C.; Stevenson, C.A.; Hilbish, T.F.; and Sosman, M.C. 1955. A roentgenologic study of a human population exposed to high fluoride domestic water: a ten year study. *Am. J. Roentgen.* 74:874-85.
73. Small, B.W., and Murray, J.J. 1978. Enamel opacities: prevalence, classifications and aetiological considerations. *J. Dent.* 6:33-42.
74. Murray, J.J., and Shaw, L. 1979. Classification and prevalence of enamel opacities in the human deciduous and permanent dentitions. *Arch. Oral Biol.* 24:7-13.
75. Newitt, G.A.; Frankel, J.M.; and Witter, D.M. 1963. Occurrence of non-fluoride opacities and non-fluoride hypoplasias of enamel in 588 children aged 9 to 14 years. *J. Amer. Dent. Assoc.* 66:65-69.
76. Al-Alousi, W.; Jackson, D.; Crompton, G.; and Jenkins, O.C. 1975. Enamel mottling in a fluoride and in a non-fluoride community. Parts I and II. *Brit. Dent. J.* 138:9-15, 56-60.
77. Fejerskov, O.; Thylstrup, A.; and Larsen, M.J. 1977. Clinical and structural features and possible pathogenic mechanisms of dental fluorosis. *Scand. J. Dent. Res.* 85:510-34.
78. Thylstrup, A. 1978. Distribution of dental fluorosis in the primary dentition. *Community Dent. Oral Epidemiol.* 6:329-37.
79. Gedalia, I. 1970. Distribution in placenta and foetus. In *Fluorides and human health,* pp. 128-134. Geneva: World Health Organization.
80. Fejerskov, O.; Silverstone, L.M.; Melsen, B.; and Moller, I.J. 1975. The histological features of fluorosed human dental enamel. *Caries Res.* 9:190-210.
81. Thylstrup, A., and Fejerskov, O. Clinical appearance of dental fluorosis in permanent teeth in relation to histologic changes. *Community Dent. Oral Epidemiol.* 6:315-28.
82. Nanda, R.S.; Zipkin, I.; Doyle, J.; and Horowitz, H.S. 1974. Factors affecting the prevalence of dental fluorosis in Lucknow, India. *Arch. Oral Biol.* 19:781-92.

83. Siddiqui, A.H. 1970. Fluorosis in areas of India with a high natural content of water fluoride. In *Fluorides and human health,* pp. 284-94. Geneva: World Health Organization.

84. Siddiqui, A.H. 1955. Fluorosis in Nalgonda district, Hyderabad-Deccan. *Brit. Med. J.* 2:1408-13.

85. Reddy. G.S., and Narasinga. B.S. 1971. Ca turnover with calcium and phosphorus balances. *Metabolism* 20:650-56.

86. Reddy, G.S., and Srikantio, S.G. 1971. Effect of dietary calcium, Vitamin C and protein in development of experimental skeletal fluorosis. *Metabolism* 20:642-49.

87. van Rensburg, B.G.J. 1972. Protein deficient diet, fluoride and amelogenesis. *J. Dent. Assoc. S. Afr.* 27:204-9.

88. Angmar-Mansson, B.; Ericsson, Y.; and Ekberg, O. 1976. Plasma fluoride and enamel fluorosis. *Calcif. Tiss. Res.* 22:77-84.

89. Suttie, J.W.; Carlson, J.R.; and Faltin, E.C. 1972. Effects of alternating periods of high- and low-fluoride ingestion on dairy cattle. *J. Dairy Sci.* 55:790-804.

90. Kruger, B.J. 1970. The effect of different levels of fluoride on the ultrastructure of ameloblasts in the rat. *Arch. Oral Biol.* 15:109-14.

91. Toth, K. 1975. Optimum and tolerated intake of fluorine. *Acta. Med. Acad. Sci. Hung.* 32:1-14.

92. Weatherell, J.A.; Deutsch, D.; Robinson, C.; and Hallsworth, A.S. 1977. Assimilation of fluoride by enamel throughout the life of the tooth. *Caries Res.* 11 (Suppl. 1):85-115

93. Brudevold, F.; Bakhos, Y.; and Aasenden, R. 1978. Dental fluorosis as related to the concentration of fluoride in teeth and bone. *J. Amer. Dent. Assoc.* 96:459-63.

94. Walker, J.S.; Margolis, F.J.; Luten, T.H.; Weil, M.L.; and Wilson, H.L. 1963. Water intake of normal children. *Science* 140:890.

95. DePaola, P.F., and Mellberg, J.R. 1973. Clinical experience and fluoride uptake in children receiving semiannual prophylaxes with an acidulated phosphate fluoride paste. *J. Amer. Dent. Assoc.* 87:155-59.

96. Mellberg, J.R., and Nicholson, C.R. 1974. Fluoride uptake *in vivo* by deciduous enamel of children from neutral fluoride and APF mouthrinses. *Caries Res.* 8:148-54.

97. Mellberg, J.R.; Nicholson, C.R.; and Law, F.E. 1972. Fluoride concentrations in deciduous tooth enamel of children chewing sodium fluoride tablets. *J. Dent. Res.* 51:551-54.

98. Mellberg, J.R.; Englander, H.R.; and Nicholson, C.R. 1967. Acquisition of fluoride *in vivo* by deciduous enamel from daily topical fluoride applications over 21 months. *Arch. Oral Biol.* 12:1139-48.

99. Mellberg, J.R.; Nicholson, C.R.; Packer, M.W.; and Laswell, H.R. 1973. Fluoride concentrations in deciduous teeth of children using fluoride mouthrinses. *Caries Res.* 7:324-31.

100. Mellberg, J.R., and Nicholson, C.R. 1974. Weekly mouthrinsing with 3000 ppm of fluoride; the effect of concentration of fluoride in the enamel. *J. Public Health Dent.* 34:2-7.

101. Mellberg, J.R.; Peterson, J.K.; and Nicholson, C.R. 1974. Fluoride uptake and caries inhibition from self-application of an acidulated phosphate fluoride prophylaxis paste. *Caries Res.* 8:52-60.

102. Mellberg, J.R.; Nicholson, C.R.; and Trubman, A. 1973. The acquisition of fluoride by tooth enamel *in vivo* from self-applied APF gel and prophylaxis paste. *Caries Res.* 7:173-78.

103. Mellberg, J.R.; Nicholson, C.R.; Miller, B.G.; and Englander, H. R. 1970. Acquisition of fluoride *in vivo* by enamel from repeated topical sodium fluoride applications in a fluoridated area: final report. *J. Dent. Res.* 49:1473-77.

104. Englander, H.R.; Mellberg, J.R.; and Engler, W.O. 1978. Observations on dental caries in primary teeth after frequent fluoride toplications in a program involving other preventives. *J. Dent. Res.* 57:855-60.

105. Mellberg, J.R.; Nicholson, C.R.; Franchi, G.J.; Englander, H.R.; and Mosley, G.W. 1977. Enamel fluoride uptake and retention from intensive APF gel applications *in vivo. J. Dent. Res.* 56:716-21.

106. Little, M.F.; Cooper, H.C.; and Rowley, J. 1971. Inorganic-organic inter-actions in human tooth enamel. In *International symposium on tooth Enamel. Tooth enamel II. Its composition, properties and fundamental structures,* ed. R. W. Fearnhead and M. V. Slack. Bristol, England: John Wright & Sons.

107. Smith, F.A., and Hodge, H.C. 1959. Fluoride toxicity. In *Fluorine and Dental Health,* eds. J.C. Muhler and M.K. Hine. Bloomington: Indiana Univ. Press.

108. Mellberg, J.R. 1977. Enamel fluoride and its anti-caries effects. *J. Prev. Dent.* 4:8-14, 16, 20.

Chapter 4

Water Fluoridation

The fluoride saga began in the early part of the 19th century with the discovery of fluoride in the enamel and dentin of fossilized elephant and human teeth. In the latter part of the same century, German and English practitioners were prescribing fluoride preparations for the prevention of dental caries.[1] At about the same time, brown defective enamel of the teeth of people living in the Chiaia region of Italy was described in a literary journal. Shortly thereafter, a brief communication describing enamel defects of the teeth of emigrants embarking from Naples for the United States was sent by a Public Health Service officer to the Surgeon General of the United States.[2] This report was of particular interest to *Dr. Frederick S. McKay,* a Colorado dentist who had observed a similar condition on the teeth of some of his patients. Thus began the long search for what was called at that time "Colorado Brown Stain," later identified as *mottled enamel* or *enamel fluorosis*. Nearly 30 years passed before excessive ingestion of fluoride during tooth development was implicated as the etiologic factor.[3]

As researchers investigated the cause of enamel fluorosis, they observed that patients with mottled teeth also had a remarkable resistance to dental caries. Studies were soon initiated to determine the relationship between mottled teeth, dental caries, and the fluoride content of communal water supplies. Led by *Dr. H. Trendley Dean* of the United States Public Health Service, extensive epidemiologic studies were conducted that demonstrated that drinking water containing fluoride in the amount of 1 ppm* provided dramatic reductions in tooth decay with none of the cosmetically disfiguring side effects of enamel fluorosis.[4] Table 4-1 demonstrates the relationship of the prevalence of dental caries in children residing in 21 United States cities and the level of natural fluoride present in the water supplies. Lower caries rates were found in the communities with higher levels of fluoride. These findings provided the basis for controlled studies of the fluoridation of communal water supplies.

Starting in the 1940s, a series of controlled fluoridation programs was initiated in the cities of Brantford, Ontario; Evanston, Illinois; Grand Rapids, Michigan; and Newburgh, New York.[5-8] The positive results from these studies, along with similar results from later studies in other parts of the world, provided the impetus and justification for the fluoridation of public water supplies deficient in natural fluoride in order to reduce the incidence of dental caries.

The recommended daily dosage of fluoride for children above 3 years of age is 1 mg. This can be obtained by drinking one liter of water with a concentration of 1 ppm fluoride ion. Since the amount of water consumed

*ppm = parts per million

Table 4-1 Caries experience of 12–to 14–year-old white children residing in communities with different levels of natural fluoride*

Community	Number of children examined	F (ppm)	DMF teeth per child
Galesburg, Ill.	273	1.9	2.4
Elmhurst, Ill.	170	1.8	2.5
Colorado Springs, Colo.	404	2.6	2.5
Maywood, Ill.	171	1.2	2.6
Aurora, Ill.	633	1.2	2.8
East Molene, Ill.	152	1.2	3.0
Joliet, Ill.	447	1.3	3.2
Kewanee, Ill.	123	0.9	3.4
Pueblo, Colo.	614	0.6	4.1
Elgin, Ill.	403	0.5	4.4
Marion, Ohio	263	0.4	5.6
Lima, Ohio	454	0.3	6.5
Evanston, Ill.	256	0.0	6.7
Middletown, Ohio	370	0.2	7.0
Quincy, Ill.	330	0.1	7.1
Oak Park, Ill.	329	0.0	7.2
Zanesville, Ohio	459	0.2	7.3
Portsmouth, Ohio	469	0.1	7.7
Waukegan, Ill.	423	0.0	8.1
Elkhart, Ind.	278	0.1	8.2
Michigan City, Ind.	236	0.1	10.4

*Data from *Dean*.[4]

will vary with the temperature, the fluoride ion concentration considered optimal for a particular locality is predicated upon the average of maximum daily air temperature (see *Myers* for a more complete exposition of the relationship between water consumption, ambient temperature, and water fluoride concentration).[9] For dental purposes, the optimal level of fluoride in the drinking water is normally given as between 0.7 and 1.2 ppm.

Community water fluoridation

Compounds used in water fluoridation

Theoretically, any compound that forms fluoride ions in aqueous solution can be utilized for the fluoridation process. However, the choice of chemical will depend on such factors as the number and accessibility of water sources, water quality, and other concurrent treatment processes. Additionally, the chemical compound must be sufficiently soluble for routine water plant practices, have no undesirable side effects from the cation moity of the fluoride compound, and be both readily available and inexpensive.

Table 4-2 Fluoride compounds used for water fluoridation: listed by range of population served, December 31, 1975

Population range of fluoridated communities	Number of places fluoridating	Sodium fluoride Dry	Sodium fluoride Solution	Sodium silicofluoride Dry	Sodium silicofluoride Solution	Hydrofluosilicic acid Solution	Calcium fluoride, ammonium fluosilicate, adjusted natural fluoride, and not specified
1,000,000 and over	7	0	0	0	0	7	0
500,000 — 999,999	14	0	0	5	1	7	1
250,000 — 499,999	23	4	0	9	0	9	1
100,000 — 249,999	81	7	5	33	0	29	7
50,000 — 99,999	156	11	4	72	5	58	6
25,000 — 49,999	392	33	31	153	21	133	21
10,000 — 24,999	864	63	105	316	44	308	28
5,000 — 9,999	854	47	114	304	35	308	46
2,500 — 4,999	951	53	175	280	40	357	46
1,000 — 2,499	1,318	52	366	283	43	511	63
Under 1,000	2,014	65	504	425	54	797	169
Not specified	121	10	8	53	2	20	28
Total	6,795	345	1,312	1,933	245	2,544	416

Data from U. S. Dept. of Health, Education, and Welfare.

Sodium fluoride was the first compound used in controlled fluoridation programs. This choice was based on the above considerations as well as the thorough study of its toxicity and physiologic effects; but once fluoridation became an established practice, other compounds were tried. Owing largely to its low cost, sodium silicofluoride replaced sodium fluoride as the chemical most often used for water fluoridation. Within the last 20 years, however, there has been an increased use of hydrofluosilicic acid as the fluoride ion source. Several factors are responsible for the selection of this compound in preference to other fluoride compounds: (1) It can be utilized with simple feed equipment, which may consist of nothing more than a positive displacement chemical feed pump. (2) Small water supplies can be easily fluoridated using only a dilution tank and transfer pump. (3) Chemical handling is uncomplicated. (4) The cost is low. Compounds currently used in community water fluoridation programs in the United States are listed in Table 4–2.

Recently, there has been some concern that in some fluoridated communities the residents are not receiving the benefits of fluoridation.[11] Surveys of fluoridation control systems in eight states revealed that of 88 water supplies checked, only 43 were actually fluoridating within a therapeutically optimal range. This finding emphasizes the need for strict surveillance procedures by fluoride monitoring agencies as well as for the careful training of plant operators in fluoridation practices.

Table 4-3 Caries experience prior to and after the introduction of controlled fluoridation

Community	Age (years)	DMFT Before F	DMFT After F	Percent reduction
Brantford, Ont.[5]	8	2.4	1.1	54.2
Newburgh, N.Y.[8]	9	3.1	1.5	51.6
Grand Rapids, Mich.[7]	10	4.9	2.3	53.1
Hastings, New Zealand[13]	11	7.2	3.6	50.0
Evanston, Ill.[6]	12-14	9.0	4.6	48.9
Hartlepool, England[12]	15	9.0	5.0	44.6

Benefits of water fluoridation—to Children

Primary dentition

The benefits of communal water fluoridation are not limited to the permanent teeth but extend to the primary teeth as well. *Ast* and coworkers[8] reported that 6- to 9-year-old children in the fluoridated city of Newburgh had almost six times as many caries-free primary cuspids and molars as children of the same age in the fluoride-deficient city of Kingston. Other studies have reported similar findings.[5,6]

Permanent dentition: Differences in caries prevalence prior to fluoridation and after the introduction of controlled fluoridation in six communities in various parts of the world are presented in Table 4-3. In all of the communities, the caries inhibition in the permanent teeth was approximately 50%. In addition to these classical studies, numerous other reports have attested to the effectiveness of community water fluoridation in reducing dental caries.

A dental health survey was recently completed in Connecticut, the first state to adopt a mandatory fluoridation law.[14] One of the assessments in the survey included the caries prevalence in 6- to 11-year-old children in urban New Haven. Since the survey was conducted ten years after the introduction of fluoride to the city's water supplies, some of the children had a lifetime exposure to waterborne fluoride while others had not. After ten years of fluoridation, children in this age group who were born in New Haven experienced a 52.4% reduction in the number of decayed, missing, and filled teeth. This is comparable to the findings of the initial controlled fluoridation studies listed in Table 4-3. Thus, the level of caries protection afforded by this method has remained constant since it was first utilized more than 35 years ago.

Benefits to be derived from fluoride are the greatest when optimal amounts are available during the period of tooth mineralization. Nevertheless, teeth that have completed mineralization and erupted prior to the start of fluoridation also receive protection. *Bushel and Smith*[15] have shown that 17-year-old Newburgh children, who had been exposed to fluoridated water for only 9 years, had 28% less caries than their counterparts in the fluoride-deficient city of Kingston.

The cariostatic effect of fluoridation is preferential since some tooth surfaces receive greater protection against caries than others. The smooth tooth surfaces, especially the proximal surfaces, derive greater protection than do the pit-and-fissured

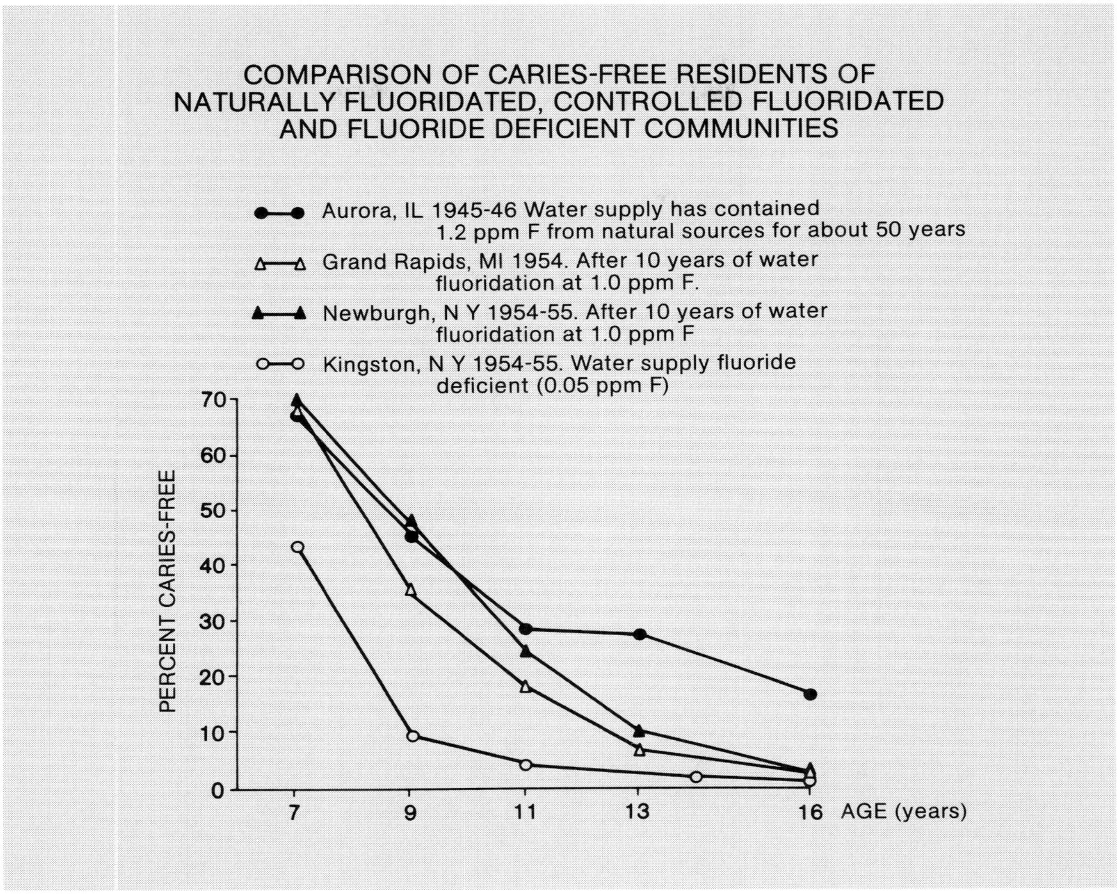

Figure 4-1 (Adapted from Ast.[17])

occlusal surfaces. Community fluoridation studies in Newburgh,[8] Evanston,[6] Hastings (New Zealand),[13] and Tiel (the Netherlands)[16] all confirm this finding. Additionally, in fluoridated communities there is a greater proportion of caries-free children and a lower incidence of extractions. Figure 4-1 presents the percentage of caries-free children by age residing in either a fluoride-deficient, naturally fluoridated, or controlled-fluoridated community.[17] The percentage of caries-free children in the fluoridated communities is considerably higher than in the fluoride-deficient community. Children, 11 years of age and older, in Grand Rapids and Newburgh did not have fluoridated water available from birth. Nevertheless, as seen in the figure, the percentage of caries-free children in these cities was still higher than in the fluoride-deficient city of Kingston.

Malocclusion

It has been suggested that untreated carious lesions and the extraction of teeth due to caries are frequent etiologic factors in the development of dental malocclusion. If this is true, the benefits of fluoridation may include a lower prevalence of malocclusion. *Ast* and co-workers[18] reported three times as many children with normal occlusion in the fluoridated community of Newburgh compared to nonfluoridated Kingston. They attributed this difference to fewer teeth, especially first permanent molars, lost per child in the Newburgh children. However, neither *Blayney* and *Hill*,[6] who examined children in Evanston, Illinois, nor *Pelton* and *Elsasser*,[19] who examined schoolchildren in Idaho, were able to detect a lower prevalence of malocclusion as a result of fluoridation. It is possible that these contradictory results represent differences in the examiners' criteria of what constitutes a malocclusion. Further evaluations using standardized criteria are indicated.

Benefits of water fluoridation—to Adults

Dental caries

Englander and *Wallace*[20] conducted one of the first studies comparing the prevalence of dental caries in young adults with lifelong exposure to naturally optimally fluoridated water to individuals of similar age in a community with fluoride-deficient water. They found over 60% fewer DMF surfaces in the 18- and 19-year-olds living in the fluoridated area. *Russell* and *Elvove*[21] examined 20- to 44-year-old residents of Colorado Springs, Colorado (2.5 ppm F), and Boulder, Colorado (0.1 ppm F). Total rates for DMF teeth were about 60% lower in Colorado Springs than in Boulder. Native residents of fluoride-deficient Boulder had lost nearly four times an many teeth as had residents of Colorado Springs. Other studies have also substantiated the caries reductions that fluoridation provides to adults.[22-24]

Osteoporosis

While the beneficial effects of optimal fluoride levels in drinking water in preventing dental caries has been well established, the role of waterborne fluoride in the prevention of osteoporosis is less clear. *Leone* and associates[25] compared radiographic evidence of osteoporosis in Framingham, Massachusetts (0.1 ppm F), with that of two communities in Texas (8.0 ppm F). The much greater frequency of osteoporosis in Framingham led them to conclude that "disadvantageous effects on bone structure of the adult population may be associated with the use of drinking water that contains an insufficient concentration of fluoride." A study conducted in North Dakota by researchers from the Harvard School of Public Health offered further evidence that fluoride deficiency may be the most important etiologic factor in the development of osteoporosis.[26] This same study also revealed a significantly lower incidence of calcification of the aorta in men living in a high fluoride area (4.0 to 6.0 ppm). It must be recognized that the adult populations in both of these studies were consuming relatively high fluoride levels from birth; thus, the fluoride was incorporated into bone as it was developing and was also available as osteoclastic-osteoblastic turnover occurred.

While both the Framingham and North Dakota studies indicate that consuming drinking water with relatively high levels of fluoride (4.0 to 8.0 ppm) may significantly lessen the incidence of osteoporosis, other investigators found no evidence of increased bone density *(osteosclerosis)* in residents of communities where the water supply had less than 4 ppm fluoride.[27,28] There is a need for continued study of the relationship between bone density and waterborne fluoride levels. Unfortunately, a study of this relationship, started in Tiel, the Netherlands, was terminated due to the discontinuation of fluoridation in that country.[29]

Effects of discontinuing community water fluoridation

Studies have evaluated the effect of the discontinuation of consuming a fluoridated water supply. When the fluoride concentration in the community water of Galesburg, Illinois, was reduced from its natural level of 2 ppm to a fluoride-deficient level (<0.1 ppm), children who had been continuous residents experienced a significant increase in caries. Additionally, the number of caries-free children decreased markedly during this same time period. In Antigo, Wisconsin, fluoride supplementation of the water supply was discontinued after 11 years.[31] A dental survey of the schoolchildren in this city was made shortly before fluoridation was discontinued. DMF counts were found to be similar to other fluoridated areas in the state. Four years later, and again just after fluoridation was reinstituted, additional dental surveys were conducted. Results of these surveys showed a marked increase in caries activity to a level approximating nonfluoridated areas in the state.

Safety of fluoridation

Dental effects

As previously discussed, early investigations of the effects of fluoride on the teeth were related not to the beneficial properties of the fluoride ion but to the detrimental effects of excessive levels on tooth development and mineralization.[32,33] Excessive levels of fluoride during the period of tooth development (i.e., to approximately 8 years of age, exclusive of the development of third molars) can cause fluorosis, or mottling, of the teeth.

Mild dental fluorosis is characterized by white flecks or white, wavy lines on the teeth. This level of fluorosis is not cosmetically detracting and may even enhance the appearance of the teeth. However, more severe forms have the appearance of paper white opaque areas or brown intrinsic stains, and hypoplasia of the tooth surface can occur. Fluoride opacities are usually symmetrically distributed in the mouth and are generally present only in the permanent dentition, although, in areas with very high concentrations of waterborne fluoride, fluorosis has been found in the primary dentition (see Chapter 3). *Dean*[34] has classified dental fluorosis into six categories according to the severity of the condition (Table 4-4). The clinical appearance of teeth with different levels of severity is shown in Figure 4-2.

Dean rated each tooth present in an individual's mouth according to the fluorosis index that he established. The individual's fluorosis score was based upon the severest form recorded for two or more teeth. In addition to the individual scores, *Dean* calculated a community fluorosis index (F_{ci}) using the following formula:

$$F_{ci} = \frac{\Sigma\ (\text{frequency} \times \text{individual fluorosis score})}{\text{number of individuals}}$$

Dean and his colleagues[35] established the relationship between the level of fluoride in a community's water supply and the community fluorosis index. These investigators examined over 5,000 children from 22 cities with different levels of fluoride in the community water supplies and found the prevalence and severity of fluorosis were directly related to the concentration of fluoride in the water. The values in Table 4-5 are excerpted from Dean's publication. As seen in the table, the teeth of the majority of residents residing in communities where the fluoride levels are 1.2 ppm or less are normal, only mild levels of fluorosis are detected, and no residents exhibit disfiguring brown spots or pitting. At approximately 2 ppm F, moderate fluorosis is observed, while severe fluorosis occurs at approximately 3 ppm. As the concentration

Fig. 4-2a to e Increasing levels of fluorosis severity
(Figs. 4a, c, and d courtesy of Dr. H. *Bohannan*, American Fund for Dental Health, National Preventive Dentistry Demonstration Program. Figs. 4b and e courtesy of Dr. H. *Horowitz*, Community Programs Section, National Caries Program, National Institute of Dental Research.)

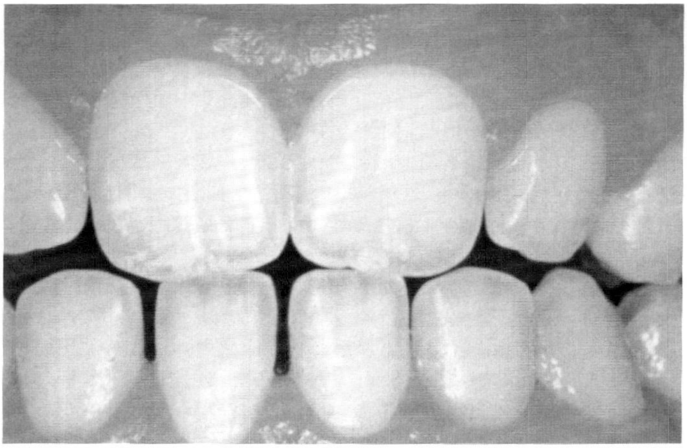

Fig. 4-2a questionable

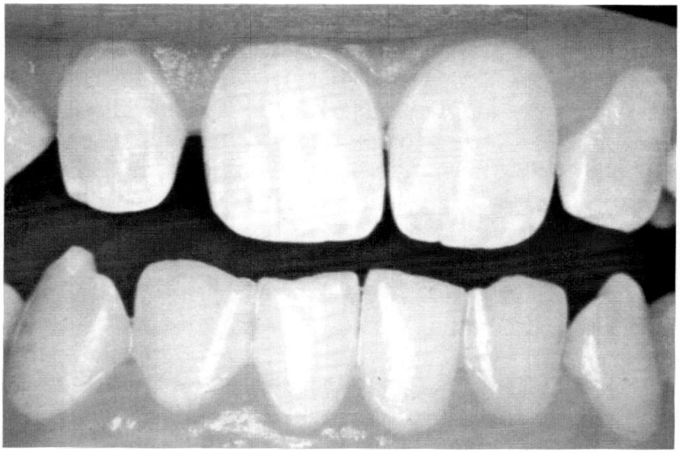

Fig. 4-2b very mild

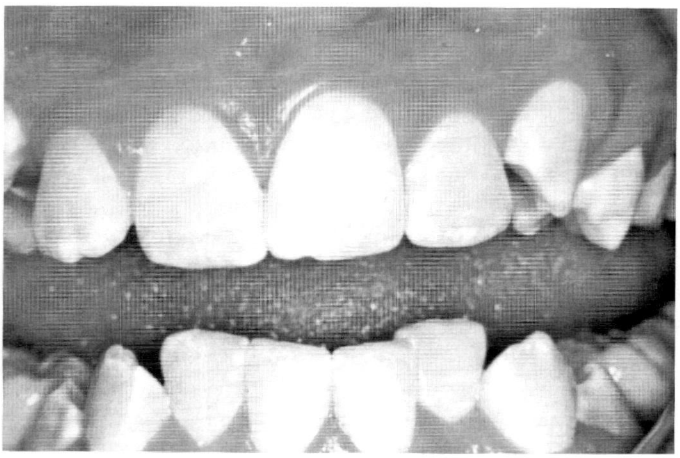

Fig. 4-2c mild

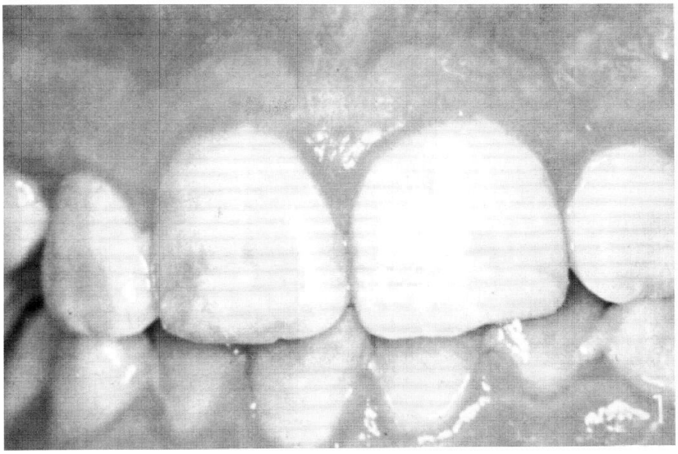

Fig. 4-2d moderate

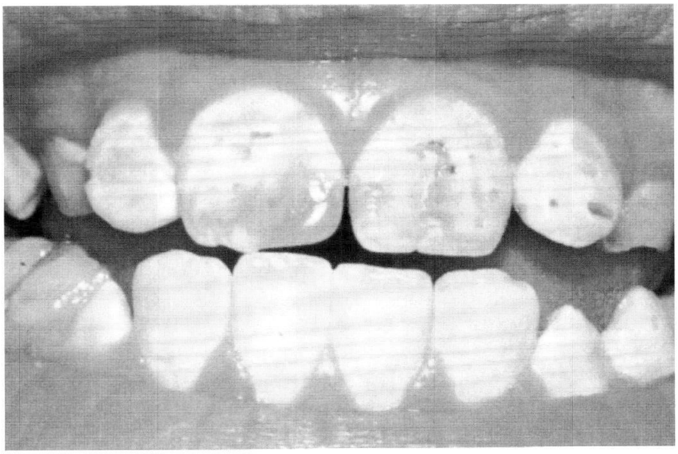

Fig. 4-2e severe

of fluoride increases above 3 ppm, the percentage of individuals with severe fluorosis increases significantly.

More recently, *Myers*[9] tabulated over 50 reports from 13 countries in which community fluorosis levels were assessed. In several instances, the prevalence and/or severity of fluorosis was higher than would be anticipated from the water fluoride concentrations. *Meyers* postulated that this might be due to an increased volume or increased frequency of drinking fluoridated water. These practices could occur when either the outdoor or indoor mean maximum temperatures are sufficiently high to encourage greater water consumption.

Systemic effects

Extensive studies have been conducted to ascertain whether the consumption of an optimally fluoridated water supply results in any systemic abnormalities. As part of the Kingston-Newburgh caries-fluoride study, a long-term medical study was also under-

Table 4-4 Dean's dental fluorosis classification

Category	Dental fluorosis score	Description of enamel
Normal	0.0	Smooth, glossy, pale creamy-white translucent surface
Questionable	0.5	A few white flecks or white spots
Very mild	1.0	Small opaque, paper-white areas covering less than 25% of the tooth surface
Mild	2.0	Opaque white areas covering less than 50% of the tooth surface
Moderate	3.0	All tooth surfaces affected; brown stain; marked wear on biting surfaces
Severe	4.0	All tooth surfaces affected; brown stain; discrete or confluent pitting

Data from *Dean.*[34] Source: Leske, G.S.; Ripa, L.W.; and Leske, M.C. Dental Public Health (chap. 43). In *Maxcy-Rosenau Public Health and Preventive Medicine.* 11th ed., J.M. Last, ed., pp. 1423-68. New York: Appleton-Century-Crofts, 1980.

taken. The growth and development of children in the two cities (Kingston F $\leqq$ 0.1 ppm; Newburgh F = 1.2 ppm) were evaluated. Comparisons were made of specific conditions in the two groups as disclosed by medical histories, physical examinations, and laboratory and roentgenographic studies. These examinations were conducted annually beginning in 1945 and continuing through 1955. No significant medical differences were found between the two groups of children.[36]

Leone and co-workers[37,38] conducted physical, laboratory, and roentgenographic examinations on residents of Bartlett, Texas, a community with excessive (8.0 ppm) levels of fluoride in the water supply. The results were compared to those obtained on residents of Cameron, Texas, with 0.4 ppm fluoride. Individuals with an average continuous residence of more than 35 years in either city were evaluated. As expected, because of the high levels of fluoride, dental fluorosis was present in all Bartlett residents. The only significant systemic difference was a higher prevalence of cardiovascular abnormalities in the fluoride-deficient community of Cameron. Another observation in Bartlett was the possible beneficial effect of fluoride on bone in counteracting age-associated osteoporotic changes.

Opponents of fluoridation have claimed that significant differences in morbidity and mortality rates exist for fluoridated and nonfluoridated communities. However, extensive studies in this country and in other parts of the world do not support this claim.[38-41] Recently, antifluoridationists have opposed the addition of fluoride to public water supplies on the grounds that it is associated with an increased incidence of cancer and cancer deaths.[42,43] Nevertheless, studies of cancer incidence and mortality in specific localities of the United States between 1950 and 1969 showed no trends that could be attributed to fluoridation.[44] *Doll* and *Kinlen*[45] reviewed cancer mortality rates for 1950 to 1970 in 10 fluoridated cities and 10 fluoride-deficient cities in the United States. After adjusting for age, sex, and ethnicity, they found a decrease in cancer rates in cities with fluoridated water, while there was no

Table 4-5 Fluorosis distribution according to natural levels of fluoride in the drinking water

Fluoride concentration (ppm)	Signs absent		White areas		Brown areas and pitting	
	Normal	Questionable	Very mild	Mild	Moderate	Severe
0.0	97.9	1.9	0.2	0.0	0.0	0.0
0.3	84.1	13.7	2.2	0.0	0.0	0.0
0.6	72.3	21.2	6.2	0.3	0.0	0.0
0.9	52.8	35.0	10.6	1.6	0.0	0.0
1.2	53.2	31.8	13.9	1.1	0.0	0.0
1.9	25.3	27.1	40.3	6.2	1.1	0.0
2.2	13.0	16.0	23.9	35.4	11.0	0.7
2.9	4.1	8.3	34.0	26.8	23.7	3.1
3.9	3.1	6.6	15.2	28.0	33.9	13.2
8.0	0.0	0.0	0.0	9.5	47.6	42.8

Data from *Dean*.[35]

change in the fluoride-deficient cities. In an extensive review of mortality trends from 1950 to 1970 in 473 United States cities, *Rogot* and co-workers[46] also failed to document a relationship between the fluoride levels of the city water supplies and either heart-related or cancer death rate trends.

In the first of a two-part investigative report, *Consumer Reports* concluded that the charge that fluoridated water causes cancer was "baseless."[47] In the second part of the report, other charges of alleged adverse effects were also reviewed.[48] The concluding statement of this consumer advocacy periodical was significant: "The simple truth is that there is no 'scientific controversy' over the safety of fluoridation. The practice is safe, economical, and beneficial. The survival of this false controversy represents, in CU's [Consumers Union] opinion, one of the major triumphs of quackery over science in our generation."

The findings cited in this chapter as well as others support the statement by the Royal College of Physicians of Britain that "there is no evidence that fluoride increases the incidence or mortality of cancer in any organ."[49] All major health organizations throughout the world support the controlled fluoridation of community water supplies as a safe and effective public health measure to reduce the incidence of dental caries.

While no problem of a chronic nature has been ascribed to the long-term consumption of optimally fluoridated water, an incident occurred in 1979 that stresses the importance of careful and continuous monitoring of the amount of fluoride added to a community's water supply. In Annapolis, Maryland, fluoride was accidently added at a level of over 30 ppm for several days.[50] As a result, a resident being treated by kidney dialysis using tap water instead of deionized water expired and seven other dialysis patients became ill. It must be stressed that these individuals were medically compromised and were not consuming water in the usual sense; no untoward effects were reported in the population at large from temporarily consuming water containing this higher level of fluoride.

Sociopolitical implications of fluoridation

With the advent of controlled water fluoridation there developed simultaneously an antifluoridation resistance that continues today and that has not only succussfully prevented the implementation of controlled fluoridation in many communities, but has also succeeded in defluoridating communities in which fluoride had been previously introduced.

A usual hallmark of successful antifluoridation activity is to make it compulsory that the decision to fluoridate be decided by referendum, thus removing a public issue from the jurisdiction of local health boards or other agencies and placing the decision in the hands of the voter. It has been shown, however, that when participatory governments allow public issues to be decided directly by the people the result tends to be more referenda.[51] These referenda provide a public platform for the antifluoridationist movement, which has been very successful in defeating attempts to fluoridate. Of the approximately 900 referenda held between 1955 and 1965, only about one-third resulted in a positive vote for fluoridation.[52] As of 1975, 6,795 localities in the United States had controlled fluoridation. Only 503, or 7%, were authorized by referenda, while most of the remainder were authorized by the governing body of the municipality. Additionally, from 1945 to 1975, 230 municipalities discontinued fluoridation, while only 121 communities reinstated fluoridation after discontinuation.[10]

Antifluoridation initiatives further escalated in the late 1970's as statewide campaigns to limit fluoridation were launched in Oregon, Washington, and Utah.[53] In Oregon and Washington, the electorate rejected the proposals. In Utah, however, a proposal was passed to make it compulsory that water fluoridation be approved by referendum.

Internationally there have also been some major setbacks in the attempt to fluoridate. In 1971, the Swedish Parliament abolished the right to fluoridate the drinking water,[54] and in 1976 the Netherlands, by royal decree, also abolished water fluoridation. In both instances, the decision rescinded previous laws that favored fluoridation.

The successful challenges by the antifluoridation movement demonstrate the unpreparedness of the health professionals who support fluoridation and who are not accustomed to having their health-related decisions challenged. One of the factors contributing to the inability of health professionals to muster public support has been their belief that the issue was a scientific, not a political one. *Knutson* brands this concept as "naive" and his statement is supported by the findings that opposition to fluoridation is linked to antiscientific and antiintellectual attitudes, ambivalence toward science and technology, and resentment of government.[52,55,56]

Experience has shown that the decision to fluoridate should be kept out of the public arena. If, however, the issue of fluoridation is to be fought with the ballot, then the proponents must recognize the reality of being in a political, rather than a scientific, debate.

The status of community water fluoridation

Fluoridation in the United States

Approximately 11 million people in the United States reside in areas in which optimal or higher levels of fluoride occur naturally in the drinking water.[10] Additionally, almost 95 million people are consuming drinking water that has been adjusted to optimal levels. Thus, 49.4% of the United States population is receiving the benefits of waterborne fluoride. Figure 4-3 indicates the percentage of state populations using fluoridated water

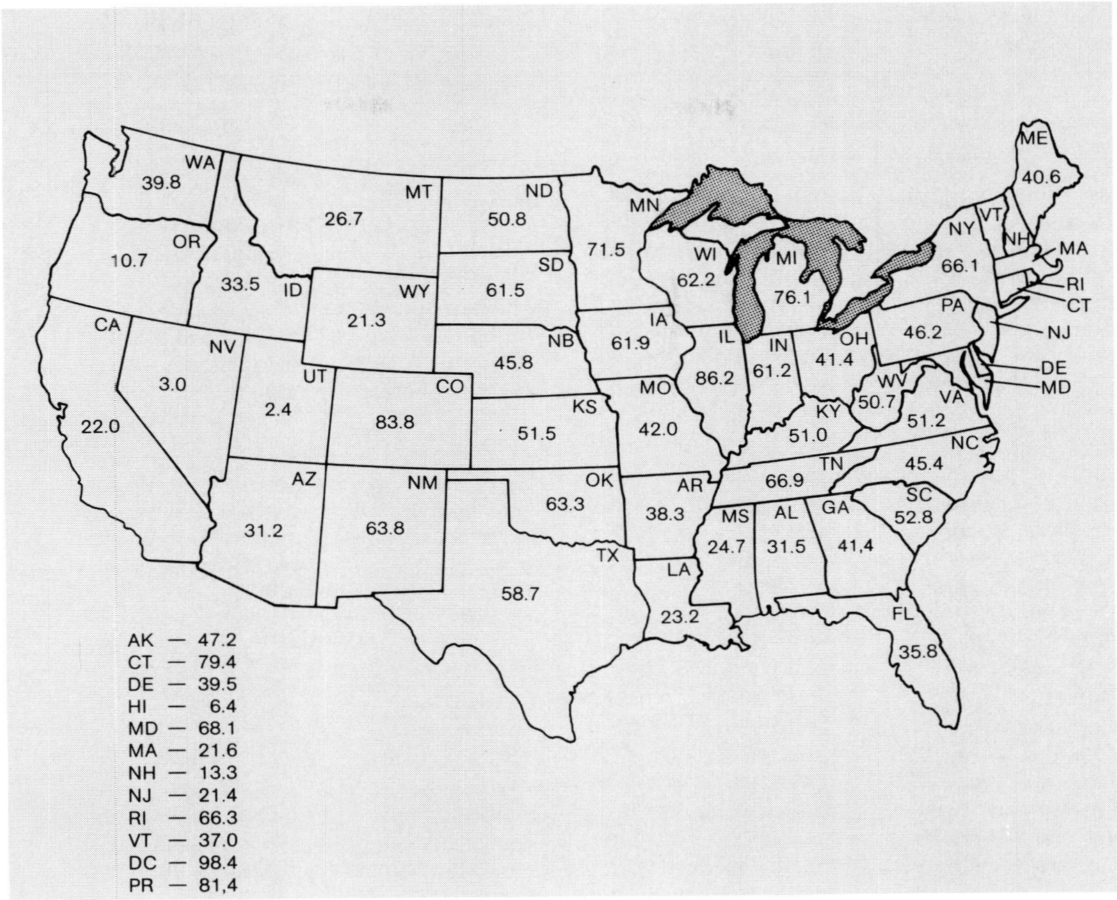

Fig. 4-3 Percent of total residents by state consuming drinking water containing fluoride at or above optimal level.

(1975). Eight states* and the Commonwealth of Puerto Rico have mandated the addition of fluoride to the water supplies of all communities with a certain minimum population; nevertheless, there are still 28 states in which less than 50% of the population consumes water with optimal levels of fluoride.

Most large United States cities are fluoridated. Of the 57 cities in the United States with populations of 250,000 or more, only 13 do not have optimal fluoride levels and, of the six largest cities, only Los Angeles' water supply is not fluoridated (Table 4-6).

*Connecticut, Georgia, Illinois, Michigan, Minnesota, Nebraska, Ohio, and South Dakota. In 1968, Delaware had mandated fluoridation; as of 1974, however, this state requires that local referenda be held.

International fluoridation

Worldwide, approximately 320 million people are consuming drinking water containing optimal levels of fluoride; of these, one-third are residents of the United States. The

Table 4-6 Status of fluoridation in the largest United States cities (population 250,000 or more)

Controlled Fluoridation

City	Population	Date
New York, N.Y.	7,647,000	1965
Chicago, Ill.	3,173,000	1956
Philadelphia, Pa.	1,862,000	1954
Detroit, Mich.	1,387,000	1967
Baltimore, Md.	878,000	1952
Dallas, Tex.	816,000	1966
San Diego, Calif.	757,000	1952*
Indianapolis, Ind.	734,000	1951
Washington, D.C.	734,000	1952
Milwaukee, Wis.	691,000	1953
San Francisco, Calif.	687,000	1952
Cleveland, Ohio	679,000	1956
Memphis, Tenn.	659,000	1970
Boston, Mass.	618,000	1978
New Orleans, La.	573,000	1974
St. Louis, Mo.	558,000	1955
Columbus, Ohio	541,000	1973
San Jose, Calif.	523,000	1965†
Denver, Colo.	516,000	1954
Seattle, Wash.	503,000	1969
Kansas City, Mo.	488,000	1962*
Pittsburgh, Pa.	479,000	1952
Atlanta, Ga.	451,000	1969
Nashville, Tenn.	449,000	1953
Cincinnati, Ohio	426,000	1976
Buffalo, N.Y.	425,000	1955
Minneapolis, Minn.	382,000	1957
Toledo, Ohio	377,000	1955
Omaha, Nebr.	377,000	1969
Oklahoma City, Okla.	374,000	1954
Fort Worth, Tex.	360,000	1965
Louisville, Ky.	356,000	1951
Miami, Fla.	354,000	1952
Oakland, Calif.	348,000	1976
Long Beach, Calif.	347,000	1971
Tulsa, Okla.	335,000	1953
Austin, Tex.	291,000	1973
St. Paul, Minn.	287,000	1952
Charlotte, N.C.	285,000	1949
Norfolk, Va	283,000	1952
Rochester, N.Y.	277,000	1952
Albuquerque, N.Mex.	274,000	1974
Akron, Ohio	266,000	1969

Natural Fluoridation

City	Population
Houston, Tex	1,320,000†
Jacksonville, Fla.	548,000†
El Paso, Tex.	353,000

NonFluoridated

City	Population
Los Angeles, Calif.	2,747,000
San Antonio, Tex.	756,000
Phoenix, Ariz.	637,000
Portland, Oreg.	378,000
Newark, N.J.	368,000
Honolulu, Hawaii	338,000
Tucson, Ariz.	308,000
Birmingham, Ala.	296,000
Tampa, Fla.	277,000
Sacramento, Calif.	267,000
Wichita, Kans.	261,000

* Discontinued fluoridation.
† Partly fluoridated.

Source: Leske, G.S.; Ripa, L.W.; and Leske, M.C. Dental Public Health (Chap. 43). In *Maxcy-Rosenau Public Health and Preventive Medicine.* 11th ed., J.M. Last, ed., pp. 1423-68. New York: Appleton-Century-Crofts, 1980.

Table 4-7 Countries in which one million or more residents receive optimally fluoridated water

Country	Population served (millions)
U.S.A.	105.3
U.S.S.R.	30.0*
Brazil	10.5
Colombia	10.0
Australia	9.0
Canada	8.5
Venezuela	5.0*
Chile	4.1
Malaysia	4.0
England and Wales	4.0
Hong Kong	3.9
Mexico	3.3
Poland	2.3
Singapore	2.2
Czechoslovakia	1.7
New Zealand	1.5
Ireland	1.4
German Democratic Republic	1.2
Panama	1.0*
Ecuador	1.0*

*Estimated.
Data from the Canadian Dental Association and the Pan American Health Organization (1978).

Republic of Ireland is the only country to adopt legislation for national water fluoridation. Table 4-7 lists the countries that are major users of fluoridated water.

Cost of community water fluoridation

The cost of fluoridation is generally computed on an annual per capita basis and varies with such factors as the size of the community, the source of the water supply, and the type of fluoride used. Based on 55 water systems in New York State, the annual cost per capita ranges from a high of $0.33, in communities having less than 5,000 people, to a low of $0.06, in communities with populations over 1,000,000.[57] The annual per capita cost of fluoridation in Hastings, New Zealand, was computed at $0.10. While some of these figures were compiled approximately 10 years ago, they indicate that fluoridation, which results in a 50 to 60% reduction in dental caries, is a very economical preventive measure.[58]

Community fluoridation produces economies in children's dental care in terms of both treatment time and costs. Fewer and less complex treatment services are required by children receiving the benefits of fluoridation. The costs of children's dental care in fluoridated areas can be less than one-half the costs in fluoride-deficient areas. It has been estimated that for every dollar spent on community fluoridation, the resultant savings will be $50.[59]

In 1979, an amendment to Sections 317 and 318 of the United States Public Health Service Act added fluoridation programs to the current regulations for state and local government agencies to qualify for grants to assist them in meeting costs of preventive health services programs.[60] This grant program makes funds available for costs associated with the promotion, installation, operation, monitoring, surveillance, and upgrading of fluoridation systems.

School water fluoridation

Of the approximately 220 million persons in the United States, slightly more than 75% live in areas served by a public water supply and can potentially benefit from community water fluoridation. However, alternative methods of caries prevention must be used for the over 50 million individuals whose water is obtained from other sources. One method for supplying systemic fluoride to children is fluoridating the individual school water supply.

A pilot school water fluoridation study was initiated in 1954 in the Virgin Islands.[61] The fluoride content of the water at two schools on the island of St. Thomas was adjusted to 2.3 ppm, slightly more than three times the optimum level recommended for community water supplies in that temperature zone. In 1962, 8 years after the start of the project, children in the test schools had a 21.9% lower caries incidence than their counterparts in control schools with unadjusted water supplies.

Further studies of school water fluoridation were begun in Pennsylvania and Kentucky in 1957.[62,63] In Pike County, Kentucky, fluoride was added to the school water supply at 3 ppm (approximately 3.3 times the level recommended for this area), while in Elk Lake, Pennsylvania, the school water supply was fluoridated at 5 ppm (approximately four and a half times the recommended level). Interim findings after 4 years in Pike County revealed a reduction of 24.5% in caries prevalence, and after 5 years in Elk Lake, there was a reduction of 28.6% in caries prevalence. Results of the final examinations in Elk Lake made in 1970, after 12 years of school water fluoridation, showed that children who had attended school continuously had 39% fewer decayed, missing, and filled teeth than did their counterparts at the baseline examinations.[64]

The most effective fluoride level for school fluoridation programs has not been established. To obtain additional information on this subject, *Heifetz* and co-workers[65] initiated a 12-year study in Seagrove, North Carolina. Fluoride was added to the school water supply at a concentration of 6.3 ppm (seven times the recommended level). Interim findings after 8 years revealed that children in grades one through eight had approximately 40% fewer DMF surfaces than did children of a similar age who were examined before the study began. This reduction is almost identical to the Elk Lake findings in which a level of 4.5 times the optimal community fluoride level was tested. In neither of these studies did any of the examined children show signs of dental fluorosis.

The results of the several studies of school water fluoridation indicate that it can be an effective public health measure to reduce dental caries in communities where the fluoridation of local water supplies is not feasible. Nevertheless, this method has some disadvantages. Most children are 5 or 6 years old upon entering school. At this age, their dental development precludes that the fluoride from a school water fluoridation program will provide preeruptive contact to the primary teeth and allows only limited preeruptive contact to the permanent teeth. In no instance will any tooth have fluoride contact during its entire developmental period. Thus, the potential benefits of waterborne fluoride are reduced because contact from birth is not possible.

Another disadvantage of school water fluoridation is the intermittent exposure of the children to fluoride. Most children attend school for 5 to 6 hours a day, and are actually in school less than 180 days during a calendar year. Thus, school-age children spend only about 20 to 25% of their waking hours in school. To compensate for this limited access to fluoridated water, the Public Health Service recommends that the fluoride content of a school water supply be adjusted to a level considerably higher than that recommended for community fluoridation in the same locale.

The most recent United States fluoridation census revealed that approximately 125,000 schoolchildren in 383 schools drink fluoridated water through school fluoridation programs.[10] The largest statewide programs are in North Carolina and Kentucky. More than 100 schools in each state have fluoridated

Table 4-8 School population and number of schools using adjusted fluoridation by state, December 31, 1976

Location	School population using fluoridated water	Number of schools
U.S.A.	124,475	383
North Carolina	43,574	105
Kentucky	36,632	123
Vermont	12,981	54
Indiana	10,115	27
Wisconsin	5,229	24
Tennessee	4,976	17
Pennsylvania	3,600	4
Maine	2,238	8
Wyoming	1,749	12
New Mexico	1,473	6
Nebraska	1,288	1
Florida	450	1
Montana	170	1

Data from U.S. Dept. of Health, Education, and Welfare.[10]

their water supplies. Table 4-8 lists the 13 states having fluoridated school water supplies.

As with community water fluoridation, the safety of school water fluoridation must be continually monitored. A case of acute fluoride overdose was reported at a rural grammar school in Stanly County, North Carolina.[66] Two hundred one students and 12 adults became ill after drinking orange juice at a morning recess. All of the individuals experienced nausea; all of the children and seven of the 12 adults vomited. The episode lasted less than an hour and no one was hospitalized. Analysis of the orange juice revealed a fluoride level of 270 mg/liter (270 ppm). The cause of the accident was shown to be a malfunctioning fluoride feeder pump that continuously fed sodium fluoride into the water system during an extended school holiday period.

Summary

The presence of optimal levels of fluoride in drinking water, whether naturally present or adjusted, results in an inhibition of dental caries of 50% or more. The beneficial effects of therapeutic levels of fluoride are accompanied by no known side effects to the general health of the population. To the contrary, there is some indication that lifetime residents of fluoridated communities may have a lower prevalence of osteoporosis than individuals who drink fluoride-deficient water.

Drinking water that contains therapeutic levels of fluoride reduces the caries prevalence in both children and adults. Likewise, beneficial effects accrue to both the primary and permanent dentitions, although the smooth surfaces of the teeth are better protected than the pit-and-fissured occlusal surfaces.

Barriers to fluoridation have included sociopolitical resistance and technical difficulties in fluoridating certain communities. Antifluoridation resistance has been strong, persistent, and organized. It has resulted not only in the defeat of proposals to fluoridate communities, but has also led to defluoridation in communities that had initially accepted the procedure. Many communities are not served by public water sources and thus community fluoridation is not feasible. One solution to this problem is the fluoridation of the water supplies of individual schools. Since children have only limited exposure to a school's drinking water, the level of fluoride introduced should be several times the level recommended for the community's water supply. School water fluoridation has been accomplished at these higher levels without the development of enamel fluorosis.

There is no evidence to indicate that the consumption of therapeutic levels of fluoride causes chronic medical or systemic problems. However, an accidental overdose can cause acute problems, emphasizing the need for strict surveillance when controlled fluoridation is introduced to either a school's or a community's water supply.

References

1. Volker, J. 1968. Introduction: symposium on fluorides in the control of caries. *N.J. Acad. Med. Bul.* 14:206-9.
2. Eager, J.M. 1901. Denti di chiaie. *Pub. Health Rep. (U.S.)* 16:2576.
3. McClure, F.S. 1970. *Water fluoridation: the search and the victory*, pp. 1-16. Washington, D.C.: U.S. Gov't. Printing Office.
4. Dean, H.T. 1946. Epidemiological studies in the United States. In *Dental caries and fluorine*, ed. F.R. Moulton, pp. 5-31. Washington, D.C.: Amer. Assoc. Adv. of Sci.
5. Brown, H.K., and Poplove, M. 1965. The Brantford-Sarnia-Stratford fluoridation study: final survey, 1963. *Med. Serv. J. Canada* 21:450-56.
6. Blayney, J.R., and Hill, I.N. 1967. Fluorine and dental caries. *J. Amer. Dent. Assoc.* 74:233-302.
7. Arnold, F.A.; Likins, R.C.; Russell, A.L.; and Scott, D.B. 1962. Fifteenth year of the Grand Rapids fluoridation study. *J. Amer. Dent. Assoc.* 65:780-85.
8. Ast, D.B.; Smith. D.J.; Wachs, B.; and Cantwell, K.T. 1956. Newburgh-Kingston caries-fluorine study XIV. Combined clinical and roentgenographical dental findings after ten years of fluoride experience. *J. Amer. Dent. Assoc.* 52:314-25.
9. Myers, H.M. 1978. Fluorides and dental fluorosis 7. In *Monographs in oral science.* New York: S. Karger.
10. U.S. Dept. Health, Education, and Welfare. 1977. *Fluoridation census, 1975.* Atlanta: Public Health Service.
11. American Dental Association. 1972. *Fluoridation reporter.* Vol. 10, No. 2.
12. Murray, J. 1969. Caries experience of 15-year-old children from fluoride and non-fluoride communities. *Brit. Dent. J.* 127:8-69, 128.
13. Ludwig, T. G. 1971. Hastings fluoridation project VI. Dental effects between 1954 and 1970. *N. Zealand Dent. J.* 67:155-60.
14. Konick, L. 1979. 1977 dental health survey of New Haven school children after ten years of fluoridation. *Connecticut Health Bulletin* 93(2):32-40.
15. Bushel, A., and Smith, D.J. 1955. Newburgh-Kingston caries fluoride study X. Dental findings for 17-year-old group after nine years of fluoride experience. *N.Y. J. Dent.* 25:215-18.
16. Backer-Dirks, O., Houwink, B.; and Kwant, G.W. 1961. The results of 6½ years of artificial fluoridation of drinking water in the Netherlands. The Tiel-Culemborg experiment. *Arch. Oral Biol.* 5:284-300.
17. Ast, D.B. 1973. Dental public health. In *Preventive medicine and public health,* ed. P. E. Sartwell, New York: Appleton-Century-Crofts.
18. Ast, D.B.; Alloway, N.; and Draker, H.L. 1962. The prevalence of malocclusion related to dental caries and lost first permanent molars in a fluoridated city and a fluoride-deficient city. *Amer. J. Orthodont.* 48:106-13.
19. Pelton, W.J., and Elsasser, W.A. 1953. Studies of dentofacial morphology III. The role of dental caries in the etiology of malocclusion. *J. Amer. Dent. Assoc.* 46:648-57.
20. Englander, H.R., and Wallace, D.A. 1962. Aurora-Rockford, Illinois Study III. Effects of naturally fluoridated water on dental caries in adults. *Pub. Health Rep.* 77:887-93.
21. Russell, A.L., and Elvove, E. 1951. Domestic

water and dental caries VII. A study of the fluoride-dental caries relationship in an adult population. *Pub. Health Rep.* 66:1389-1401.

22. Murray, J.J. 1971. Adult dental health in fluoride and non-fluoride areas. I. Mean DMF values by age. *Brit. Dent. J.* 131:391-95.
23. Murray, J.J. 1971. Adult dental health in fluoride and non-fluoride areas. II. Caries experience in each tooth type. *Brit. Dent. J.* 131:437-42.
24. Murray, J.J. 1971. Adult dental health in fluoride and non-fluoride areas. III. Tooth mortality by age. *Brit. Dent. J.* 131:487-92.
25. Leone, N.C.; Stevenson, C.A.; Besse, B., Hawes, L.E.; and Dawber, T.C. 1960. The effects of the absorption of fluoride. II. A radiological investigation of 546 human residents of an area in which the drinking water contained only a minimum trace of fluoride. *A.M.A. Arch. Industr. Health* 21:326-27.
26. Bernstein, D.S.; Sadowsky, N.; Hegsted, D.M.; Guri, C.D.; and Stare, F.S. 1966. Prevalence of osteoporosis in high- and low-fluoride areas of North Dakota. *J.A.M.A.* 198:499-504.
27. Geever, F.F.; Leone, N.C.; Geiser, P.; and Liebermann, J. 1958. Pathological studies in man after prolonged ingestion of fluoride in drinking water. II. Findings in bones in communities with water levels from 1.0 to 4.0 ppm fluoride. *Pub. Health Rep.* 73:721-31.
28. Zipkin, I.; McClure, F.J.; Leone, N.C.; and Lee, W.A. 1958. Fluoride deposition in human bones after prolonged ingestion of fluoride in drinking water. *Pub. Health Rep.* 73:8:732-40.
29. Groot, E.R. 1977. Water fluoridation-dental caries-osteoporosis. Old and new views on the fluoridation of drinking water. *Nut. Metal.* 21 (Suppl. 1):208-11.
30. Way, R.M. 1964. The effect on dental caries of a change from a naturally fluoridated to a fluoride-free communal water. *J. Dent. Child.* 31(2):151-57.
31. Lemke, C.W.; Doherty, J.M.; and Arra, M.C. 1970. Controlled fluoridation: the dental effects of discontinuation in Antigo, Wisconsin. *J. Amer. Dent. Assoc.* 80:782-86.
32. Black, G.V.; and McKay, F.S. 1916. Mottled teeth: an endemic developmental imperfection of the teeth heretofore unknown in the literature of dentistry. *Dent. Cosmos* 58:129-56.
33. Churchill, H.V. 1931. The occurrence of fluorides in some waters of the United States. *J. Amer. Water Works Assoc.* 23:1399-1407.
34. Dean, H.T. 1934. Classification of mottled enamel diagnosis. *J. Amer. Dent. Assoc.* 20:319-33.
35. Dean, H.T. 1942. Geographic distribution of endemic dental fluorosis (mottled enamel). In *Fluoride and dental health*, ed. F.R. Moulton. Washington, D.C.: Amer. Assoc. Adv. Sci., Pub. No. 19.
36. Schlesinger, E.R.; Overton, D.E.; Chase, H.C.; and Cantwell, K.T. 1956. The Newburgh-Kingston caries fluoride study XIII. Pediatric findings after ten years. *J. Amer. Dent. Assoc.* 52:296-306.
37. Leone, N.C.; Stevenson, C.A.; Hilbush, T.F.; and Sosman, M.C. 1955. A roentgenologic study of a human population exposed to high fluoride domestic water. A ten year study. *Amer. J. Roentgenol.* 74:874-85.
38. Leone, N.C.; Shimkin, M.B.; Arnold, F.A., Jr.; Stevenson, C.A.; Zimmerman, E.R.; Geiser, P.B.; and Liebermann, J.E. 1954. Medical aspects of excessive fluoride in a water supply. *Pub. Health Rep.* 69:925-36.
39. Hagan, T. 1957. *Effects of fluoridation on general health as reflected in mortality data.* Amer. Assoc. Adv. Sci. Symposium, Indianapolis.
40. Gabovich, R.D., and Ovrutskiy, G.D. 1977. *Fluorine in stomatology and hygiene.* DHEW Pub. No. (NIH)78-785, U.S. Dept. of Health, Education, and Welfare, Public Health Service, Bethesda, Md.
41. Hagan, T.L.; Pasternack, M.; and Scholz, G.C. 1954. Water-borne fluorides and mortality. *Pub. Health Rep.* 69:450-54.
42. Yiamouyiannis, J.A. 1975. Fluoride and cancer. *Nat. Health Fed. Bul.* 21:9.
43. Burk, D., and Yiamouyiannis, J. 1975. *Congressional Record.* 191, H7171-7176, July 21st.
44. Hoover, R.W.; McKay, F.W.; and Fraumeni, J. F., Jr. 1970. Fluoridated drinking water and the occurence of cancer. *J. Natl. Cancer Inst.* 57:757-68.
45. Doll, R., and Kinlen, L. 1977. Fluoridation of water and cancer mortality in the U.S.A. *Lancet* 1:1300-2.
46. Rogot, E.; Sharrett, A.R.; Feinleib, M.; and Fabsitz, R.R. 1978. Trends in urban mortality in relation to fluoridation status. *Amer. J. Epidemiol.* 107:104-12.
47. Fluoridation—the cancer scare, part 1. *Consumer Reports,* July 1978:392-96.
48. Six ways to mislead the public—the attack on fluoridation, part 2. *Consumer Reports,* August 1978:480-82.
49. Fluoride, teeth, and health. *Report of Royal College of Physicians.* London: Pitmans, 1976.
50. Anderson, R.; Beard, J.H.; and Sorley, D. 1980. Fluoride intoxication in a dialysis unit. *Maryland Morbidity and Mortality Weekly Report* 29(12):134-36.

51. Crain, R.L., and Rosenthal, D.B. 1963. *The fluoridation decision. Report #2: the community confronts an innovation,* pp. 17-30. Philadelphia: National Analysts, Inc.
52. Knutson, J.W. 1970. Water fluoridation after 25 years. *J. Amer. Dent. Assoc.* 80:765-69.
53. Evans, C.A., and Pickles, T. 1978. Statewide antifluoridation initiatives: a new challenge to health workers. *Amer. J. Pub. Health* 68:59-62.
54. Petterson, E.O. 1972. Abolition of the right of local Swedish authorities to fluoridate drinking water. *J. Pub. Health Dent.* 32:243-47.
55. Kirscht, J.P., and Knutson, A.L. 1961. Science and fluoridation: an attitude study. *J. Soc. Issues* 17:37-46.
56. Simmel, A. 1961. A signpost for research on fluoridation; the concept of relative deprivation. *J. Soc. Issues* 17:26-36.
57. *Fluoridation of public water supplies in New York State.* Albany: New York State Department of Health, August 1968.
58. Carlos, J.P. 1975. Delivery of preventive methods to the public. In *Prevention and oral health,* pp. 61-68. Fogarty International Center Series on Preventive Medicine, Vol. 1. Washington, D.C.: U.S. Gov't. Printing Office, DHEW Pub. No. (NIH) 74-707.
59. Horowitz, H.S. 1980. The assessment of cost-effectiveness of caries preventive agents and procedures. In *Final technical report: dental caries studies of the commission on oral health.* Fédération Dentaire Internationale, Research and epidemiology (CORE).
60. U.S. Dept. of Health, Education, and Welfare. *Grants for preventive health services; grants for fluoridation.* 55378 Federal Register, Vol. 44, No. 88, Wednesday, September 26, 1979, Rules and Regulations.
61. Horowitz, H.S.; Law, F.E.; and Pritzker, T. 1965. Effect of school water fluoridation on dental caries, St. Thomas, V.I. *Pub. Health Rep.* 80:381-88.
62. Horowitz, H.S.; Heifetz, S.B.; and Law, F.E. 1965. School fluoridation studies in Elk Lake, Pennsylvania and Pike County, Kentucky: interim report. *J. Amer. Dent. Assoc.* 71:1124-28.
63. Horowitz, H.S.; Heifetz, S.B.; Law, F.E.; and Driscoll, W.S. 1968. School fluoridation studies in Elk Lake, Pennsylvania and Pike County, Kentucky: results after eight years. *Amer. J. Pub. Health* 58:2240-50.
64. Horowitz, H.S.; Heifetz, S.B.; and Law, F.E. 1972. Effect of school water fluoridation on dental caries: final results in Elk Lake, Pennsylvania after 12 years. *J. Amer. Dent. Assoc.* 84:832-38.
65. Heifetz, S.B.; Horowitz, H.S.; and Driscoll, W.S. 1978. Effect of school water fluoridation on dental caries: results in Seagrove, North Carolina after eight years. *J. Amer. Dent. Assoc.* 97:193-96.
66. Clarke, R.; Welch, J.; Leiby, G.; Cobb, W.Y.; and MacCormack, J.N. 1974. Acute fluoride poisoning. *North Carolina Morbidity and Mortality Weekly Report,* June 1:199.

Chapter 5

Dietary Fluoride Supplementation

Approximately one-half of the American population is consuming drinking water containing natural or supplemented therapeutic levels of fluoride. For those children lacking fluoride in their drinking water or in which their schools do not contain individual fluoridation systems (see Chapter 4), alternative methods of providing *systemic* fluoride supplementation must be found.

The most common method of systemic, or dietary, supplementation is through the prescription of fluoride-containing vitamins, fluoride drops, tablets, or oral rinse supplements. Such regimens may be recommended, usually by a dentist or physician, to individual patients, or may be part of a school- or home-based public health preventive dentistry program. Adherence to a conscientious schedule of systemic supplementation will produce caries reductions in the primary and permanent dentitions similar to those derived from drinking optimally fluoridated water.[1] Since the regimen must be continued for many years, in some countries fluoride has been added to milk or table salt in order of offset the possible waning interest of individuals in continuing the program.

Systemic effects of fluoride supplements

Absorption, retention, and excretion

When an individual consumes a fluoride tablet, fluoride-vitamin drops, or other fluoride preparations, the ingested fluoride is absorbed through the stomach and small intestine into the bloodstream. Fluoride is absorbed as the ion (F^-), and, provided it is ingested in solution or easily soluble form, absorption will be rapid and relatively complete. Within an hour after ingestion, over 75% of the fluoride is absorbed and maximum blood levels are reached.[2-4]

Once in body fluids, the pattern of fluoride distribution is relatively simple. It will either be excreted, principally by the kidneys, or it will be deposited in the calcified portions of the body. Peak urinary fluoride concentrations are reached within two hours after ingestion of a single dose of sodium fluoride.[5] Since fluoride is not retained in significant amounts by the soft tissues, the bones and teeth represent the principal sites of fluoride retention. In a young child, about one-half of ingested fluoride deposits in calcifying tissues, while the other half is excreted. In the adult under continuous exposure, such as a resident of an optimally fluoridated community, the skeleton will ultimately reach a steady state in which a small amount of ingested fluoride will be utilized in the osteo-

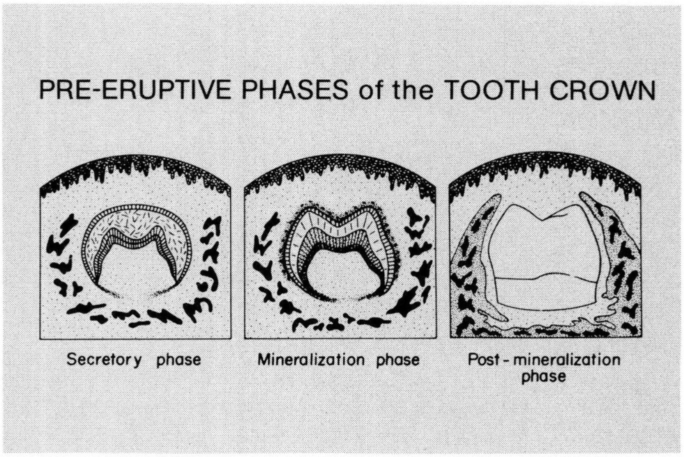

Fig. 5-1 The three phases of a developing tooth. At each phase, fluoride can deposit into the enamel. During the secretory phase, fluoride is bound to the enamel protein. Much of this is eventually lost as the protein concentration decreases. During the mineralization and postmineralization phases, fluoride is incorporated into and on the hydroxyapatite crystals.

clastic-osteoblastic reworking of the skeleton, while most will be excreted in the urine.[6]

The skeleton is the principal site of fluoride retention. Newbrun[7] has indicated that the body of an adult contains about 2.6 gm of fluoride, 95% of which is in the skeleton. Thus, while only a small amount of fluoride is retained in the teeth, it nevertheless has a profound effect on the teeth's susceptibility to decay.

Pre-eruptive deposition of fluoride into teeth

The absorbed fluoride will be transported through the body via the circulatory system and will be present in the extracellular fluid that bathes the teeth. It is important to remember that teeth do not erupt immediately after the completion of mineralization of the tooth crown; instead they remain in the jaws until approximately two-thirds of their roots are formed. The preeruptive period of crown formation may actually be divided into three phases: a phase of organic matrix deposition (also called the secretory phase); a phase of rapid mineralization (the postsecretory or maturation phase); and a postmineralization phase where crown formation is complete and the root or roots are developing (Fig. 5-1).

It is interesting that the highest concentrations of fluoride in developing enamel have been found during the first stage of organic matrix deposition.[8-10] This fluoride appears to be bound to the enamel protein and, as maturation progresses, there is a decrease in both the amount of protein and the concentration of fluoride in the developing tooth. The clinical significance of the initial accumulation and subsequent reduction of fluoride during this phase of tooth development is not currently understood. However, *Spiers*[11] has demonstrated in tooth germs of the domestic pig that the lost fluoride may concentrate in the follicle surrounding the developing tooth and, he believes, some may actually be recycled into the crown as development continues.

During the phase of mineralization, fluoride becomes incorporated into the precipitating apatite crystals of the teeth (see Chapter 2). Even after mineralization is complete, fluoride continues to be deposited from the tissue fluids into the outer layer of enamel.[9,12,13] It is important, therefore, that fluoride supple-

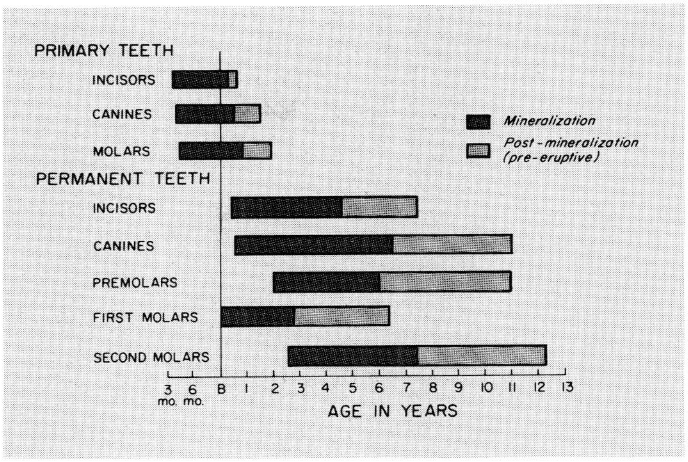

Fig. 5-2 Preeruptive chronology of the mineralization and postmineralization phases of the primary and permanent teeth.

ments be continued until all the permanent teeth, exclusive of third molars, have erupted.*

Figure 5-2 presents an approximate chronology of the two preeruptive periods of *mineralization* and *postmineralization* for the primary and permanent dentitions. Notice that for the permanent teeth, the postmineralization period is frequently as long as the period of mineralization. By age 8, all of the permanent teeth will usually have completed mineralization of the crown; however, intraoral eruption is not completed for all teeth until ages 12 or 13. *Therefore, systemic fluoride supplements should be continued until age 13, or until all of the teeth have erupted.* As seen in Figure 5-2, continual supplementation from birth will also provide preeruptive fluoride contact to the primary teeth, which have begun mineralization before birth, but which erupt between 6 months and 2 years of age.

*The discussion in this chapter excludes third molars, which are often congenitally absent, impacted, or require extraction because of insufficient arch length.

Topical effects of fluoride supplements

Clinical studies of systemic fluoride supplements have shown that teeth that had erupted *before* the studies began benefited from the fluoride regimen.[14-22] The anticariogenic effect of ingested fluoride on *erupted* teeth must be a local one involving the tooth surface, dental plaque, or both (see Chapter 2). Therefore, the fluoride must either contact the tooth surface before it is swallowed or pass through the circulation and be secreted in the saliva. Since stimulated duct saliva contains very low levels of fluoride (approximately 0.01 to 0.02 ppm F, which may be elevated to 0.05 ppm), it is unlikely that fluoride supplements have a significant local effect through this circuitous route. Rather, the topical effect most likely occurs before the fluoride is swallowed.

It is highly desirable, therefore, when prescribing a fluoride supplement, that the potential benefits of the regimen be maximized by recommending a preparation that can provide both a topical benefit to teeth that have erupted and a systemic benefit to teeth that are unerupted. For example, fluoride-vitamin drops are meant to be quickly

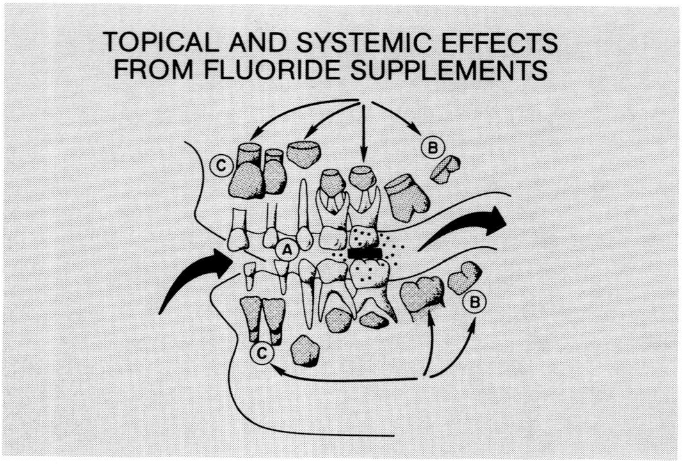

Fig. 5-3 Chewing and swishing a fluoride dietary supplement will provide topical contact to erupted teeth (a). Swallowing will allow fluoride contact to teeth in the mineralization (b) and postmineralization (c) preeruptive phases.

swallowed and will presumably provide only a systemic benefit; however, fluoride tablets may be chewed, dissolved in the saliva, and swished before swallowing, thus providing both topical and systemic benefits to the patient. Fluoride rinse supplements, which may be swished and then swallowed, will do the same. The topical and systemic relationships of fluoride supplements to the teeth are diagramed in Figure 5-3.

Considerations in determining proper fluoride dosage

There has been considerable controversy concerning when fluoride supplements should begin and what should be the dosage.[23,24] The American Dental Association, the American Academy of Pediatrics, federal agencies, and individuals have proposed dosage schedules, all of which are not in agreement.[24-30] A suitable dosage schedule must be predicated upon several factors:

—concentration of fluoride in the drinking water
—total amount of bioavailable fluoride
—age of the child
—dosage forms commercially available

Concentration of fluoride in the drinking water

The level of fluoride in drinking water that is necessary to produce a reduction of dental caries has been established in numerous epidemiological studies. From these studies, it has been deduced that for children 3 years of age or older, a controlled daily consumption of 1 mg F will provide optimal benefits to the teeth. This can be obtained by drinking one liter of water containing a concentration of 1 ppm fluoride ion. Since the amount of water consumed by individuals varies with the temperature, the fluoride concentration in the drinking water that is considered optimal for a particular locality is predicated upon the average maximum daily temperature.[31] For dental purposes, the optimal level of fluoride in drinking water is normally listed as between 0.7 and 1.2 ppm (Table 5-1).

The Council on Dental Therapeutics of the American Dental Association recommends that fluoride supplements be prescribed when the concentration of natural fluoride in

Table 5-1 Recommended levels of fluoride in drinking water relative to climate

Annual average of maximum daily air temperature		Recommended level of fluoride (ppm)	
°F	°C	Optimum	Range
79.3–90.5	26.3–32.5	0.7	0.6–0.8
70.7–79.2	21.5–26.2	0.8	0.7–1.0
63.9–70.6	17.8–21.4	0.9	0.7–1.2
58.4–63.8	14.7–17.7	1.0	0.8–1.3
53.8–58.3	12.2–14.6	1.1	0.8–1.5
50.0–53.7	10.0–12.1	1.2	0.9–1.7

Source: U.S. Public Health Service.
Reference: U.S. Public Health Service. Public Health Service Drinking Water Standards 1962. Washington, Government Printing Office, 1962 (P.H.S. Pub. No. 956)

the drinking water is "no higher than 60 percent of the optimal level recommended for community water fluoridation in a geographical area."[25] *Thus, dietary fluoride supplements are indicated where waterborne natural fluoride levels are 0.7 ppm or less,* depending on the geographic area.

Total amount of bioavailable fluoride

Excessive levels of fluoride during the period of tooth development can cause enamel *fluorosis,* or mottling of the teeth.[31,32] Therefore, one must recommend a fluoride supplement at a level that will produce optimum dental benefits without causing undesirable fluorosis. The potential for ingestion of excessive levels of fluoride exists because it is available not only from fluoride supplements and from the drinking water, but also from foods and beverages.[33] In small children, fluoride may also be consumed by swallowing a fluoride-containing dentifrice after brushing[34-36] (see Chapter 8).

To prescribe the proper amount of fluoride, it is necessary to know what constitutes the optimal safe dosage of fluoride and what is the total amount of bioavailable dietary fluoride. While there is no definite consensus, the optimal dosage for infants and young children, in whom teeth are developing and therefore are sensitive to excessive levels of fluoride, has been set at 0.05 to 0.07 mg F/kg body weight.[31] However, the determination of the total dietary fluoride, especially in infants (birth to 6 months) has proven to be difficult.

The amount of fluoride in cow's milk or in human milk, even when the fluoride in the drinking water is 1 ppm, is only 0.1 ppm or less.[37,38] *Schwab* and *Schwartz*[39] found that 68% of 50 children, 2 years and under, residing in communities where the fluoride content of the water averaged 1 ppm, were receiving less than 0.5 mg F/day* from liquid ingestion. All of the breast-fed children and two-thirds of the children whose principal milk source was cow's milk were included in this group. Thus, it is generally accepted that there is little danger of fluorosis if a fluoride supplement is administered to infants being breast-fed or bottle-fed with whole milk.

However, infant feeding patterns quickly

*The daily dosage then recommended by the American Academy of Pediatrics.

Table 5-2 Fluoride content of milk-based commercial baby formula

Brand	F content (ppm) Reported by Adair and Wei[41]	Reported by Tinanoff and Mueller[42]
Similac (ready-to-feed)	0.12	0.86
Similac (concentrate)	0.68	0.13
Similac Powder and deionized water	0.29	
Enfamil (ready-to-feed)	0.70	0.20
Enfamil (concentrate)	$<$0.10	$<$0.10
Enfamil Powder and deionized water	0.27	
SMA (ready-to-feed)	0.27	0.18
SMA (concentrate)	0.33	0.17
SMA Powder and deionized water	0.10	

change.[40] While during the first month of life 20% of infants in the United States are breast-fed and 2% are fed cow's milk, by 6 months only 5% are breast-fed while the percentage drinking cow's milk increases. At infancy, 64% of infants are fed commercially prepared milk-based formulas, but by 6 months less than one-third of all children are fed commercial preparations. The consistency of the diet also changes to one that gradually includes more solids. Usually these are commercially prepared baby foods.

In the late 1970s, several investigators showed that commercial milk-based formulas (whether prepared, concentrates, or powders) and commercial baby foods processed in areas where fluoridation existed had relatively high levels of fluoride[41-43] (Tables 5-2 and 5-3). In addition, the reconstitution of powdered milk or milk concentrates with fluoridated water at home was found to further increase the level of fluoride being consumed by the infant.[41]

The level of fluoride in processed baby foods was also found to vary depending upon whether the processing plant was located in a fluoridated or nonfluoridated area,[42,43] or whether water from a fluoridated source was added at home.[41] Once alerted to the problem, baby food processors voluntarily began, in 1978 and 1979, to take corrective steps to reduce the fluoride concentrations in baby foods and formulas. Nevertheless, because of the levels of fluoride that had been analyzed in these products, a number of reports indicated that infants and young children might have been exposed to a total fluoride intake that could cause fluorosis and advised moderation when recommending fluoride supplements for very young children.[29,30,41,43-46]

The degree of fluorosis can vary. *Dean*[47] described five levels of fluorosis: questionable, very mild, mild, moderate, and severe. *Questionable fluorosis* appears as only a few white flecks or white spots on the teeth. This form of fluorosis is not unesthetic and, in fact, may be cosmetically pleasing. *Very mild* and *mild* forms involve the presence of opaque white areas covering less than 25 or 50% of the tooth surface respectively, while *moderate* to *severe fluorosis* is associated with brown stains and finally with pitting.

Driscoll and *Horowitz*[24] reviewed the question of the amount of fluoride to prescribe for infants and young children. They noted that the dosage schedule recommended by the American Dental Association had not

Table 5-3 Fluoride content of processed infant foods*

Semisolid foods	Mean of food group (ppm)	Range (ppm)
Strained Meats	0.99	0.14-10.64
Vegetables	0.24	0.02- 0.67
Fruits	0.05	0.01- 0.23
Dry cereals	**Processed using non-F water**	**Processed using F water**
Mixed cereal	0.93	3.85
Oatmeal	0.98	4.87
Rice	2.11	6.35
Barley	1.99	4.30
Juices	**Processed using non-F water**	**Processed using F water**
Orange	0.029	0.15
Mixed fruit	0.014	0.38
Apple-cherry	0.14	1.48

*Reported by *Singer* and *Ophaug*.[43]

been shown to produce any objectionable fluorosis. Only one study that evaluated the effect of dietary fluoride supplements reported a high level of enamel fluorosis. In this study, by *Aasenden* and *Peebles*,[48] 67% of the participants, who had consumed fluoride supplements from birth, had very mild, mild, or moderate levels of fluorosis. The dosage from birth to age 2 used in this study was 0.5 mg. of fluoride per day. This was the amount recommended by the American Academy of Pediatrics at the time of the study and is twice that recommended by the American Dental Association. The Committee on Nutrition of the American Academy of Pediatrics has since revised their dosage recommendation downward, to conform to that of the American Dental Association.[26] In addition, as indicated above, once the major baby food processors were aware of the problem of unmonitored levels of fluoride in their products, steps were taken to limit the fluoride content of baby formulas to less than 0.1 mg per liter of formula. It was the assumption of the Committee on Nutrition of the American Academy of Pediatrics that "by the time of publication [of their report in January, 1979] no commercial formula will be manufactured with fluoridated water." As of November, 1978, Mead Johnson is using deionized water in the processing of their infant formula.

Since objectionable fluorosis has not been reported in infants receiving supplements at 0.25 mg per day, and because the baby food industry has taken steps to control the concentration of fluoride in processed baby formulas, the dosage presented later in this

Table 5-4 Fluoride content of dietary fluoride supplements

Product	Fluoride dosage
Fluoride drops	
Luride Drops (Hoyt)	0.125 mg/drop
Pacemaker Nafeen Solution (Pacemaker)	0.125 mg/drop
Karidium Liquid (Lorvic)	0.125 mg/drop
Fluoritab Liquid (Fluoritab)	0.25 mg/drop
Flura-Drops (Kirkman)	0.25 mg/drop
Pediaflor Drops (Ross)	0.5 mg/drop
Fluoride drops with vitamins	
Poly-Vi-Flor 0.25 mg (Mead Johnson)	0.25 mg/1.0 ml
Tri-Vi-Flor 0.25 mg (Mead Johnson)	0.25 mg/1.0 ml
Vi-Daylin/F ADC Drops (Ross)	0.25 mg/1.0 ml
Vi-Daylin/F ADC Plus Iron Drops (Ross)	0.25 mg/1.0 ml
Vi-Daylin/F Drops (Ross)	0.25 mg/1.0 ml
Vi-Daylin/F Plus Iron Drops (Ross)	0.25 mg/1.0 ml
Adeflor Drops (Upjohn)	0.5 mg/0.6 ml
Poly-Vi-Flor Drops (Mead Johnson)	0.5 mg/1.0 ml
Poly-Vi-Flor with Iron (Mead Johnson)	0.5 mg/1.0 ml
Tri-Vi-Flor (Mead Johnson)	0.5 mg/1.0 ml
Vi-Penta F Multivitamin Drops (Roche)	0.5 mg/0.6 ml
Vi-Penta F Infant Drops (Roche)	0.5 mg/0.6 ml
Fluoride tablets and lozenges	
Luride 0.25 Lozi Tabs (Hoyt)	0.25 mg/tablet
Luride 0.5 Lozi Tabs (Hoyt)	0.5 mg/tablet
Adeflor Chewable Tablets (Upjohn)	0.5 mg/tablet

chapter for infants residing in communities with negligible levels of fluoride in the drinking water is consistent with the recommendations of the American Dental Association and the American Academy of Pediatrics.

Age of child

Dosage recommendations for fluoride supplements are based, in part, upon the age of the child. Three age categories have generally been designated:

—below 2 years
—2 to 3 years
—3 years and older

These age ranges parallel changes in body weight during infancy and childhood.

Wei and his co-workers[29,30,41] have recommended that fluoride supplements not be given before 6 months of age because of the danger of fluorosis to the developing teeth. This question has already been discussed in the previous section. By starting fluoride supplementation from birth, as recommended by the American Dental Associa-

Table 5-4 (Continued)

Product	Fluoride dosage
Adeflor Chewable Tablets (Upjohn)	1.0 mg/tablet
Fluritab Tablets (Fluoritab)	1.0 mg/tablet
Luride Lozi Tabs (Hoyt)	1.0 mg/tablet
Luride-SF Lozi Tabs (Hoyt)	1.0 mg/tablet
Flura-Loz (Kirkman)	1.0 mg/tablet
Flura-Tablets (Kirkman)	1.0 mg/tablet
Karidium Tablets (Lorvic)	1.0 mg/tablet
Nufluor Chewable Tablets (Janar)	1.0 mg/tablet
Pacemaker Nafeen Tablets (Pacemaker)	1.0 mg/tablet
Fluoride tablets with vitamins	
Cari-Tab Softab Tablets (Stuart)	0.5 mg/tablet
Adeflor Chewable Tablets (Upjohn)	0.5 mg/tablet
Adeflor Chewable Tablets (Upjohn)	1.0 mg/tablet
Mulvidren-F Softab Tablets (Stuart)	1.0 mg/tablet
Poly-Vi-Flor Chewable Tablets (Mead Johnson)	1.0 mg/tablet
Poly-Vi-Flor With Iron Chewable Tablets (Mead Johnson)	1.0 mg/tablet
Tri-Vi-Flor Chewable Tablets (Mead Johnson)	1.0 mg/tablet
Vi-Daylin With Fluoride Chewable (Ross)	1.0 mg/tablet
Vi-Penta F Chewables (Roche)	1.0 mg/tablet
Rinse supplements	
Phos-Flur Oral Rinse/Supplement (Hoyt)	1.0 mg/5 ml

Sources: Physician's Desk Reference, 33rd ed., 1979; *Accepted Dental Therapeutics,* 37th ed., 1977; product literature.

tion, or at 2 weeks after birth, which is the American Academy of Pediatrics' recommendation, fluoride will contact the primary teeth while they are still mineralizing (Figure 5-2). Both agencies concur that by starting fluoride supplementation early, greater protection will be imparted to the primary teeth.[25,26,49] It is not certain whether caries protection will be enhanced in the permanent dentition by starting fluoride supplementation at birth rather than 6 months later. Nevertheless, since first permanent molars, the most caries-susceptible teeth, usually begin mineralization in the neonatal period, it seems advisable to start fluoride supplementation as soon after birth as possible.

As already discussed, supplementation should continue until all permanent teeth have erupted. Excluding third molars, this is until approximately 13 years of age. The American Academy of Pediatrics recommends supplementation until age 16.[26] This schedule will include the stage of mineralization of third molars; however, development of these teeth can be quite variable and they are often congenitally missing.

Table 5-5 Daily dosage of fluoride according to age and fluoride content of water supply

	Age		
Fluoride in water (ppm)	Birth to 24 months	25 to 36 months	37 months to 13 years
0.3 or less	0.25 mg	0.5 mg	1.0 mg
Greater than 0.3 to 0.7	0.0 mg*	0.25 mg	0.5 mg

*Unless breast-fed; during the period of breast feeding, use 0.125 mg.

Dosage forms of fluoride supplements

Fluoride supplements are available as drops, tablets and lozenges, fluoride-vitamin preparations, and oral rinse supplements. All are prescription items. When prescribing oral rinses one must be aware that all fluoride rinses are not supplements; some are meant to be rinsed and *expectorated,* achieving a topical effect only. Table 5-4 lists the dosages in which the various forms of fluoride supplements are supplied.

It is recommended that a child consume no more than 1 mg of fluoride per day from fluoride supplements and from the drinking water. The American Dental Association's Council on Dental Therapeutics has recommended prescribing fluoride supplements on a sliding scale to accommodate the suboptimal level of fluoride that may be present in a water supply.[25] For instance, if there is 0.2 ppm F in the water, the dose prescribed should be 0.8 mg F per day; if there is 0.4 ppm F, the dose should be 0.6 mg F per day, etc. This approach is not practical. Because of the dosage forms in which fluoride supplements are available, they cannot be easily divided to meet this precise adjustment. In 1974, *Ripa*[28] recommended that the dosage should be divided less precisely in order to make prescribing fluoride supplements less complicated. According to *Ripa,* the appropriate marketed dosage forms may be given full strength or half-strength, depending upon the patient's age and level of fluoride in the drinking water. The American Academy of Pediatrics has subsequently adopted this approach.[26*]

Recommended dosage schedule

It is the recommendation of the authors that fluoride supplements be started at birth or as soon as possible thereafter, and that they continue until all permanent teeth, exclusive of third molars, have erupted. This will be to approximately 13 years of age.

Fluoride supplements should be prescribed in communities for which the level of fluoride in the drinking water is 0.7 ppm or less. For purposes of supplementation, communities with suboptimal levels of natural fluoride are divided into two categories: those having 0.3 ppm F or less and those having more than 0.3 ppm to 0.7 ppm. The latter communities will generally receive a daily fluoride supplement that is half that of the former communities relative to the patient's age. The dosage schedule is described below and reproduced in Table 5-5. It should be noted that the

*During the preparation of this book, the American Dental Association also adopted a full or half-strength fluoride dosage schedule.

dosage forms of fluoride drops or vitamins, tablets, and oral rinse supplements (Table 5-4) easily accommodate these recommendations.

Communities where the level of fluoride in the drinking water is 0.3 ppm or less

Birth to 24 months

The recommended dosage is 0.25 mg F per day. Because of the age of the child, fluoride must be prescribed in liquid form. Until recently, no fluoride-vitamin drops were available that contained less than 0.5 mg F per drop. Products are now available in which fluoride-vitamin drops or fluoride drops alone may be administered in 0.25 mg per drop.

25 to 36 months

The recommended dosage is 0.5 mg F per day. Because of the age of the child, a liquid vehicle is still recommended. Fluoride drops or fluoride-vitamin preparations may be used, which have droppers calibrated to release 0.5 mg per drop, or the liquid supplement recommended from birth to age 2 may be increased to two drops.

37 months to 13 years

The recommended dosage is 1 mg F per day. In order to provide both a *topical* benefit to the already erupted teeth and a *systemic* benefit to teeth that are unerupted, the dosage form should be changed to a tablet or lozenge that can be chewed or sucked and then swallowed, or to an oral rinse supplement that can be swished and then swallowed.*

*Note that all oral rinses are not meant to be swallowed. (Oral rinses will be discussed in Chapter 9.)

Communities where the level of fluoride in the drinking water is greater than 0.3 ppm to 0.7 ppm

Birth to 24 months

Fluoride supplementation is not recommended unless the child is breast-fed. During the period of breast feeding, the child may receive 0.125 mg F per day. The prescriber, however, must weigh the benefit of recommending a fluoride supplement against the risk of not being informed when the child is weaned.

25 to 36 months

The recommended dosage is 0.25 mg F per day. This can be achieved by using fluoride drops or fluoride-vitamin drops.

37 months to 13 years

The recommended dosage is 0.5 mg F per day. Half-strength fluoride tablets or fluoride-vitamin tablets are available, or a 1 mg scored tablet may be halved. Fluoride drops or fluoride-vitamin supplements with droppers releasing 0.5 mg per drop are also available. A dosage form that allows both a topical and systemic effect, however, is more desirable.

Sample prescriptions for dietary fluoride supplements are presented at the end of this chapter.

Prenatal supplements

Prior to 1966, fluoride was prescribed in prenatal supplements for potential caries prevention in teeth whose development began before birth. This assumed that fluoride would cross the placental barrier and that it would be acquired by the developing teeth sufficiently to provide caries protection.

Several studies have shown that fluoride can pass the placental barrier and be incorporated into the mineralizing bones and teeth of the fetus.[50-56] However, the importance of this transfer to caries resistance of the teeth is equivocal. Since only the primary teeth begin mineralization before birth (except, perhaps, for the cusp tips of first permanent molars in some individuals), the only cariostatic benefit of prenatal supplements can be to the primary dentition.

Arnold et al.,[57] *Blayney* and *Hill,*[58] and *Tank* and *Storvick*[59] all concluded that prenatal exposure to waterborne fluoride could benefit the primary teeth. Conversely, *Carlos* et al.,[60] *Horowitz* and *Heifetz,*[61] *Katz* and *Muhler,*[62] and *Lemke* and co-workers[63] reported that prenatal fluoride had no effect on the caries incidence of primary teeth. *Glen,* in a private dental practice, followed children whose mothers had taken prenatal fluoride supplements.[64,65] She felt that the exposure to prenatal supplements provided a high degree of caries immunity to the teeth. However, she included in her analysis many patients with a mixed or full permanent dentition. Since the permanent teeth are generally not developing prenatally, her conclusions may be questioned. Four clinical trials comparing the effects of pre- and postnatal supplements all reported greater benefits to children exposed to the prenatal supplements.[66-69] *Driscoll,*[1] in a comprehensive review, discussed these studies and concluded that they were not sufficiently conclusive to recommend the use of prenatal supplements.

The United States Food and Drug Administration also concluded that sufficient evidence did not exist to support claims of efficacy of prenatal fluoride supplements, although their safety was not in question. In 1966, the Food and Drug Administration banned advertising claiming that prenatal fluoride supplements provided a dental benefit, but it did not ban their sale by prescription.[70]

Effect of fluoride supplements on the primary teeth

In one of the first studies testing the efficacy of systemic fluoride supplements on caries in the primary dentition, Arnold and co-workers[71] reported that the reduction obtained when supplementation was begun at birth was comparable to that achieved with community water fluoridation. Since then, additional studies have evaluated the effect to the primary teeth of systemic fluoride supplements.[14-16,48,66-69,72-83] As seen in Table 5-6, most of these studies were positive. Some, such as the report by *Margolis* and co-workers,[72] compared the efficacy of systemic supplements from birth to that achieved by consuming optimally fluoridated water and found similar reductions in dental caries. This substantiated *Arnold* and co-workers' original finding and emphasized that the benefits of systemic fluoride therapy were similar, whether the fluoride was consumed as a single daily dose or in small, frequent amounts received through water intake.

The caries reductions listed in Table 5-6 range from no effect to reductions as high as 70 to 80%. Wide ranges of effectiveness are not unusual when comparing clinical trials of cariostatic agents, and can result from differences in the baseline characteristics of the participating children, their initial caries susceptibility, different examiners' criteria of caries, and other factors. Nevertheless, the fact that the majority of studies listed in Table 5-6 are positive, with reductions of 30% or more reported, indicates the general level of efficacy that can be achieved with this technique.

In a series of reports by *Hennon* and co-workers[14,15,75] in which the initial age of the children using fluoride supplements ranged from birth to 5.5 years, the greatest caries reductions occurred in those children in whom supplementation was begun at birth. This finding is generally supported by reviewing the results presented in Table 5-6. The

Table 5-6 Caries preventive effects of neutral sodium fluoride supplements on the primary teeth

Study	Daily dosage (mg F)	Age supplementation began (years)	Duration (years)	Percent reduction DEFT	Percent reduction DEFS
Margolis et al.[72]	0.5-1.0+V*	B	5	70	
Margolis et al.[73]	0.5-1.0+V	B	6	76	
Prichard[68]	?	B	6	44	
			7	42	
			8	33	
Hamberg[74]	0.5+V	B	3	57	
			4	54	
			5	50	
			6	49	
Schutzmannsky[69]	0.25-1	B	9	14	
Aasenden and Peebles[48]	0.5-1.0±V**	B	7-12	78***	
Hoskova[66]	0.25-1.0	B-1	4	54	
Hennon et al.[14]	0.5-1.0+V	B-5.5	3	55	63
Hennon et al.[15]	0.5-1.0+V	B-5.5	4	60	68
Hennon et al.[75]	0.5-1.0+V	B-5.5	5.5	49	56
Kailis et al.[67]	?	"after birth"	4-6	56	
Fanning et al.[76]	?	< 1	3-4	58	
			4-5	34	
			5-6	33	
Hennon et al.[77]	0.5-1.0+V	< 1	7	16.7§	21.6
	0.5 + V	< 1	7	27.2§	42.4
Hennon et al.[16]	1.0 + V	1.5-3	1	58	57
			2	68	66
	1.0	1.5-3	1	55	55
			2	55	63
Ziemnowicz-Glowaka[78]	0.8	3	2		26
Stolte[79]	1.0†	3	3	11	
Pollak[80]	1.0 + V	3	2	80	
		4	2	20	
Kamocka et al.[81]	0.75	3	3	0	
		4	3	0	
Leonhardt[82]	1.0 + V	3	2	38	
		4	2	30	
Lutomska and *Koninska*[83]	0.6	3-4	2	"no significant effect"	

*V = vitamins. **An F-V supplement was given to age 3 to all participants, after which some children received F without V and others with V. ***Approximate percentage for primary cuspids and molars. §Level of F in water supply = 0.6-0.8 ppm. †Type of fluoride used not known. Foreign language citations from *Driscoll*.[1]

Table 5-7 Caries preventive effects of neutral sodium fluoride supplements on the permanent teeth

Study	Daily dosage (mg F)	Age supplementation began (years)	Duration (years)	Percent reduction DMFT	Percent reduction DMFS
Aasenden and *Peebles*[48]	0.5-1.0 ± V* **	B	7-12		80
Hamberg[74]	0.5 + V	B	7	70	
Schutzmannsky[69]	0.25-1.0	B	9	39	
Hennon et al.[14]	0.5-1.0 F + V	B-5.5	3	36	43
Hennon et al.[15]			4	41	46
Hennon et al.[75]			5.5	52	64
Minoguchi et al.[86]	0.25 + V	B-6	6	36	
Margolis et al.[73]	0.5-1.0+V	B	10	58	
		4	6	14	
Stolte[79]	1.0***	3	3	69	
Kamocka et al.[81]	0.75§	3	3	17	
	0.75§	4	3	60	
Ziemnowicz-Glowacka[78]	0.8§	3-6	2		33
	0.8§	3-5	3		28
Binder[87]	1.0§	6	4	35	
Hippchen[88]	1.0***	6	3	32	
Schutzmannsky[89]	0.75§	6	4		25
	0.75§	6	6		27
Leonhardt[82]	1.0	6	4	32	
	1.0	7	3	25	
Pollak[80]	1.0 + V	6-7	2	38	
Marthaler[18]	0.5-1.0§	6-7	1-8	36	
Niedenthal[90]	1.0§	6-7	3	22	
Wrzodek[91]	1.0§	6-9	3	21	
	1.0§	6-9	4	22	
Grissom et al.[92]	1.0§	6-11	2		34
Plasschaert and *Konig*[93]	1.0	7	2		32
Berner et al.[94]	1.0§	7-9	4	16	
	1.0§	7-9	6	20	
	1.0§	7-9	7	24	

*V = vitamins.

**An F-V supplement was given to age 3 to all participants, after which some children received F without V and others with V.

***Type of fluoride used not known.

§Supplements given on school days only.
Foreign language citations from *Driscoll*.[1]

reports are listed according to the age of the children when supplementation began. Greater effects to the primary dentition were found to accrue when fluoride supplements are started at birth. Conversely, supplementation beginning at age 3 or 4 is generally less effective or ineffective. This suggests that the mechanism whereby fluoride supplements prevent caries in the primary teeth is mainly through preeruptive or early posteruptive contact.

All of the crowns of the primary teeth are mineralizing at birth, and eruption of these teeth occurs between 6 months and approximately 2 years (see Fig. 5-2). Therefore, supplementation begun at birth will provide systemic contact to the primary teeth during both preeruptive stages of mineralization and postmineralization. Additionally, there will be daily topical fluoride contact as the teeth are erupting into the mouth; although the degree of contact will depend on the fluoride vehicle used.

As seen in Table 5-6, positive benefits from fluoride supplements were obtained when the fluoride was taken alone or combined with vitamins. *Hennon* and co-workers[16] compared the efficacy of fluoride-vitamin supplements to that of systemic fluoride without vitamins. Almost identical caries reductions were achieved, one and two years after supplementation, and the investigators concluded that caries inhibition was not altered when sodium fluoride and vitamins were used in a common vehicle. This conclusion is consistent with the findings that neither the retention nor metabolism of fluoride appears to be affected by the inclusion of vitamins.[84,85]

Most of the studies listed in Table 5-6, which provided supplements at birth, initially employed liquid drops and then switched to fluoride tablets when the children could chew. The daily dose from birth to age 2 or 3 was either 0.25 mg or 0.5 mg F, and 1 mg thereafter. The only indication of fluorosis of the primary teeth was the report of *Aasenden and Peebles*[48] in which four children exhibited fluorosis of the very mild type. Thus, there does not appear to be significant danger of fluorosis to the *primary dentition* from this regimen, even though 0.5 mg F per day is twice the dosage currently recommended for infants by the American Dental Association and the American Academy of Pediatrics.

Effect of fluoride supplements on the permanent teeth

Both neutral and acidulated sodium fluoride supplements have been studied for their effect on dental caries in the permanent dentition. The results of these studies (Tables 5-7 and 5-8) indicate that both are effective in reducing caries incidence in the permanent teeth.[14,15,18,19,21,48,69,73-75,78-82,86-98]

The caries reductions listed in Tables 5-7 and 5-8 vary over a wide range. As discussed in the previous section, variation in the results of clinical trials is not unusual. Nevertheless, when the studies are arranged according to the age of the children when supplementation began, as was done in Table 5-7, it can be seen that higher caries reductions in the permanent dentition occurred when supplementation was instituted before age 6. In fact, in two studies in which the supplements were started at birth, caries reductions of 70 and 80% were reported.[48,74]

The fact that early supplementation results in maximum caries reductions in the permanent dentition indicates that systemic contact during the developmental period of the teeth is important. The cariostatic mechanisms of systemic fluoride supplements, such as fluoride drops and tablets, have been discussed in Chapter 2. Preeruptive mechanisms include an increase in the level of fluoride in the developing enamel and an alteration of tooth morphology. In the study by *Aasenden*

Table 5-8 Caries preventive effects of acidulated sodium fluoride (APF) supplements on permanent teeth

Study	Daily* dosage (mg F)	Age supplementation began (years)	Duration (years)	Percent reduction DMFS
De Paola and *Lax* [95]	1.0	6-8	2.0	23
Driscoll et al.[19]	1.0	6-7	3.5	2
	2.0	6-7	3.5	27
Driscoll et al.[96]	1.0	6-7	5.5	20
	2.0	6-7	5.5	30
Driscoll et al.[21]	1.0	6-7	6.0	28
	2.0	6-7	6.0	29
Horowitz et al.[97]	1.0**	6-11	2.0	34***
Horowitz et al.[98]	1.0**	6-11	4.0	41***

*Supplements given on school days only.
**Preventive regimen also included weekly supervised rinsing with a 0.2% NaF mouth rinse and ad libitum use of a fluoride-containing dentifrice.
****Estimated* DMFS increment.

and *Peebles,*[48] in which fluoride supplements were provided from birth, in addition to evaluating the caries status of the subjects (see Table 5-7), the occlusal morphology and level of fluoride in the outer enamel of the permanent teeth were also studied. They reported atypically shallow pits and fissures, in which the occlusal fissure angle was wide and there was no explorer catch, in 47% of the children receiving fluoride supplements compared to similar findings in 4% of children who had no fluoride contact. Using enamel biopsy techniques, they found that the fluoride concentrations of the outer enamel of maxillary central incisors was approximately twice as high in the fluoride-supplemented children compared to the non-supplemented group. Interestingly, *van Houte* and co-workers[99] could find no marked difference in the frequency of isolation or proportions of *Streptococcus mutans* in plaques removed from fissures and smooth surfaces of teeth of 31 adolescents who participated in this study compared to nine adolescents who did not, suggesting that a local antimicrobial mechanism might not be involved.

A number of trials listed in Tables 5-7 and 5-8 were initiated when the children were 6 years of age or older. These programs were conducted in the children's schools and this, therefore, was the earliest age at which contact was possible. Fluoride supplementation begun at age 6 will provide preeruptive contact to many of the permanent teeth. However, the length of preeruptive contact will vary, being minimal for the first permanent molars and incisors. Additionally, some teeth will still be undergoing mineralization, while for others mineralization will be complete (see Fig. 5-2).

In these school-based studies, teeth that erupted during the course of the study[95] or late-erupting teeth[19,21,96] received the most benefit from supplementation. In the study by *De Paola* and *Lax*[95] (Table 5-8), an overall caries reduction of approximately 23% was achieved; however, the caries reduction of teeth that erupted during the course of the study was 53%. Similarly, *Driscoll* and coworkers[19,21,96] reported that twice as much protection was afforded to late-erupting teeth, which received both preeruptive and posteruptive fluoride exposure, compared to early-erupting teeth, which mainly received only posteruptive exposure. In contradistinction to *Aasenden* and *Peebles'* findings, enamel biopsies of maxillary incisors in the study of *Driscoll* and co-workers, evaluated 30 months after the program began, failed to show a higher level of fluoride in the outer enamel when compared to that of children taking placebo tablets.[100] This finding, however, should not be unexpected, since the incisors would have had little preeruptive contact with the fluoride supplements, although some posteruptive acquisition of fluoride might have been expected.

The school-based studies involving 6-year-old children or older were usually conducted following an academic time schedule. Thus, the average participant received approximately 150 tablets a year, or less than half of what might be expected if the regimen were faithfully practiced at home.[21] It is not known to what extent, if at all, this reduced frequency affected the efficacy of the method; however, it should not be overlooked when comparing the results of different studies.

Enamel fluorosis

No study known to the authors has reported *cosmetically disfiguring* enamel fluorosis of the permanent teeth from controlled dietary fluoride supplementation, even though some daily regimens were higher than those usually recommended. In the study by *Driscoll* and co-workers[19,21,96] (Table 5-8), one group of children, initially 6 to 7 years of age, received two sodium fluoride tablets each school day, one in the morning and one in the afternoon, releasing a total of 2 mg fluoride. Of 77 children evaluated after 55 months, 16 were diagnosed as having questionable fluorosis and one as having mild fluorosis.[96] Neither of these categories is cosmetically detracting. Additionally, the degree of dental fluorosis found in this group of children was not very different from that found in other children receiving either one sodium fluoride tablet a day or a nonfluoride placebo tablet. This study is significant in that it is the only one in which the dosage was twice the 1 mg F per day maximum recommended by the American Dental Association for children residing in a fluoride-deficient community.

Hennon and co-workers[77] placed children under one year of age on a daily regimen of vitamin supplements with 0.5 mg F until age 3 and then either 0.5 or 1.0 mg thereafter. The children resided in Indiana communities with 0.6 to 0.8 ppm F in the drinking water, which was considered suboptimal for these areas. Seven years after supplementation was begun, caries in the primary teeth was evaluated (Table 5-6), together with the fluorosis status of the erupted permanent teeth. Despite the relatively high level of fluoride consumption (from that which was waterborne together with that from the vitamin supplement), no clinically significant amount of fluorosis was noted in any of the groups of children under investigation, and no child demonstrated a degree of fluorosis that was considered to be moderate or severe.

The *Aasenden* and *Peebles*[48] study involved children residing in several fluoride-deficient communities in Massachusetts who received fluoride supplements from birth to ages 7 and 12. The dosage was 0.5 mg F per day from birth to age 3, and 1 mg F per day thereafter. The 0.5 mg F per day was consistent with the dosage recommended by the American Academy of Pediatrics at the time, but was twice that currently recommended by the American Academy of Pediatrics and

Table 5-9 Change in severity of enamel fluorosis in the permanent teeth of children on systemic fluoride supplements: evaluation made in the same children after a five year interval

Fluorosis level	First examination (Age: 7 to 12 Years)		Second examination (Age: 12 to 17 Years)*	
	Number	Percent	Number	Percent
Normal	8	23	15	43
Questionable	5	14	4	11
Very mild	13	37	13	37
Mild	6	17	1	3
Moderate	3	9	2	6
Severe	0	0	0	0
Total	35	100	35	100
Group fluorosis index**	0.74 ± 0.13		0.40 ± 0.10	

*Fluoride supplementation not continued by all children. **M ± S.E. Source: *Aasenden* and *Peebles*.[102]

the American Dental Association. A high incidence of enamel fluorosis was found. Sixteen percent of the children had clinically normal enamel, 51% exhibited questionable or very mild fluorosis, while the rest had mild or moderate fluorosis. No child, however, exhibited either brown discoloration or pitting. The higher incidence and severity of fluorosis of the permanent teeth, compared to that reported for the primary teeth in the same study, as discussed previously, is consistent with the general observation that primary teeth are less susceptible to fluorosis.[101]

Approximately one-third of the children were evaluated 5 years later.[102] The group index of fluorosis in the permanent teeth was less than that observed for the same children at the previous examination (Table 5-9). Individually, in only one child was the severity of fluorosis higher at the second examination, while in all other cases it remained the same or was less. The investigators felt that the degree of fluorosis had faded with time, possibly due to posteruptive mineralization or abrasion.

Recently, a case was described in which the son of a dentist received 1 mg of fluoride a day from shortly after birth until 6.5 years of age.[103] Even though this dosage was up to four times that currently recommended, the degree of enamel fluorosis of the permanent teeth, according to *Dean*'s criteria, was classified as mild (Fig. 5-4).

Safety of dietary fluoride supplements

Chronic toxicity

Chronic toxicity associated with fluoride supplements must be considered in relation to the total bioavailable fluoride consumed. It is possible that fluoride supplements at therapeutic levels of 1 mg F per day or less, coupled with ingested fluoride from foods, water, and beverages, can result in enamel

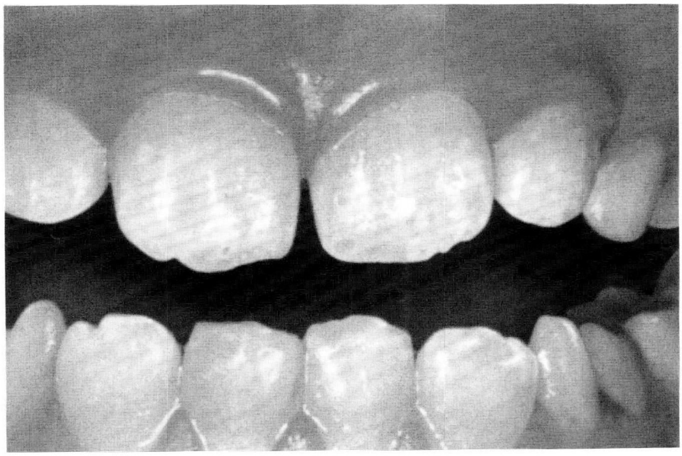

Fig. 5-4 Mild enamel fluorosis associated with excessive fluoride supplementation. The child resided in a suboptimally fluoridated community (F = 0.2 ppm). Until 4 months of age, he had consumed water that was prepared by adding a 2.2 mg NaF tablet to a liter of water. Thereafter, he was given one NaF tablet a day until 6.5 years, when his family moved to an optimally fluoridated community. Despite the excessive supplementation between 4 months and 3 years of age, the degree of fluorosis is not considered unesthetic.
(Compliments of Dr. B. A. *Burt*.)

fluorosis during the period of tooth development. The question of fluorosis associated with controlled studies of fluoride supplementation was addressed in previous sections. It was noted that even at twice the currently recommended levels for infants or older children, cosmetically detracting levels of fluorosis were never observed.[19,21,48,77,96] Therefore, fluorosis from controlled dietary supplementation does not appear to be a significant clinical problem.

In a Department of Health, Education, and Welfare newsletter, the United States Public Health Service cited the findings of a study conducted in 1978 by the Michigan Departments of Public Health and Agriculture.[104] The purpose of the study was to assess the degree of fluoride ingestion in Michigan residents and its effects. The report stated that evidence of an increase in background fluoride intake due to the general use of fluoride in commercial food processing was scanty. While it would seem reasonable to surmise that an increase had occurred, it was estimated that the increase was less than 0.5 mg per day. No evidence was found of any adverse health effects from this slight increase, and the possibility that such would occur was "remote."

Acute toxicity

Acute toxicity from fluoride supplements can occur if a large amount of fluoride is deliberately or accidentally consumed. The acute fatal dose for a 150-pound (70-kg) man is 5 to 10 grams of *sodium fluoride* or approximately 2.3 to 4.5 grams of *fluoride.*[105] On a weight basis (e.g., 70 to 140 mg NaF/kg body weight), the lethal dose for a 20-pound (9-kg) child is approximately 0.7 to 1.5 grams of sodium fluoride. Since the usual sodium fluoride tablet contains 2.2 mg NaF, a preschool child would have to ingest over 300 tablets to receive an acute fatal dose. The American Dental Association's Council on Dental Therapeutics recommends that no more than 264 mg of sodium fluoride be dispensed at one time, which is the equivalent of 120 tablets, each containing 2.2 mg sodium fluoride. This is well below the fatal dose, though it could be toxic if taken at one time. For individual patients, fluoride tablets are supplied in bottles of 100 or 120 tablets, in conformance with the American Dental Association's safety recommendation.

Usually death will occur within 2 to 4 hours after ingestion of a lethal dose of fluoride; however, it can occur in a matter of minutes.

Survival for 24 hours bodes a favorable prognosis.[105] While fluoride is a general protoplasmic poison, which inactivates proteolytic and glycolytic enzymes, the mechanism by which it causes death is not known. Fluoride will bind calcium, forming insoluble calcium fluoride, and the clinical picture of overdosage is partially due to hypocalcemia.[105,106]

The initial symptoms of acute poisoning are salty and soapy taste, salivation, nausea and vomiting, severe abdominal pain, and diarrhea, which may be bloody. This is followed by increasing excitability of skeletal muscles, painful spasms, weakness, and full-blown tetanic contractures. Death has been variously ascribed to respiratory paralysis, shock, and cardiovascular collapse.

The most practical immediate first aid measure for acute fluoride poisoning is the ingestion of soluble calcium in any form in order to bind the fluoride in the gastrointestinal tract. In the home, copious amounts of milk should be given. While milk does not reduce the amount of fluoride absorbed by the gastrointestinal tract, it does slow the rate of absorption. Vomiting should be immediately induced using an emetic such as ipecac. In case of a large overdose, the patient must be hospitalized and 10 ml of a 10% solution of intravenous calcium gluconate should be slowly administered and repeated at the first sign of muscular spasm. Gastric lavage should also be instituted using 1% calcium chloride. Shock should be treated in the usual manner.[106,107]

Implementation of dietary fluoride programs

Fluoride supplements are administered in school-based public health programs and in either public health or individual caries prevention programs conducted in the children's homes. Both school- and home-based programs have their own unique advantages and disadvantages.

School-based programs have the advantage of being conducted under relatively regimented, supervised conditions. Thus, it is usually assured that the participating children are regularly receiving their supplements. However, because the program must conform to a school calendar, children receive only about 150 tablets a year, compared to the maximum 365 that they could receive in a program conducted daily in the home.[21] Additionally, supplementation does not start until approximately age 6, so that no systemic benefit is provided to the primary teeth, and the systemic benefit to the permanent teeth is limited. Conversely, home programs not only have the advantage of being able to administer the fluoride for the entire calendar year, they also allow supplementation to begin at birth so that maximum protection can be afforded to both the primary and permanent teeth.

However, for either public health or individual home-based programs to be successful, they must be conducted conscientiously for up to 13 years. Few parents are so motivated. A home-based public health program in Australia, which distributed free sodium fluoride tablets, failed because only 12% of 26,800 eligible children participated.[108] In some communities in British Columbia, fluoride tablets were supplied at cost. Only 1 out of 13 children, 14 years of age or younger, participated.[109] In addition, up to 50% of the participants left the program in 2.5 years. It has been observed that many parents lack the motivation to ensure regular continuance of a fluoride supplementation program.[76,77,110] The potential benefit that can be derived from daily use of fluoride supplements is, therefore, seriously compromised because of a general lack of motivation by parents to overcome the personal inconvenience associated with carrying out the program.[110]

Fluoride as a food additive

Fluoride is found naturally in relatively high concentrations in certain foods such as fish and tea.[31] In some countries, it has been added in controlled amounts to table salt or milk in order to provide a cariostatic benefit.

Wespi first promoted the use of table salt as a vehicle for fluoride in the mid-1940s. Since then, controlled studies on the effect of fluoride-supplemented salt have been conducted in Switzerland, Columbia, Hungary, and Spain.[111] Initially, supplementation was at the level of 90 mg F/kg of salt.[112] However, more recently the concentrations used have ranged from 200 to 350 mg F/kg salt.[113,114] Reviewing the several studies in this area, *Marthaler* and his associates[111] concluded that the cariostatic effectiveness of fluoride-supplemented salt can equal that reported for water fluoridation, provided the concentration in the salt produces a urinary fluoride excretion level similar to that associated with optimally fluoridated water. This level is 0.8 to 1.0 mg F/l urine and can be achieved using salt supplemented at 250 mg F/kg.

Equipment for fluoridating milk is available through the Borrow Dental Milk Foundation of England. Using small milk fluoridation plants, fluoridated milk can be made available to individual schools. A caries reduction, less than that provided by water fluoridation, has been reported with the use of fluoridated milk.[115] Animal studies have shown that milk does not reduce the availability of fluoride, and human studies using calcium fluoride solutions have shown that most of the fluoride is absorbed by the gastrointestinal tract.[13,116] It is likely, therefore, that calcium binding does not significantly inhibit the absorption of fluoride from fluoridated milk.

The addition of controlled amounts of fluoride to foods is a convenient method for providing systemic fluoride supplements. However, there are inherent disadvantages associated with this approach. Dietary preferences can significantly influence the amount of fluoride ingested, and it is difficult to adjust the fluoride concentration when suboptimal levels of natural fluoride are present in water supplies.

Summary

The use of dietary fluoride supplements in the form of sodium fluoride drops or tablets, with or without vitamins, can result in a significant reduction in dental caries in both the primary and permanent dentitions.

While it is unclear whether prenatal fluoride supplements provide a significant cariostatic benefit, an analysis of the results of numerous clinical trials demonstrates that dietary fluoride supplements are most effective when therapy is begun early. For optimal results, it is recommended that supplementation begin at birth and continue to approximately 13 years of age when all teeth, exclusive of third molars, have erupted. Since both a systemic and topical effect is possible from the use of fluoride supplements, a vehicle should be used that will allow both mechanisms. Sodium fluoride tablets that can be chewed, mixed with the saliva, swished, and then swallowed provide such a vehicle and can be prescribed when the child is sufficiently mature to use tablets. Conversely, fluoride drops are quickly swallowed. While liquid drops must be used for infants and young children, they are not expected to provide a significant topical effect.

In order to prescribe an amount of daily fluoride that will produce an optimal reduction in dental caries, yet will not cause fluorosis, several factors must be considered: the concentration of natural fluoride in the drinking water, the total amount of bioavailable fluoride being ingested, the child's age, and the dosage forms of fluoride supplements commercially available. Based upon these considerations, a dosage schedule has been recommended in Table 5-5, which generally conforms to the recommendations of the American Academy of Pedodontics and the American Dental Association. While chronic toxicity, in the form of enamel fluorosis, should not constitute a serious problem when using dietary fluoride supplements, acute toxicity can result from an accidental or deliberate overdose. Because of the potential hazard from overdose, the American Dental Association recommends that no more than 264 mg sodium fluoride be prescribed at any one time. This is the equivalent of 120 2.2 mg NaF tablets, each releasing 1 mg F.

While dietary fluoride supplementation programs may be conducted in school or at home, each locale has inherent advantages and disadvantages. Because they are super-

Sample prescriptions for dietary fluoride supplements

Communities where the level of fluoride in the drinking water is 0.3 ppm or less

Birth to 24 months	℞ *Sodium fluoride drops 0.25 mg F/drop* *Dispense 19 ml* *Sig. One drop each day* Caution: Keep out of Reach of Children
25 to 36 months	℞ *Sodium fluoride drops 0.5 mg F/dropper full* *Dispense 50 ml* *Sig. One dropper full each day* Caution: Keep out of Reach of Children
37 months to 13 years	℞ *Sodium fluoride tablets 2.2 mg NaF* *Dispense 120 tablets* *Sig. Chew one tablet before bedtime. Swish for 60 seconds and swallow.* Caution: Keep out of Reach of Children

Communities where the level of fluoride in the drinking water is greater than 0.3 ppm to 0.7 ppm

Birth to 24 months (if breast-fed)

℞ Sodium fluoride drops
0.125 mg F/drop
Dispense 60 ml
Sig. One drop each day

Caution: Keep out of Reach of Children

25 to 36 months

℞ Sodium fluoride drops
0.25 mg F/drop
Dispense 19 ml
Sig. One drop each day

Caution: Keep out of Reach of Children

37 months to 13 years

℞ Sodium fluoride tablets
1.1 mg NaF
Dispense 120 tablets
Sig. Chew one tablet before bedtime. Swish for 60 seconds and swallow.

Caution: Keep out of Reach of Children

vised, participant compliance in the daily regimen is assured in school-based programs; however, such programs are generally run on an academic schedule and the actual number of fluoride contacts is about 150. Additionally, school-based programs start when children are 6 years of age, which limits the extent of preeruptive fluoride contact. Home-based programs can be conducted daily and can begin at birth; however, daily compliance for the 12 or 13 years of tooth development and eruption is an unrealistic expectation. Despite these disadvantages, dietary fluoride supplementation offers an alternate mode of systemic fluoride therapy for children residing in communities having suboptimal levels of natural fluoride in the drinking water.

References

1. Driscoll, W.S. 1974. The use of fluoride tablets for the prevention of dental caries. In *International workshop on fluorides and dental caries reductions,* eds. D.J. Forrester and E.M. Schulz, Jr., pp. 25-93. Baltimore: University of Maryland.
2. Carlson, C.H.; Armstrong, W.D.; and Singer, L. 1960. Distribution and excretion of radiofluoride in the human. *Proc. Soc. Exp. Biol. Med.* 104:235-9.
3. Wallace-Durbin, P. 1954. Metabolism of fluorine in the rat using F^{18} as a tracer. *J. Dent. Res.* 33:789-800.
4. Hodge, H.C. 1961. Metabolism of fluoride. *J.A.M.A.* 177:313-16.
5. Hennon, D.K.; Stookey, G.K.; and Muhler, J.C. 1969. Blood and urinary fluoride levels in humans associated with ingestion of sodium fluoride-containing vitamin tablets. *J. Dent. Res.* 48:1211-15.
6. Hodge, H.C., and Smith, F.A. 1965. Biological properties of inorganic fluorides. In *Fluorine chemistry.* Vol. 4, ed. J.H. Simons, p. 145. New York: Academic Press.
7. Newbrun, E. 1976. Fluoride metabolism and mechanisms of action. In *Fluorides: an update for dental practice,* ed. S.J. Moss, pp. 30-39. New York: Medcom, Inc.
8. Spiers, R.L. 1975. Fluoride incorporation into developing enamel of permanent teeth in the domestic pig. *Arch. Oral Biol.* 20:877-83.
9. Weatherell, J.A.; Deutsch, D.; Robinson, C.; and Hallsworth, A.S. 1977. Assimilation of fluoride throughout the life of the tooth. *Caries Res.* 11 (Suppl. 1): 85-115.
10. Crenshaw, M.A.; Wennberg, A.; and Bawden, J.W. 1978. Fluoride-binding by the organic matrix of developing bovine enamel. *Arch. Oral Biol.* 23:285-87.
11. Spiers, R.L. 1978. Fluoride concentration in tooth germs of permanent teeth of the domestic pig. *Arch. Oral Biol.* 23:1019-21.
12. Brudevold, F.; Steadman, L.T.; and Smith, F.A. 1960. Inorganic and organic components of tooth structure. *Ann. N.Y. Acad. Sci.* 85:110-32.
13. Spiers, R.L. 1978. Incorporation of a dietary fluoride supplement into bone and developing teeth of the domestic pig. *Arch. Oral Biol.* 23:1013-17.
14. Hennon, D.K.; Stookey, G.K.; and Muhler, J.C. 1966. The clinical anticariogenic effectiveness of supplementary fluoride-vitamin preparations. Results at the end of three years. *J. Dent. Child.* 33:3-12.
15. Hennon, D.K.; Stookey, G.K.; and Muhler, J.C. 1967. The clinical anticariogenic effectiveness of supplementary fluoride-vitamin preparations. Results at the end of four years. *J. Dent. Child.* 34:439-43.
16. Hennon, D.K.; Stookey, G.K.; and Muhler, J.C. 1972. Prophylaxis of dental caries: relative effectiveness of chewable fluoride preparations with and without added vitamins. *J. Pediatr.* 80:1018-21.
17. Bibby, B.G.; Wilkens, E.; and Witol, E. 1955. A preliminary study of the effects of fluoride lozenges and pills on dental caries. *Oral Surg.* 8:213-16.
18. Marthaler, T.M. 1969. Caries inhibiting effect of fluoride tablets. *Helv. Odont. Acta* 13:1-13.
19. Driscoll, W.S.; Heifetz, S.B.; and Korts, D.C. 1974. Effect of acidulated phosphate-fluoride chewable tablets on dental caries in school children: results after 30 months. *J. Amer. Dent. Assoc.* 89:115-20.
20. Aasenden, R.; DePaola, P.F.; and Brudevold, F. 1972. Effects of daily rinsing and ingestion of fluoride solutions upon dental caries and enamel fluoride. *Arch. Oral Biol.* 17:1705-14.
21. Driscoll, W.S.; Heifetz, S.B.; and Korts, D.C. 1978. Effect of chewable fluoride tablets on dental caries in school children: results after six years of use. *J. Amer. Dent. Assoc.* 97:820-24.
22. Stephen, K.W., and Campbell, D. 1978. Caries reduction and cost benefit after 3 years of sucking fluoride tablets daily at school. A double-blind trial. *Brit. Dent. J.* 144:202-6.
23. Concern about dietary fluoride supplementation. 1978. *J. Amer. Dent. Assoc.* 96:1158.
24. Driscoll, W.S., and Horowitz, H.S. 1978. A discussion of optimal dosage for dietary fluoride supplementation. Report of the Council on Dental Therapeutics. *J. Amer. Dent. Assoc.* 96:1050-53.
25. Prescribing fluoride supplements. 1977. In *Accepted dental therapeutics.* 37th ed. pp. 293-96. Chicago: American Dental Association.
26. American Academy of Pediatrics, Committee on Nutrition. Fluoride supplementation: revised dosage schedule. *Pediatrics* 63:150-52.
27. Newbrun, E. 1978. Dietary fluoride supplementation for the prevention of caries. *Pediatrics* 62:733-37.
28. Ripa, L.W. 1974. The role of the pediatrician in dental caries detection and prevention. *Pediatrics* 54:176-82.
29. Wei, S.H.Y.; Wefel, J.S.; and Parkins, F.M. 1977. Fluoride supplements for infants and preschool children. *J. Prev. Dent.* 4(3):28-32.
30. Fomon, S.J., and Wei, S.H.Y. 1976. Prevention of dental caries. In *Nutritional disorders in chil-*

dren. *Prevention, screening and followup,* ed. S.J. Fomon, pp. 82-95. Washington, D.C.: U.S. Government Printing Office, DHEW Pub. No. (HSA)76-5612.

31. Myers, H.M. 1978. Fluorides and dental fluorosis. *Monographs in oral science 7.* New York: S. Karger.
32. Fejerskov, O.; Thylstrup, A.; and Larson, M.J. 1977. Clinical and structural features and possible pathogenic mechanisms of dental fluorosis. *Scand. J. Dent. Res. 85:510-34.*
33. Kramer, L.; Osis, D.; Wiatrowski, E.; and Spencer, H. 1974. Dietary fluoride in different areas in the United States. *Am. J. Clin. Nutr.* 27:590-94.
34. Hargreaves, J.A.; Ingram, G.S.; and Wagg, B.J. 1970. Excretion studies on the ingestion of a monofluorophosphate toothpaste by children. *Caries Res.* 4:256-68.
35. Hargreaves, J.A.; Ingram, G.S.; and Wagg, B.J. 1972. A gravimetric study of the ingestion of toothpaste by children. *Caries Res.* 6:237-43.
36. Ericsson, Y., and Forsman, B. 1969. Fluoride retained from mouthrinses and dentifrices in preschool children. *Caries Res.* 3:290-99.
37. Ericsson, Y. 1969. Fluoride excretion in human saliva and milk. *Caries Res.* 3:159-66.
38. Backer-Dirks, O.; Jongeling-Eijundhoven, J.M.; Fliessebalje, T.O.; and Gedalia, I. 1969. Total and free ionic fluoride in human and cow's milk as determined by gas-liquid chromatography, and the fluoride electrode. *Caries Res.* 3:181-86.
39. Schwab, J.G., and Schwartz, A.D. 1975. Fluoridated water supplies; an inadequate source of fluoride for children. *J. Pediatr.* 86:735-36.
40. Fomon, S.J. 1975. What are infants fed in the United States? *Pediatrics* 56:350-54.
41. Adair, S.M., and Wei, S.H.Y. 1978. Supplemental fluoride recommendations for infants based on dietary fluoride intake. *Caries Res.* 12:76-82.
42. Tinanoff, N., and Mueller, B. 1978. Fluoride content in milk and formula of infants. *J. Dent. Child.* 45:53-55.
43. Singer, L., and Ophaug, R. 1979. Total fluoride intake of infants. *Pediatrics* 63:460-66.
44. Ericsson, Y., and Wei, S.H.Y. 1979. Fluoride supply and effects in infants and young children. *Pediatric Dent.* 1:44-54.
45. Farkas, C.S., and Farkas, E.J. 1974. Potential effect of food processing on the fluoride content of infant foods. *Sci. Total Environ.* 2:399-405.
46. Wiatrowski, B.S.; Kramer, L.; Osis, D.; and Spencer, H. 1975. Dietary fluoride intake of infants. *Pediatrics* 55:517-22.
47. Dean, H.T. 1934. Classification of mottled enamel diagnosis. *J. Amer. Dent. Assoc.* 21:1421-26.
48. Aasenden, R., and Peebles, T.C. 1974. Effects of fluoride supplementation from birth on human deciduous and permanent teeth. *Arch. Oral Biol.* 19:321-26.
49. Marthaler, T.M. 1967. The value in caries prevention of other methods of increasing fluoride ingestion, apart from fluoridated water. *Int. Dent. J.* 17:606-18.
50. Zipkin, I., and Babeaux, W.L. 1965. Maternal transfer of fluoride. *J. Oral Ther.* 1:652-65.
51. Babeaux, W.L., and Zipkin, I. 1966. Dental aspects of the prenatal administration of fluoride. *J. Oral Ther.* 3:124-35.
52. Gedalia, I.; Brzezinski, A.; Protuguese, N.; and Bercovici, B. 1964. The fluoride content of teeth and bones of human fetuses. *Arch. Oral Biol.* 9:331-40.
53. Gedalia, I.; Brzezinski, A.; Zukerman, H.; and Mayersdorf, A. 1964. Placental transfer of fluoride in human fetus at low and high F-intake. *J. Dent. Res.* 43:669-71.
54. Gedalia, I.; Zukerman, H.; and Leventhal, H. 1965. Fluoride content of teeth and bones of human fetuses: in areas with about 1 ppm of fluoride in drinking water. *J. Amer. Dent. Assoc.* 71:1121-23.
55. Gedalia, I. 1967. Fluoride tablets. *Int. Dent. J.* 17:18-30.
56. Gedalia, I.; Brzezinski, A.; Bercovici, B.; and Lazarov, E. 1961. Placental transfer of fluorine in the human fetus. *Proc. Soc. Exp. Biol. Med.* 106:147-49.
57. Arnold, F.A.; Dean, H.T.; Jay, P.; and Knutson, J.W. 1956. Effect of fluoridated public water supplies on dental caries prevalence — tenth year of Grand Rapids-Muskegan study. *Public Health Rep.* 71:652-57.
58. Blayney, J.R., and Hill, I.N. 1964. Evanston dental caries study. XXIV. Prenatal fluorides — value of water borne fluorides during pregnancy. *J. Amer. Dent. Assoc.* 69:291-94.
59. Tank, G., and Storvick, C.A. 1964. Caries experience of children one to six years old in two Oregon communities (Corvallis and Albany). I. Effect of fluoride on caries experience and eruption of teeth. *J. Amer. Dent. Assoc.* 69:749-57.
60. Carlos, J.P.; Gittelsohn, A.M.; and Haddon, W., Jr. 1962. Caries in deciduous teeth in relation to maternal ingestion of fluoride. *Public Health Rep.* 77:658-60.
61. Horowitz, H.S., and Heifetz, S.B. 1967. Effects of prenatal exposure to fluoridation on dental

caries. *Public Health Rep.* 82:297-304.

62. Katz, S., and Muhler, J.C. 1968. Prenatal and postnatal fluoride and dental caries experience in deciduous teeth. *J. Amer. Dent. Assoc.* 76:305-11.
63. Lemke, C.W.; Doherty, J.M.; and Arra, M.C. 1970. Controlled fluoridation. The dental effects of discontinuation in Antigo, Wisconsin. *J. Amer. Dent. Assoc.* 80:782-86.
64. Glenn, F.B. 1977. Immunity conveyed by a fluoride supplement during pregnancy. *J. Dent. Child.* 44:391-95.
65. Glenn, F.B. 1979. Immunity conveyed by sodium fluoride supplement during pregnancy: part II. *J. Dent. Child.* 46:17-24.
66. Hoskova, M. 1968. Fluoride tablets in the prevention of tooth decay. *Cesk. Pediatr.* 23:438-41.
67. Kailis, D.G.; Taylor, S.R.; Davis, G.B.; Bartlett, L.G.; Fitzgerald, D.J.; Grose, I.J.; and Newton, P.D. 1968. Fluoride and caries: observations on the effects of prenatal and postnatal fluoride on some Perth pre-school children. *Med. J. Aust.* 2:1037-40.
68. Prichard, J.L. 1969. The prenatal and postnatal effects of fluoride supplements on West Australian school children, aged 6, 7, and 8, Perth, 1967. *Aust. Dent. J.* 14:335-38.
69. Shutzmannsky, G. 1971. Fluoride tablet application in pregnant females. *Dtsch. Stomatol.* 21:122-29.
70. Food and Drug Administration. 1966. Statements of general policy or interpretation, oral prenatal drugs containing fluorides for human use. *Fed. Reg.* October 20.
71. Arnold, F.A.; McClure, F.J.; and White, C.L. 1960. Sodium fluoride tablets for children. *Dent. Progress* 1 (Oct.):8-12.
72. Margolis, F.J.; Macauley, J.; and Freshman, E. 1967. The effects of measured doses of fluoride. A five-year preliminary report. *Am. J. Dis. Child.* 113:670-72.
73. Margolis, F.J.; Reames, H.R.; Freshman, E.; Macauley, J.C.; and Mehaffey, H. 1975. Fluoride. Ten-year prospective study of deciduous and permanent dentition. *Am. J. Dis. Child.* 129:794-800.
74. Hamberg, L. 1971. Controlled trial of fluoride in vitamin drops for prevention of caries in children. *Lancet* 1 (Feb.):441-42.
75. Hennon, D.K.; Stookey, G.K.; and Muhler, J.C. 1970. The clinical anticariogenic effectiveness of supplementary fluoride-vitamin preparations. Results at the end of five and a half years. *Pharmacol. Ther. Dent.* 1:1-6.
76. Fanning, E.A.; Cellier, K.M.; Leadbeater, M.M.; and Somerville, C.M. 1975. South Australian kindergarten children: fluoride tablet supplements and dental caries. *Aust. Dent. J.* 20:7-9.
77. Hennon, D.K.; Stookey, G.K.; and Beiswanger, B.B. 1977. Fluoride-vitamin supplements: effects on dental caries and fluorosis when used in areas with suboptimum fluoride in the water supply. *J. Amer. Dent. Assoc.* 95:965-71.
78. Ziemnowicz-Glowacka, W. 1960. Prevention of caries by means of "Fluodar" tablets. *Czas. Stomatol.* 13:719-28.
79. Stolte, G. 1968. Results of three years of caries prophylaxis by oral fluoride application in Solingen kindergartens. *Zahnaerztl. Mitt.* 58:380-82.
80. Pollak, H. 1960. Caries prophylaxis with Mulgatum F. Results of an investigation over a period of two years in Nordheim-Westphalia. *Dtsch. Zahnaerztebl.* 14:363-65.
81. Kamocka, D.; Sebastyanska, Z.; and Spychalska, M. 1964. The effect of administration of "Fluodar" tablets on the appearance of caries in children of pre-school age in Szczecin. *Czas. Stomatol.* 17:299-303.
82. Leonhardt, H. 1964. Results of fluorine tablet applications in Salzburg school children. In *Advances in fluorine research and dental caries prevention.* Vol. 2, eds. J.L. Hardwick, J.P. Dustin, and H.R. Held, pp. 49-56. New York: MacMillan.
83. Lutomska, K., and Koninska, D. 1962. Effect of fluoride tablets. *Czas. Stomatol.* 15:493-501.
84. Margolis, F.J., and Nagler, R.C. 1967. Short-term fluoride excretion in young children. *Am. J. Dis. Child.* 113:673-76.
85. Stookey, G.K. 1970. The supply of fluorine to man. Ingestion from drugs. In *Fluorides and human health,* pp. 40-59. Geneva: World Health Organization.
86. Minoguchi, G.; Oni, T.; and Tamai, S. 1963. Prophylactic application of fluoride for dental caries in Japan. *Int. Dent. J.* 13:510-15.
87. Binder, K. 1967. Caries prevention with fluoride and its problems. *Mitt. Ost. Sanit.-Verwalt.* 68:144-46.
88. Hippchen, P. 1965. Caries prevention with fluorides in Dusseldorf children. *Zahnarztl. Mitt.* 55:897-98.
89. Schutzmannsky, G. 1965. Further results of our tablet fluoridation in Halle. *Dtsch. Stomatol.* 15:107-14.
90. Niedenthal, A. 1957. Caries prophylaxis with sodium fluoride tablets in Offenbach school children. *Zahnaerztl. Mitt.* 45:576-87.
91. Wrzodek, G. 1959. Does the prevention of caries by means of fluorine tablets promise suc-

cess? *Zahnaerztl. Mitt.* 47:1-5.

92. Grissom, D.K.; Dudenbostel, R.E.; Cassel, W.J.; and Murray, R.T. 1964. A comparative study of systemic sodium fluoride and topical stannous fluoride applications in preventive dentistry. *J. Dent. Child.* 31:314-22.

93. Plasschaert, A.J.M., and Konig, K.G. 1973. The effect of motivation and information and the effect of fluoride tablets on the incidence of dental caries in school children. *Ned. Tijdschr. Tandheelkd.* 80:21-35.

94. Berner, L.; Fernex, E.; and Held, A.J. 1967. Study of the anticarious effect of sodium fluoride tablets (Zymafluor). Results recorded in the course of 13 years of observation. *Schweiz. Mschr. Zahnheilk.* 77:528-39.

95. DePaola, P.F., and Lax, M. 1968. The caries-inhibiting effect of acidulated phosphate-fluoride chewable tablets: a two-year double-blind study. *J. Amer. Dent. Assoc.* 76:554-57.

96. Driscoll, W.S.; Heifetz, S.B.; Kortz, D.C.; Meyers, R.J.; and Horowitz, H.S. 1977. Effect of acidulated phosphate-fluoride chewable tablets in school children: results after 55 months. *J. Amer. Dent. Assoc.* 94:537-43.

97. Horowitz, H.S.; Heifetz, S.B.; Meyers, R.J.; Driscoll, W.S.; and Korts, D.C. 1977. Evaluation of a combination of self-administered fluoride procedures for control of dental caries in a non-fluoride area: findings after two years. *Caries Res.* 11:178-85.

98. Horowitz, H.S.; Heifetz, S.B.; Meyers, R.J.; Driscoll, W.S.; and Korts, D.C. 1979. Evaluation of a combination of self-administered fluoride procedures for the control of dental caries in a non-fluoride area: findings after four years. *J. Amer. Dent. Assoc.* 98:219-23.

99. van Houte, J.; Aasenden, R.; and Peebles, T.C. 1978. Oral colonization of *Streptococcus mutans* in human subjects with low caries experience given fluoride supplements from birth. *Arch. Oral Biol.* 23:361-66.

100. Shern, R.J.; Driscoll, W.S.; and Korts, D.C. 1977. Enamel biopsy results of children receiving fluoride tablets. *J. Amer. Dent. Assoc.* 95:310-14.

101. Thylstrup, A. 1978. Distribution of dental fluorosis in the primary dentition. *Community Dent. Oral Epidemiol.* 6:329-37.

102. Aasenden, R., and Peebles, T.C. 1978. Effects of fluoride supplementation from birth on dental caries and fluorosis in teenaged children. *Arch. Oral Biol.* 23:111-15.

103. Corpron, R.E., and Burt, B.A. 1978. Fluorosis from supplementation with fluoride tablets: a case report. *J. Mich. Dent. Assoc.* 60:615-18.

104. U.S. Dept. of Health, Education, and Welfare. 1979. *Total fluoride intake.* FL-108, March.

105. Gleason, M.N.; Gosselin, R.E.; Hodge, H.C.; and Smith, R.H. 1976. Clinical toxicology of commercial products. 4th ed. pp. 159-63. Baltimore: Williams & Wilkins.

106. Arena, J.M. 1974. Poisoning: toxicology-symptoms-treatments. 3rd ed., pp. 122-23. Springfield: Charles C. Thomas.

107. Dreisbach, R.H. 1974. Handbook of poisoning: diagnosis and treatment. 8th ed., pp. 189-92. Los Altos, Calif.: Lange Medical Publications.

108. Royal Commission on Fluoridation. 1968. *Report into the fluoridation of public water supplies in Tasmania, 1967-68.* p. 216. Hobart: Govt. Printer.

109. Gray, A.S., and Gunther, D.M. 1976. Supplemental fluorides: a community health centre project in preventive dentistry. *Can. J. Public Health* 67:55-58.

110. Richardson, A.S. 1967. Parental participation in the administration of fluoride supplements. *Can. J. Public Health* 58:508-13.

111. Marthaler, T.M.; Mejia, R.; Toth, K.; and Vines, J.J. 1978. Caries-preventive salt fluoridation. *Caries Res.* 12 (suppl. 1):15-21.

112. Marthaler, T.M., and Schenardi, C. 1962. Inhibition of caries in children after 5½ years' use of fluoridated table salt. *Helv. Odontol. Acta* 6:1-6.

113. Toth, K. 1970. Increment of dental caries over two years of fluoridation of domestic salt. A preliminary report. *Caries Res.* 4:293-95.

114. Toth, K. 1976. Fluoridated domestic salt and its effect on dental caries over a 5-year period. *Caries Res.* 10:394-99.

115. Rusoff, L.L.; Konikoff, B.S.; Frye, J.B., Jr.; Johnston, J.E.; and Frye, W.W. 1962. Fluoride addition to milk and its effect on dental caries in school children. *Am. J. Clin. Nutr.* 11:94-101.

116. Largent, E.J., and Heyroth, F.F. 1949. The absorption and excretion of fluorides. III. Further observations on metabolism of fluorides at high levels of intake. *J. Indust. Hyg. & Toxicol.* 31:134-38.

Chapter 6

Chemistry of Topical Fluoride Treatment

Resistance of the tooth to dental caries is increased through the interaction of fluoride with its mineral phase. When fluoride is present during the long preeruptive stage of enamel, some is incorporated into the hydroxyapatite crystal lattice forming fluorapatite or hydroxyfluorapatite. Fluorapatite crystals are larger, more perfectly formed[1,2] and less soluble in acid[3,4] than hydroxyapatite and, as discussed in Chapter 2, fluorapatite is responsible for the increased resistance of enamel to dental caries. Topical fluoride treatments are obviously much shorter than preeruptive fluoride exposure and utilize much higher fluoride concentrations, but for the most part, the intention of topical applications has been to convert hydroxyapatite to fluorapatite. Formation of insoluble coatings on enamel surfaces has been another aim of some fluoride treatments, particularly by agents possessing heavy metal cations such as tin, zirconium, or titanium.

The chemical products formed by the interaction of fluoride and tooth mineral must be considered one of the primary factors in determining the effectiveness of topical fluoride therapy. The identity of these products will vary depending on the particular fluoride agent used, its concentration, and the pH of the preparation. Similarly, the amount of fluoride deposited, the degree of fluoride penetration, and its retention will also vary. It is the intention of this chapter to present the fluoride-mineral reactions that occur during and following topical fluoride exposure, the factors that affect the extent of reaction, and the amounts of fluoride deposited in dental enamel from various topical preparations.

Enamel-fluoride reactions

General reactions

When fluoride is applied to an enamel surface it diffuses inward by way of the less dense interprismatic spaces to a depth related to its concentration, the treatment time, pH, and the type of fluoride agent. When the fluoride source is removed and replaced with water or saliva, a large part rapidly diffuses back out,[5] while another part diffuses out more slowly, probably as a result of absorption into the hydration layer of the crystals.[6,7] The fluoride that remains has reacted to form one or more of several compounds, depending on the conditions present.

The reaction of solutions containing low fluoride concentrations (approximately 75 to 100 ppm or less) with hydroxyapatite yields fluorapatite by replacement of surface hydroxyl groups. Since not all hydroxyl groups need to be replaced by fluoride, hydroxyfluorapatite is also formed:

$$\underset{\text{hydroxyapatite}}{Ca_{10}(PO_4)_6(OH)_2} \xrightarrow{F^-} Ca_{10}(PO_4)_6(OH)F \xrightarrow{F^-} \underset{\text{fluorapatite}}{Ca_{10}(PO_4)_6F_2} \quad (1)$$

Because short-term fluoride exposures result in exchange of hydroxyl groups on the crystal surfaces, the crystals may become covered with a coating of fluorapatite. Exchange of hydroxyl groups in the interior of the crystal will necessitate diffusion of fluoride ions through a solid. Because this is a solid state reaction, it would be expected to be very slow and not of clinical significance. Longer exposure of hydroxyapatite to solutions of low fluoride concentration in the laboratory has shown incorporation of fluoride by crystal growth and by the reprecipitation of dissolved hydroxyapatite.[8]

Exposure of hydroxyapatite to solutions of high fluoride concentration (> 100 ppm) favors dissolution of the crystal and formation of calcium fluoride.[6,9]

$$Ca_{10}(PO_4)_6(OH)_2 + 20\ F^- \rightarrow 10\ CaF_2 + 6\ PO_4^{\equiv} + 2\ OH^- \quad (2)$$

The relative amounts of hydroxyfluorapatite and calcium fluoride formed by hydroxyapatite powder treated at pH 7.0 with various fluoride concentrations up to 1,000 ppm are shown in Figure 6-1. Although hydroxyfluorapatite (and fluorapatite) formation increases with an increase in the fluoride concentration in the treatment solution, the amount of calcium fluoride increases more rapidly. Other laboratory experiments have shown that the proportion of calcium fluoride that forms depends on the ratio of treatment solution to hydroxyapatite solid. At pH 7.0 and low solution to solid ratios, fluorapatite may be the principal product, even when the treatment solution contains 1,000 ppm F or more.[10,11]

Because saliva is unsaturated with respect to calcium fluoride,[12] it has been thought that calcium fluoride precipitated on the enamel surface from a topical fluoride treatment would rapidly dissolve in the mouth. However, because much of the precipitate may exist well below the enamel surface and out of direct contact with saliva, it may be expected to remain for a longer time and, under favorable conditions, result in the formation of fluorapatite. This may occur simply by the slow dissolution of calcium fluoride, which will supply fluoride ions for subsequent substitution of the hydroxyl groups of hydroxyapatite.

$$CaF_2 \rightarrow Ca^{++} + 2F^- \xrightarrow{Ca_{10}(PO_4)_6(OH)_2} Ca_{10}(PO_4)_6F_2 + 2OH^- \quad (3)$$

Also, if calcium fluoride dissolves in the presence of a solution containing calcium and phosphate (as may be supplied by saliva), fluorapatite may form in this way.[13]

$$CaF_2 \rightarrow Ca^{++} + 2F^- \xrightarrow{6PO_4^{\equiv} + 9Ca^{++}} Ca_{10}(PO_4)_6F_2 \quad (4)$$

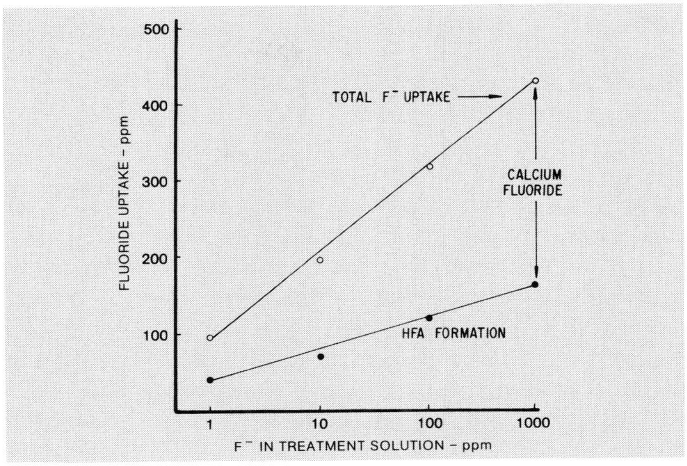

Fig. 6-1 Total F^- uptake and hydroxyfluorapatite formation by hydroxyapatite powder following one minute treatment with fluoride solutions at pH 7. (*Duke* and *Forward*.[100] Reproduced with permission of the authors and *Caries Res.*)

The formation of dicalcium phosphate dihydrate on the surface of enamel equilibrated with weak acid buffers has been reported,[14] and it is conceivable that this may also occur during a cariogenic challenge in the mouth.

$$Ca_{10}(PO_4)_6(OH)_2 + 8H^+ \longrightarrow 6\ CaHPO_4{\cdot}2H_2O + 4\ Ca^{++} \quad (5)$$

In the presence of fluoride, however, dicalcium phosphate dihydrate is not stable and forms either calcium fluoride or fluorapatite, or mixtures of the two.[15,16]

$$CaHPO_4{\cdot}2H_2O \xrightarrow{F^-} \begin{cases} CaF_2 \\ Ca_{10}(PO_4)_6F_2 \end{cases} \quad (6)$$

Chow and *Brown*[15] suggested that fluorapatite formation may be increased by the intentional formation of dicalcium phosphate dihydrate and subsequent treatment with fluoride. They pointed out that fluorapatite coatings on hydroxyapatite crystals prevent reaction with crystal interiors but that reaction of fluoride with dicalcium phosphate dihydrate causes loss of water and phosphate, resulting in a shrinkage of the crystal, which allows additional fluoride to penetrate to the interior of the crystal and thus a more complete conversion to fluorapatite.

Reactions of acidulated-phosphate-fluoride

Clinical applications of fluoride are usually given annually or semiannually and require that a relatively large amount of fluoride be deposited in enamel within a relatively short time. Because high fluoride concentrations and low pH favor fluoride deposition, several small clinical trials with high fluoride, low pH solutions, acidified with acetic acid or hydrofluoric acid, were undertaken with the expectation that an improved anticaries effect would be found.[17-19] Contrary to the expected results, the acidified solutions were ineffective. *Brudevold* et al.[20] suggested that the poor clinical results were due to adverse effects of the particular acid used, but that acidification of the fluoride solution with phosphoric acid would suppress the dissolution of enamel, as well as the formation of calcium fluoride, and provide a more effective treatment. The result of successful laboratory[20] and clinical[21,22] studies with this combination was "acidulated-phosphate-fluoride" (APF). The original APF solution contained 1.2% F from sodium fluoride and 0.1 M phosphate at pH 3.2. Some manufacturers, however, have increased the pH to near 4.0 to improve the flavor.

Although the use of phosphoric acid probably does supress enamel dissolution and calcium fluoride formation, the reactions of APF with enamel are essentially those of a high fluoride, low pH solution, and calcium fluoride is the principal reaction product[23-25] (equations 2, 5, 6), except when the fluoride concentration is below about 0.04% when fluorapatite is the principal product.[26] The finding that calcium fluoride is the principal product of APF was determined from laboratory studies with powdered enamel of various particle sizes ranging from 37 to 176 μ.[24] The largest amount of calcium fluoride was formed when the enamel particle size was small and therefore had a proportionally greater surface area and rate of dissolution. However, because the solution to solid ratios were high in comparison to the situation below an enamel surface, where reactions occur *in vivo,* the amount of calcium fluoride that formed *in vitro* might have been higher than would have formed *in vivo* from a topical fluoride application.

The calcium fluoride that forms during a topical treatment is partly lost by dissolution in the saliva, but there is evidence that a substantial amount is retained, probably by transformation to fluorapatite via the reactions shown by equations (3), (4), and (6).[5,27] The state of the fluoride acquired by the enamel during an APF treatment and its degree of retention will be discussed in a later section.

Reactions of stannous fluoride

The use of stannous fluoride as a topical anticaries agent is based on the finding that it greatly reduces the solubility of powdered enamel in acid.[28] Stannous fluoride solutions are naturally acidic, ranging from pH 3.2 for a 0.4% solution to 2.3 for an 8% solution.[29] Therefore, they produce large amounts of calcium fluoride (equation 2) as well as a number of compounds containing the tin ion. Although the tin compounds resulting from short-term applications (a few minutes) have not been identified clearly, analysis of a very thin layer, 0.4 μ thick, by electron spectroscopy for chemical analysis (ESCA), suggested the presence of calcium fluoride, fluorapatite, tin oxide, tin hydroxide, and tin hydroxyphosphate.[30] This is the only report found in the literature suggesting fluorapatite formation in enamel by stannous fluoride.

Longer reaction times (more than 8 minutes) result in the formation of $Sn_3F_3PO_4$ (equation 7).[31-33]

$$Ca_{10}(PO_4)_6(OH)_2 + 19\ SnF_2 \longrightarrow 6\ Sn_3F_3PO_4 + 10\ CaF_2 + SnO \cdot H_2O \quad (7)$$

Wei and *Forbes*[34] studied the reactions of stannous fluoride with enamel after various times and suggested that, initially, the surface dissolves and reacts to form $Sn_3F_3PO_4$ and calcium fluoride. As the reaction proceeds, additional precipitates, which include hydrated stannous oxides, accumulate on the surface and inhibit further diffusion into the enamel, thus limiting both fluoride and tin deposition. The depth of tin penetration into the enamel was approximately 20 μ after 30 seconds, and although the tin concentration increased significantly with time, its penetration increased only slightly. High concentrations of tin have been found to accumulate in circumscribed areas of enamel thought to be demineralized.[35] The formation of Sn_2PO_4OH,[30,36,37] hydrated stannous oxides (SnO_xH_2O),[38,39] and $Ca(SnF_3)_2$[37] after long reaction times has also been reported.

The deposition of tin compounds onto enamel from stannous fluoride causes the formation of a brownish-black pigmentation in early lesions, the margins of restorations,[40,42] and in the plaque of subjects with poor oral hygiene.[43-46] The colored compounds apparently arise from a change of the originally deposited colorless compounds to dark colored stannous sulfides.[47,48] However, these compounds are not stable in the oral environment and slowly disappear with time.[40,49]

Aqueous solutions of stannous fluoride are not stable and react according to the following equations:[29]

$$Sn^{++} + 2OH^- \longrightarrow Sn(OH)_2 \tag{8}$$

$$Sn(OH)_2 \longrightarrow SnO + H_2O \tag{9}$$

In the presence of oxygen, the stannous ion will undergo further oxidation to form the stannic ion. Although clinical evidence is lacking, it has been thought that fresh stannous fluoride solutions must be used for topical treatments. However, it has been shown that aged stannous fluoride solutions, which undoubtedly contain stannic ions, and solutions of stannic fluoride were equal to, or more effective than, fresh stannous fluoride solutions in reducing enamel solubility *in vitro*.[50,51] Stannic fluoride has also been shown to be effective in preventing experimental caries *in vivo*.[52]

Stable solutions have been prepared by dissolving stannous fluoride in anhydrous glycerol.[53] Although glycerol solutions of stannous fluoride will not provide the same degree of enamel protection[54,55] as aqueous solutions, dilution with at least 70% water will restore most of the effect.

Reactions of monofluorophosphate

Sodium monofluorophosphate differs from all other agents used for topical fluoride therapy in that its fluorine atom is covalently bonded to a phosphorus atom.

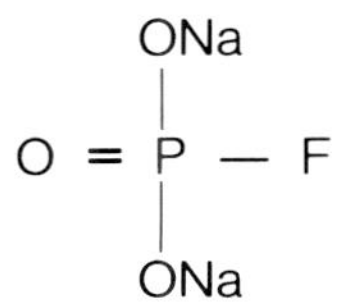

sodium monofluorophosphate

It is also unique because only fluorapatite forms even when it is applied to enamel in high concentrations or at low pH.[56,57] Although total fluoride uptake by enamel is lower from monofluorophosphate than other topical fluoride agents, the exclusive formation of fluorapatite may be the reason why it is equally effective as an anticaries agent. This may also be the reason why monofluorophosphate-treated enamel has been reported to be less soluble in acid than sodium fluoride-treated enamel when compared to enamel *of the same fluoride content*.[58,59]

Several mechanisms for the reaction of monofluorophosphate with enamel have been suggested, but a consensus as to which reaction predominates has not been reached. The mechanisms include direct incorporation of the $PO_3F^=$ anion into hydroxyapatite or first its hydrolysis to phosphate and fluoride ions, which then react to form fluorapatite.

Ericsson[60] proposed that the $PO_3F^=$anion was directly incorporated into apatite by exchange with orthophosphate, which was followed by an intracrystalline transposition where $PO_3F^=$ and OH^- of the apatite interacted to form orthophosphate, fluoride, and hydrogen ions.

$$PO_3F^= + OH^- \longrightarrow PO_4^= + F^- + H^+ \quad (10)$$

The fluoride thus released would replace another hydroxyl in the apatite lattice to form a fluoridated hydroxyapatite.

Ingram[58] suggested that $PO_3F^=$ was permanently incorporated into the surfaces of apatite crystals by exchange with $HPO_4^=$. He pointed out that enamel is a calcium-deficient apatite and could undergo the following reaction:

$$Ca_9(HPO_4)(PO_4)_5(OH)_2 \cdot H_2O + PO_3F^= \longrightarrow Ca_9(PO_3F)(PO_4)_5(OH)_2 \cdot H_2O + HPO_4^= \quad (11)$$

He further showed that addition of orthophosphate or bicarbonate, two ions that would compete for sites on the crystal surface, inhibited fluoride uptake from a monofluorophosphate solution.[61] Lowering the pH of the solution increases the fluoride uptake,[57,61] possibly by reducing the amount of the competing $HPO_4^=$ ion in solution.

It has also been proposed that monofluorophosphate is initially acquired intact by enamel, but that during a caries attack it is released and hydrolyzed to fluoride ion, which then reacts to form fluorapatite.[62]

Gron et al.[63] concluded that $PO_3F^=$ is first hydrolyzed at the crystal surface and the released fluoride ion is subsequently incorporated into the apatite lattice by replacing hydroxyl groups. This reaction clearly occurs in two steps since a slow accumulation of fluoride ion is found in monofluorophosphate solutions in contact with apatite.[57,63] Because of the greater surface area of demineralized enamel, the surface-activated hydrolysis should be greater in incipient carious lesions. Hydrolysis of monofluorophosphate is also catalyzed by salivary enzymes.[63,64] Because plaque can accumulate monofluorophosphate, it can serve as a depot where slow hydrolysis can occur, thus slowly releasing fluoride ions to react with enamel. When the pH is lowered during a caries attack, the rate of hydrolysis is increased[57] at a time when fluoride is best utilized.

Reactions of amine fluoride

Amine fluoride is used in some European countries, primarily Switzerland, for topical applications and in dentifrices. Amine fluoride preparations contain a mixture of two long chain aliphatic amine hydrofluorides at pH 4.5.

The amine fluoride preparations were developed to utilize the protection of both fluoride ions and long chain amines.[65] Reduction of enamel solubility from amine fluoride was

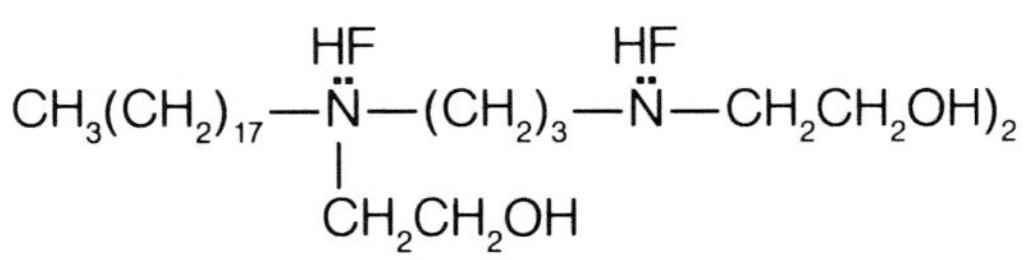

N-octadecyl—N,N′,N′-tris(2-hydroxyethyl) propane diamine dihydrofluoride

$$CH_3(CH_2)_7CH{=}CH(CH_2)_8NH_2 \cdot HF$$

oleylamine hydrofluoride

reported to be better than from stannous fluoride,[65] and fluoride deposition in enamel was similar to or perhaps better than that from acidulated phosphate fluoride.[66,67] Fluoride deposition occurs primarily by formation of calcium fluoride.[66] However, the calcium fluoride precipitates formed on the enamel surface are different from those formed by sodium fluoride, possibly because of adsorption of the amine moiety.

The amine portion of the agent has both surfactant and antimicrobial properties.[68] When used in a mouthwash, it was found to suppress plaque glycolysis.[69]

Permanence of topically acquired fluoride

In the foregoing discussion of the reactions of different fluoride agents with hydroxyapatite and enamel, the formation of a number of compounds was described. Because some of these compounds are soluble in saliva, they will not be permanently retained in the teeth. However, because they are formed, at least in part, below the enamel surface, they are protected from direct salivary contact and may persist for periods of up to many months. During this time the continuous availability of a low concentration of fluoride in solution brought about by slow dissolution of the soluble compounds will provide the conditions favorable to formation of fluorapatite, the only known physiological fluoride compound insoluble under normal oral conditions.

When a solution with a high fluoride concentration is applied to a tooth, some of the fluoride diffuses into the enamel where part reacts according to the equations discussed earlier and part remains unreacted or, at most, bound loosely by electrostatic forces. Upon removal of the fluoride preparation from the tooth surface, the unreacted and loosely bound fluoride begins to diffuse back out. To this is added the fluoride resulting from dissolution of soluble compounds on or near the enamel surface. The most rapid loss occurs during the first few minutes. Two-thirds or more of the fluoride initially acquired is lost within the first 24 hours.[5,70,71] A slower loss occurs for longer periods in cases where a potent fluoride application has been given. Figure 6-2 shows fluoride concentrations found in saliva after topical applications of acidulated phosphate fluoride solution and after use of a neutral sodium fluoride mouth rinse solution.[72] Loss of fluoride into saliva from the teeth (and other oral tissues) was noted for up to one week with the more concentrated topical solution. The rinse solution increased salivary fluoride for about one day, but it is likely that much of this was from the soft tissues rather than the teeth.

The slow loss of fluoride by dissolution of soluble fluoride compounds has been studied by analysis of primary teeth that were exfoliated at various times after the use of topical fluoride preparations. Figure 6-3 shows the amount of acquired fluoride remaining in the anterior teeth of children who had self-applied an acidulated phosphate fluoride prophylactic paste by toothbrush.[73] In this study, a major part of the acquired fluoride was lost within 4 to 6 months.

Fluoride retention and loss from more intensive fluoride applications are shown in Figure 6-4. This figure shows the fluoride concentrations at a depth of 5 μ in primary teeth during and after a treatment period when acidulated phosphate fluoride gel was given by custom-fitted mouthpiece on 5, 10, or 25 consecutive school days.[27] The period of fluoride loss was longest for those teeth that received the greatest number of treatments, ranging from about 100 days for those that received five treatments to about 250 days for those that received 25 treatments. Analysis of teeth exfoliated at later times showed

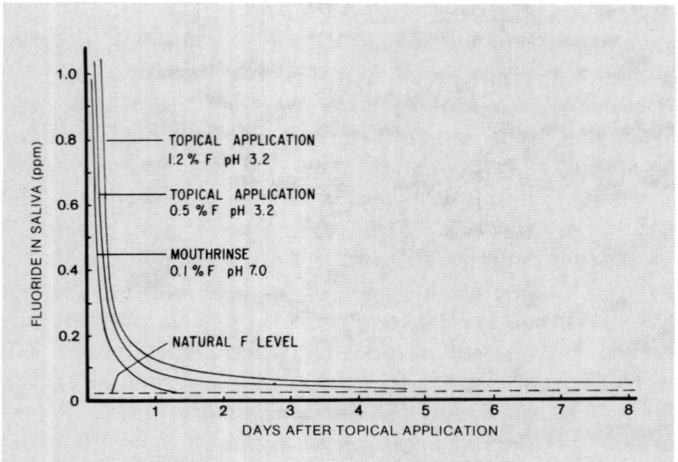

Fig. 6-2 Fluoride concentrations in saliva after topical fluoride applications or mouth rinsing with fluoride solutions. (Adapted from *Aasenden* et al.[72])

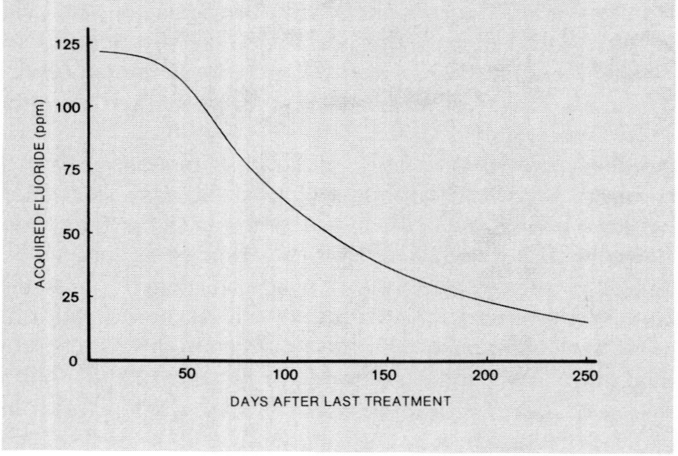

Fig. 6-3 Loss of enamel fluoride acquired from self-applied prophylaxis paste *in vivo*.
(Adapted from *Mellberg* et al.[73])

that the fluoride remaining in the teeth was permanently bound. This is highly significant because it shows that not all of the fluoride initially acquired was lost, suggesting that a large part of the calcium fluoride formed by these treatments was ultimately utilized in the formation of fluorapatite. This is in agreement with the results of an earlier study where an increase in enamel fluoride from a series of four applications of neutral 2% sodium fluoride was found to persist unchanged for at least 7 years.[74]

Although fluoride loss after treatment occurs similarly from sodium fluoride,[5] stannous fluoride,[5] and amine fluoride,[67] the loss of tin compounds deposited from stannous fluoride has not received much study. It has been shown, however, that there is a gradual loss of tin from sound and carious enamel[75] and that, as previously noted, the stain formed in carious and demineralized enamel is gradually lost with time.[40,49]

The enamel solubility-reducing effect of stannous fluoride applications has also been found to diminish with time. The decrease in acid solubility of rat molars produced by

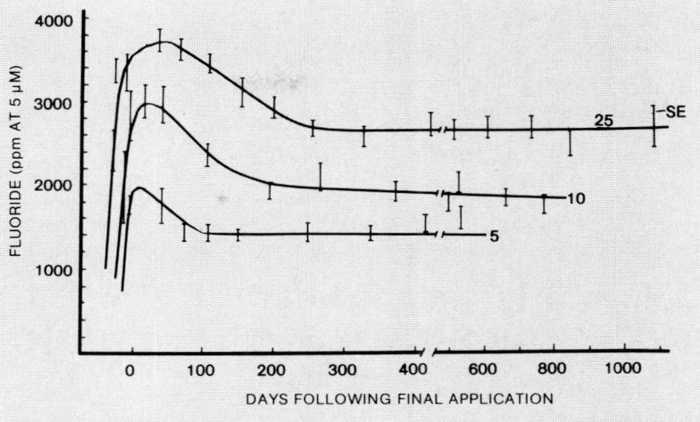

Fig. 6-4 Enamel fluoride concentrations in primary teeth at a depth of 5μ after 5, 10, or 25 self-applications of APF gel (1.2% F, pH 3.2). (*Mellberg* et al.[27] Reproduced with permission of *J. Dent. Res.*)

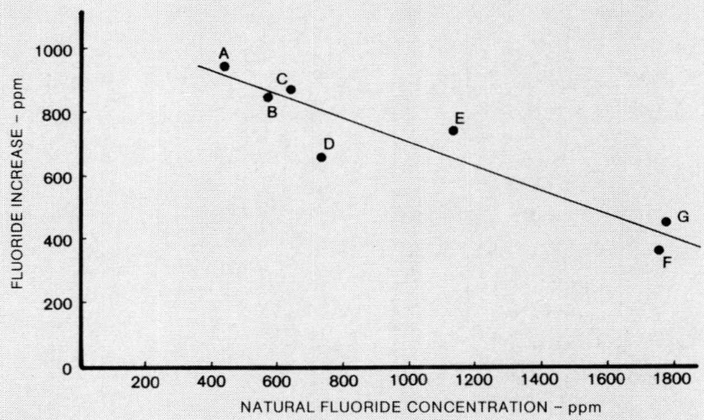

Fig. 6-5 Mean increase in enamel fluoride concentration at a depth of 5 μ in fluoride-treated teeth.

A primary, age 9-11
B primary, age 11-13, low natural F
C permanent, under age 25, low natural F
D permanent, over age 25, low natural F
E primary, age 11-13, high natural F
F permanent, over age 25, high natural F
G permanent, under age 25, high natural F

(Adapted from *Nicholson* and *Mellberg*.[86])

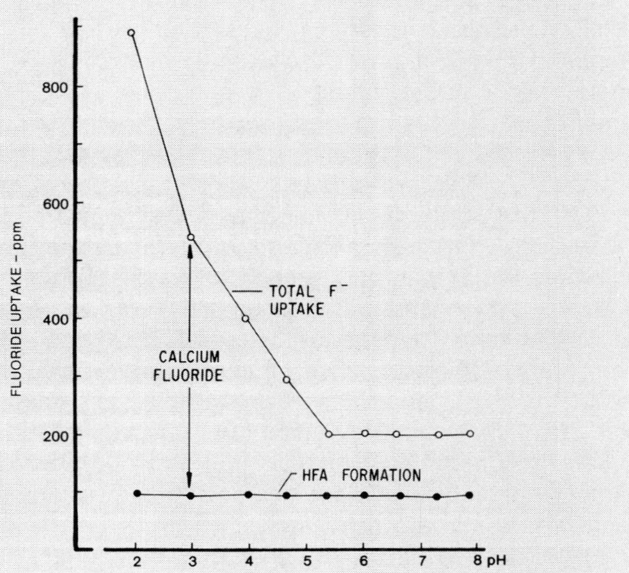

Fig. 6-6 Total F^- uptake and hydroxyfluorapatite formation by hydroxyapatite powder following one-minute treatment with 200 ppm F^- at varying pH. (*Duke* and *Forward*.[100] Reproduced with permission of the authors and *Caries Res.*)

application of 8% stannous fluoride *in vivo* was substantially lost after 5[76] or 10[77] days. Two-thirds of the initial solubility reduction attained by enamel of human teeth treated *in vitro* with 10% stannous fluoride was lost after exposure to saliva for 24 hours.[78]

Factors affecting topical fluoride deposition in teeth

The amount of fluoride taken up posteruptively by tooth mineral is affected by many factors, some of which have been used in attempts to improve the clinical effectiveness of the agents. These factors can be grouped into three broad areas:

—tooth condition
—treatment formulation
—application procedure

Tooth condition

Tooth age

As the tooth erupts into the mouth it is not yet fully mineralized. Enamel mineralization is completed during a posteruptive maturation period when calcium, phosphate, and trace elements fill in the spaces between the hydroxyapatite crystals and decrease the porosity.[79,80] This decrease in porosity reduces the amount of fluoride able to diffuse into the enamel and therefore decreases the amount that can be taken up. An inverse relationship between enamel fluoride uptake and the age of the tooth has been shown in data from several studies.[81-84]

Table 6-1 shows the amount of fluoride acquired by unerupted or mature permanent enamel and mature primary enamel from a typical treatment with acidulated-phosphate-fluoride solution *in vitro*.[85] The unerupted permanent enamel acquired about eight times more fluoride than the mature permanent enamel. The mature primary enamel acquired twice the fluoride compared to the less porous mature permanent enamel.

Natural fluoride concentration

Much of the fluoride acquired by enamel from concentrated, low pH, topical fluoride solutions is probably the result of an increase in the available surface area and soluble calcium following slight dissolution of hydroxyapatite crystallites. Because fluorapatite is less soluble than hydroxyapatite, enamel with a high natural fluoride content will dissolve less and therefore will acquire slightly less fluoride. The relationship between the natural enamel fluoride concentration (i.e., preeruptively acquired) and the amount of fluoride acquired from a topical application of acidulated phosphate fluoride is shown in Figure 6-5. In this study,[86] teeth that contained 400 to 600 ppm F in the outer 10 μ of enamel acquired more than 800 ppm F from the treatment. Teeth that contained about 1,800 ppm acquired only about half as much. (A small effect of age can also be seen in the data.)

Enamel defects

Enamel defects such as open carious lesions, incipient caries (white spots), microcracks, hypomineralized areas, and the margins of some restorations acquire larger amounts of fluoride than sound enamel because of their greater porosity and surface area[83,87,88] (see also Fig. 2-7). Hypomineralized areas or arrested incipient lesions are often evident as stained enamel. Table 6-2 shows that the fluoride concentration is greater in white spots and discolored enamel and increases with age.[89] This study also shows that the fluoride concentration was highest near the enamel surface, thus demonstrating that it was acquired topically.

Table 6-1 Fluoride concentrations (ppm) at a depth of 5μ in teeth of different ages before and after treatment with APF solutions

Teeth	Pretreated	Treated	Difference
Unerupted permanent	1,140	2,780	1,640
Erupted primary	720	1,140	420
Erupted permanent (over age 25 years)	720	930	210

Data from *Mellberg* and *Nicholson*.[85]

Table 6-2 Fluoride in sound and defective human permanent enamel

Type of enamel	Fluoride concentration (ppm)* Age group (years) 20	40–49
Sound	250	430
White spot	873	1,100
Diffusely discolored	808	3,043
Brown	1,075	2,035

*Enamel layer approximately 50μ thick.

Data from *Little*, *Cooper*, and *Rowley*.[89]

Weatherell et al.[90] found that fluoride near the gingival margins of teeth increases with age. They suggested that the periodic formation of acid by plaque causes a dissolution and then reprecipitation of enamel mineral. In the presence of fluoride, the reprecipitated mineral becomes enriched in fluorapatite. Well-defined "trapping regions" in enamel, probably corresponding to areas of partial demineralization or hypomineralization, have also been reported to acquire large amounts of tin from stannous fluoride applications.[35]

Another type of nonnormal enamel is the surface that is exposed by severe abrasion, for example by stripping interproximal areas.[91] This enamel has not posteruptively matured in saliva and therefore will acquire more fluoride.[87] Similarly, acid-etched enamel acquires very large amounts of fluoride because of greatly increased porosity and dissolved minerals. Enamel that had been etched by agitation in 0.5 N $HClO_4$ until approximately 200 μ had been removed, and which was then well washed under running water before fluoride treatment, acquired five times more fluoride than unetched enamel.[92]

Dentin/cementum

Dentin and sometimes cementum are also treated with fluoride. These may include exposed root surfaces, cavity preparations, or the entire roots of teeth to be replanted or transplanted. Much more fluoride is acquired by dentin or cementum than by enamel from a topical application. For example, a four-minute application of acidulated phosphate fluoride to the roots of extracted premolars produced an uptake of approximately 4,000 ppm F in a thin, outer layer.[93] This is approximately 10 times the uptake by enamel. Roots that were similarly treated, but which were not washed free of unreacted fluoride, contained as much as 200,000 ppm F near the surface, showing the great capacity that roots have for absorbing fluoride. Dentin powder has also been shown to take up more fluoride than enamel powder.[6,94]

Treatment formulation

Fluoride agent

Fluoride agents in common use have different natural or adjusted pHs, different fluoride concentrations, and result in the formation of different fluoride-containing compounds. Furthermore, the compounds that are formed may influence the penetration of fluoride into enamel and the amount eventually retained. Fluoride uptake by enamel from a particular agent is dependent upon a summation of the effects of these factors. Measurements of fluoride uptake reported by various investigators usually are not identical because the test conditions, and frequently the formulations, were different. For example, if the posttreatment rinse was short, fluoride uptake will be higher because it will include a large amount of fluoride that would eventually have been lost *in vivo*.

Table 6-3 lists the fluoride uptake findings from a number of studies with commonly used agents. Because the treatment conditions and formulations differ, the uptake from different agents should only be compared within a single study. Nevertheless, taken as a whole, the table provides a general review of the relative effectiveness of the agents in depositing fluoride in enamel.

Occasionally it is implied that the magnitude of enamel solubility reduction obtained in laboratory experiments is directly proportional to fluoride uptake. To some degree this is valid if different formulations of the same agent are being compared; however, it is not valid when the formulations contain different agents. For example, stannous fluoride provides better enamel solubility reduction than APF formulations but results in less fluoride uptake.

pH

Lowering the pH of a fluoride treatment solution results in partial dissolution of enamel crystal surfaces. The ionic calcium thus formed readily reacts to form calcium fluoride and, therefore, an increased total fluoride uptake. *Duke* and *Forward*[100] treated enamel powder with fluoride solutions adjusted to various pHs with hydrochloric acid and found that below a pH of about 5.5 total fluoride uptake increased, but the amount of fluorapatite formed remained constant (Fig. 6-6). They also found a similar result when using an APF solution diluted tenfold with water. However, because the diluted solution contained only 0.01 M phosphate and the phosphate in APF is intended to prevent enamel dissolution and enhance fluorapatite formation,[20] it cannot be assumed that fluorapatite formation will also be unaffected by a change in pH when the full 0.1 M phosphate concentration contained in undiluted APF solutions is present.

Fluoride concentration

The fluoride uptake by sound, intact enamel increases almost linearly with an increase in the fluoride concentration of the treatment solution, although there is some lessening of the increase as the treatment solution concentration rises. This has been shown for neutral sodium fluoride and sodium monofluorophosphate concentrations ranging from 10 to 1,000 ppm F[101] and for APF solutions

Table 6-3 Fluoride uptake by enamel from various fluoride agents

Study reference number	Estimated depth in enamel (μ)	APF	SnF_2	NaF	Amine F	Na_2PO_3F
67*	3	1,003 (1.2–3.2)**			978 (1.0–5.5)	
5	5	919 (1.2–3.2)	63 (1.2–2.5)			
95	4	890 (1.2–3.2)	390 (2.5–2.3)	210 (1.8–9.3)	2,910 (1.0–4.5)	
96*	5	190 (1.2–3.2)	30 (2.5–2.3)			
97	6	1,498 (1.2–2.3)	286 (1.9–2.4)	810 (0.9–7.0)	360 (1.0–5.5)	193 (1.0–7.0)
98	5	854 (1.2–4.0)			645 (1.0–4.8)	
99*	5	379 (0.9–4.5)	267 (1.9–2.4)	461 (0.9–7.0)		123 (0.7–7.0)

*In vivo studies.
**Values in parentheses are (% F-pH).

prepared with ammonium silicofluoride and ranging from 10,000 to 100,000 ppm F (i.e., 1 to 10%).[102] Figure 6-7 shows the near linearity of fluoride uptake versus treatment fluoride concentration. The figure also shows that almost a tenfold increase in treatment concentration is required to double the fluoride uptake.

Formulation Components

Thickening agents — Materials such as hydroxyethylcellulose are frquently added to formulations to increase their thickness. This tends to reduce the rate of fluoride diffusion[103] and may reduce fluoride uptake.[104,105] A high fluoride concentration in the preparation can overcome this effect,[106,107] but if the viscosity is high enough, fluoride uptake can be prevented entirely.[108] Although fluoride diffusion through thixotropic gels is much slower than through most other gels,[103] fluoride uptake has been reported to be similar.[109]

Humectants — These agents, which include glycerol, sorbitol, and propylene glycol, are used to prevent gel and paste formulations from losing water and drying out. Although it has been reported that fluoride uptake by powdered enamel is increased by glycerol,[110] most investigators report reduced uptake. Fifty percent glycerol solutions were found to reduce fluoride uptake approximately 50% from sodium fluoride and sodium monofluorophosphate,[105] and to lower the enamel solubility-reducing effect of stannous fluoride.[111] Although 30% glycerol in an aqueous solution did not reduce uptake from sodium fluoride, when it was used with 2% hydroxyethylcellulose, uptake was completely prevented.[108] Sorbitol (40 to 47%) has also been shown to inhibit fluoride uptake.[105-108]

Abrasives — Some abrasives used in pro-

Table 6-4 Mean fluoride concentration at 5μ depth in untreated teeth and uptake in homologous teeth treated with fluoride solution or paste

Treatment	Mean subject age (years)	Mean F (ppm) untreated teeth	Mean F (ppm) uptake
APF solution	28.4	894	190
SnF_2 solution	28.1	1,246	30
APF paste	28.9	712	91
SnF_2 paste	29.5	800	-4

Data from *Heifetz* et al.[96]

phylaxis pastes and dentifrices react with fluoride, thereby reducing the amount available for reaction with the enamel[105,108,112] (Fig. 6-8) and frequently changing the pH of the preparation.[108,113-115]

Abrasives can be broadly categorized as those that react rapidly with fluoride (e.g., calcium carbonate), those that react slowly (e.g., sintered aluminum oxide), and those that either do not react (insoluble sodium metaphosphate) or react to form active fluoride compounds (silica). For example, the reaction of acidic fluoride solution with silica is as follows:

$$6HF + SiO_2 \longrightarrow H_2SiF_6 + 2H_2O \qquad (12)$$

Because H_2SiF_6 is an active fluoride source that is frequently used in drinking water fluoridation, there is no loss in effectiveness. The stability and effectiveness of a silicofluoride-silica prophylaxis paste has been shown in several studies.[73,108,116]

Ericsson[105] used radioactive fluoride and investigated its compatability with calcium carbonate, tricalcium carbonate, calcium pyrophosphate, insoluble sodium metaphosphate, silica, and silica gel. Heat-treated tricalcium phosphate and calcium pyrophosphate were also evaluated. He found that all abrasives except insoluble sodium metaphosphate adsorbed some fluoride, but that prior heat treating of the abrasive reduced the adsorption. In another study,[117] he found that several aluminum-containing abrasives also adsorbed fluoride, but that under appropriate pH conditions some were sufficiently compatible to be considered for use in prophylaxis pastes.

Fluoride uptake from prophylaxis pastes has been investigated *in vivo* in adults and children. The results in adults are shown in Table 6-4, where fluoride uptake from two prophylaxis pastes is compared to uptake from aqueous solutions.[96] The acidulated-phosphate-fluoride paste (silica abrasive) deposited approximately half as much fluoride as the acidulated-phosphate-fluoride solution but more than the stannous fluoride solution. The stannous fluoride paste (zirconium silicate abrasive) deposited no detectable fluoride in the enamel.

Four professional applications of the acidulated-phosphate-fluoride paste listed in Table 6-4 to children at six-month intervals provided an uptake of 300 ppm F in the outer 2 μ of enamel of permanent teeth and 275 ppm F in the outer 10 μ of primary teeth.[116] Fluoride deposition from self-applied acidulated-phosphate-fluoride paste has also been shown. In one study, a mean uptake of 201 ppm F at a depth of 5 μ was found after six applications given at three-month intervals.[118] In another study, fluoride uptake at

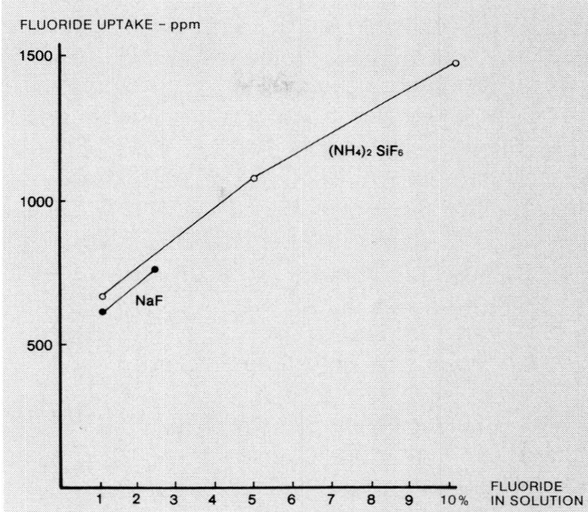

Fig. 6-7 Fluoride uptake by human enamel from acidulated phosphate fluoride solutions prepared with NaF or $(NH_4)_2SiF_6$.
(*Mellberg* and *Loertscher*.[102] Reproduced with permission of *Arch. Oral Biol.*)

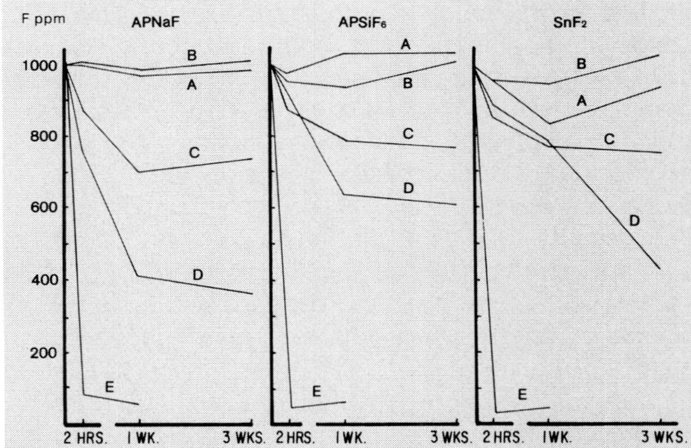

Fig. 6-8 Fluoride concentrations in filtrates of abrasive-fluoride slurries after 2 hours, 1 week, or 3 weeks.
A silicon dioxide
B insoluble sodium metaphosphate
C zirconium silicate
D flour of pumice
E calcium carbonate
APNaF, APS_1F_6 = acidulated phosphate fluoride slurries prepared with NaF and $(NH_4)_2S_1F_6$ respectively.
(*Mellberg* and *Nicholson*.[108] Reproduced with permission of *Arch. Oral Biol.*)

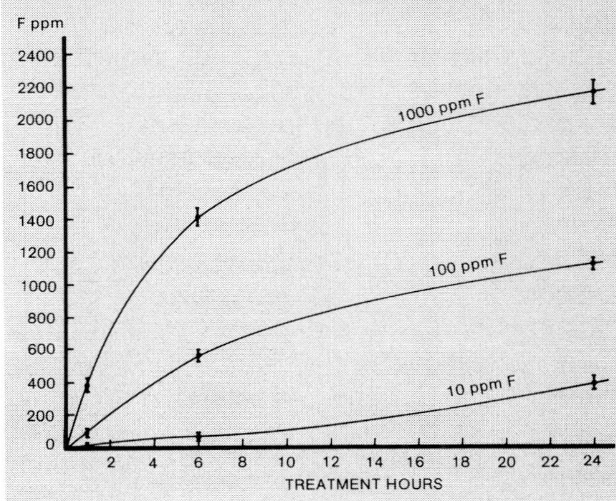

Fig. 6-9 Rate of fluoride uptake by the outer enamel layer from 10, 100, and 1,000 ppm F as monofluorophosphate.
(*Mellberg*.[101] Reproduced with permission of *Caries Res.*)

5 μ was 121 ppm F in anterior teeth and only 14 ppm F in posterior teeth.[73] This suggests that the paste was not effectively applied to the posterior surfaces.

Obviously, fluoride uptake from prophylaxis pastes will differ greatly depending on the abrasive used, the amount of humectant and thickening agent present, and the pH of the system. Although fluoride uptake from prophylaxis pastes is not likely to be as great as from topical solutions or gels, a well-formulated paste can be used to provide some benefit when solutions or gel treatments are not given.

Fluoride also reacts with the abrasives used in dentifrices, however, the formulation can be adjusted to slow the reaction to acceptable rates. In addition, the abrasives can be modified in manufacturing to improve their fluoride compatability, and sodium monofluorophosphate, a fluorine source more compatible with dentifrice abrasives than the other commonly used fluorides, can be used. Modern fluoride dentifrices are all adequately stable to provide caries protection.

Other agents — Agents added to formulations, not necessarily to modify their physical characteristics but instead intended to be active components, frequently have an effect on fluoride uptake. In most cases, these components have been studied only in experimental formulations and are not present in commercial products.

The addition of phosphate to acidic sodium fluoride preparations was discussed earlier. Phosphate has also been added to stannous fluoride solutions[119] and pastes.[115] In these systems the phosphate precipitates most of the tin,[71] producing a system resembling the acidulated-phosphate-fluoride solution prepared with sodium fluoride. *Muhler* et al.[119] however, reported that the stannous fluoride-phosphate solution provided better enamel solubility reduction and caries inhibition.

Diphosphonates, added to fluoride solution or given as a pretreatment, strongly inhibit fluoride uptake,[120] presumably because the diphosphonate molecules coat the hydroxyapatite crystals. However, diphosphonate also results in improved retention of fluoride in enamel,[121] probably because the diphosphonate protects the apatite crystals from the local environment.

Polyvalent metal ions (e.g., aluminum) added to a fluoride solution may increase fluoride deposition in enamel through complexation. This is discussed more fully in the section dealing with pretreatment.

Application procedure

Prophylaxis

It is commonly assumed that thorough cleaning of the teeth is necessary to obtain maximum fluoride uptake from a topical fluoride application. This assumption is based on the finding of a single clinical trial[122] where topical application of sodium fluoride was found to be only half as effective as in other studies where similar applications were preceded by a pumice prophylaxis. The assumption was also supported by laboratory studies showing greater fluoride uptake by teeth given a pumice prophylaxis[81,87] and by an inhibition of uptake when a film of saliva was present.[123] It was also shown that the microscopic appearance of an enamel surface treated with 0.1% fluoride when a salivary flim was present was different.[124] These studies all used dilute fluoride solutions, usually much less than 0.1%. Although the studies suggest that plaque and saliva may have an adverse effect on uptake from dilute fluoride preparations such as dentifrices or rinses, other studies have shown that plaque or pellicle has no effect on the uptake from the more concentrated preparations used for professional topical applications.

Bruun and *Stoltze*[125] found that fluoride uptake from amine fluoride was similar on clean teeth and on those covered with a five-day accumulation of plaque. In an *in vitro* study, *Joyston-Bechal* et al.[126] found that artificial plaque had no effect on the amount of fluoride deposited in enamel from acidulated-phosphate-fluoride, and *Tinanoff* et al. could find no improvement in uptake when natural[127] or artificial[128] pellicle was removed by a prophylaxis before application of acidulated-phosphate-fluoride.

Effect of time

As the duration of the fluoride treatment increases, the amount of fluoride deposited in enamel also increases. The rate of penetration of fluoride from neutral sodium fluoride solutions into sound enamel is proportional to the square root of time; that is, its rate is diffusion controlled.[129] The rate of fluoride penetration from acidulated-phosphate-fluoride is also diffusion controlled, but only after the first 5 minutes, during which its reaction with enamel is very rapid.[129]

The penetration of fluoride into enamel, however, cannot be taken as a measure of fluoride deposition, since a major part of the fluoride that diffuses into the enamel during the application diffuses back out during the subsequent 24 hours.[5] The amount of fluoride that remains after the application will be the sum of fluoride diffusion into enamel, reaction of imbibed fluoride with enamel, back diffusion of unreacted fluoride out of the enamel, dissolution of soluble reaction products (e.g., CaF_2), and back diffusion of dissolved products. Fluoride uptake in surface enamel measured after a 24-hour washing period to allow the back diffusion processes to occur showed that uptake from sodium fluoride and sodium monofluorophosphate is directly proportional to time from 10 ppm fluorine, but not from 100 or 1,000 ppm fluorine solutions.[101] With the higher concentrations, uptake is rapid at first but slows with time (Fig. 6-9). Fluoride uptake in deeper enamel is directly proportional to time at all three of the fluoride concentrations (Fig. 6-10).

Fluoride uptake from 10% stannous fluoride has also been shown to increase during treatment times as long as 5 days.[130]

Temperature

An increase in the temperature of the fluoride treatment preparation increases the amount of fluoride deposited in enamel.[102,130-133] Approximately twice as much fluoride is deposited *in vitro* from acidulated-phosphate-fluoride at 35°C than is deposited at room temperature.[102] Stannous fluoride treatments given at higher temperatures were also found to deposit more fluoride, but a greater temperature increase was needed to show the effect on sound enamel. Etched enamel responded more directly to a temperature increase.[133]

Number of applications

Repeated applications of concentrated solutions and gels of sodium fluoride increase enamel fluoride in an incremental fashion. For example, repeated applications of 0.5% F as neutral sodium fluoride or acidulated-phosphate-fluoride (pH 4.5) produced the effect shown in Figure 6-11.[134] Likewise, an even more highly concentrated acidulated-phosphate-fluoride gel (1.2% F, pH 3.2) produced the effect shown in Figure 6-12.[27]

Penetration of fluoride is also increased by repeated applications of potent preparations. Figure 6-13 shows that self-application of acidulated-phosphate-fluoride containing 0.5% F results in greatly increased fluoride levels in subsurface enamel. At 80 μ from the surface, teeth given a mean of 172 self-applications contained 1,400 ppm F compared to 65 ppm in untreated teeth. High levels extended beyond 300 μ, where the enamel still contained about 200 ppm F.[134] Penetration of fluoride into teeth treated with the neutral 0.5% F gel increased much less and did not extend beyond 80 μ.

Less concentrated fluoride solutions used as

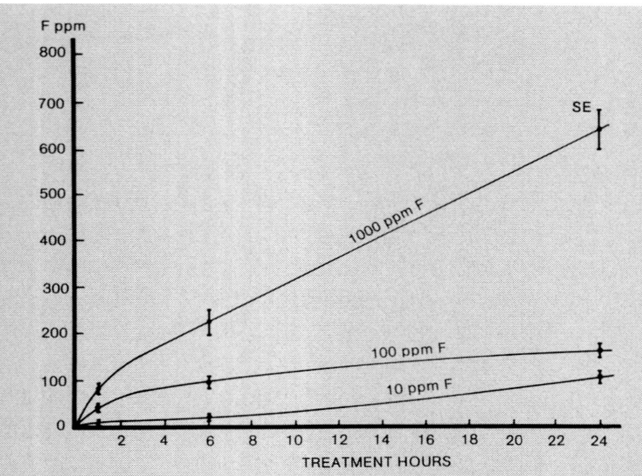

Fig. 6-10 Rate of fluoride uptake by enamel at a depth of approximately 23 μ from 10, 100, or 1,000 ppm F as monofluorophosphate.
(*Mellberg.*[101] Reproduced with permission of *Caries Res.)*

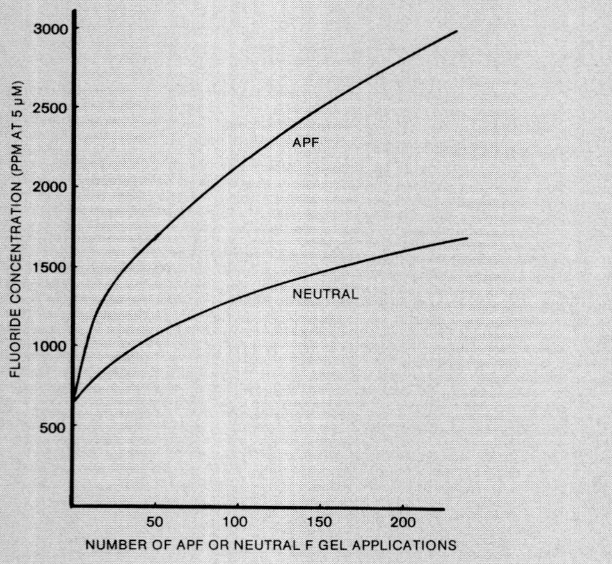

Fig. 6-11 Rate of fluoride uptake *in vivo* by primary enamel from APF (0.5% F, pH 4.5) and neutral fluoride (0.5% F, pH 7) gels.
(Data from *Mellberg* et al.[134])

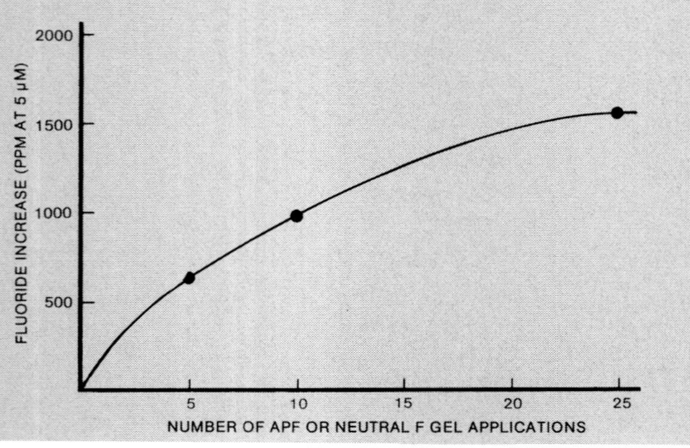

Fig. 6-12 Rate of fluoride uptake *in vivo* by primary enamel from APF gels (1.2% F, pH 3.2) in mouthpieces.
(Data from *Mellberg* et al.[27])

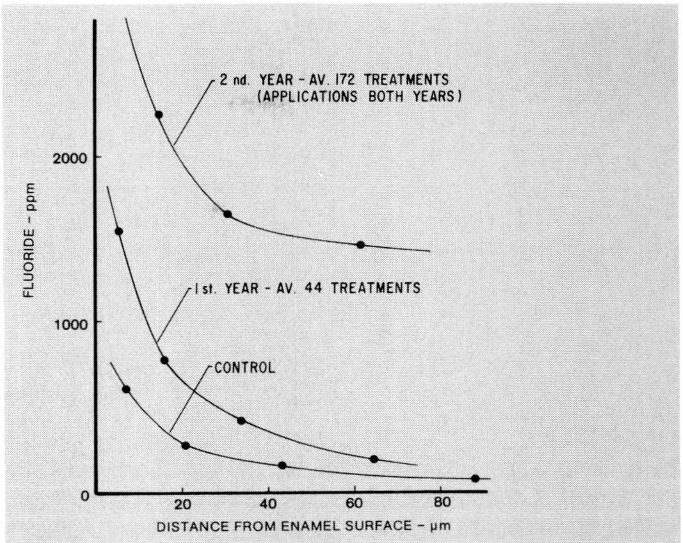

Fig. 6-13 Penetration of fluoride into primary enamel *in vivo* from daily applications of acidulated phosphate fluoride gel (0.5% F, pH 4.5) during two school years.
(*Mellberg* et al.[134] Reproduced with permission of *Arch. Oral Biol.*)

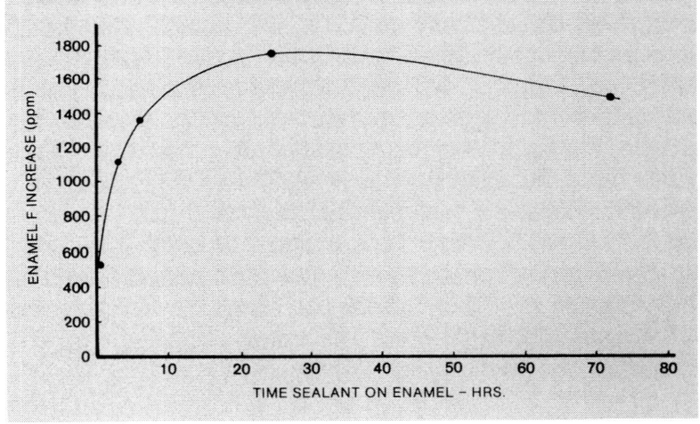

Fig. 6-14 Effect of a sealant applied after an APF treatment *in vitro* on fluoride retention by enamel.
(Data from *Mellberg* et al.[70])

mouth rinses do not result in significant, continuous increases over prolonged periods of frequent rinsing.[135-137] During a three-year period of daily rinsing with an acidulated-phosphate-fluoride rinse containing 200 ppm F at pH 4, an increase in enamel fluoride was observed only during the first part of the study.[135] Fluoride uptake by enamel from a neutral sodium fluoride solution containing 200 ppm F in the same study was not found at 5 μ. However, analysis of thinner layers showed that there was an increase at 2 μ.[138] This shows that there is a very shallow depth of penetration even after many applications from dilute preparations, particularly those with a neutral pH.

Daily use of 1 mg fluoride tablets increased the fluoride concentration of the outer 10 μ of enamel slabs mounted in a dental appliance by about 50 ppm per day up to 6 days.[139] Discontinuation of tablet use was followed by complete loss of the acquired fluoride. Using an enamel biopsy technique, the outer 2 μ of enamel of permanent incisors was shown to increase 29 ppm F and 55 ppm F after use of one or two 1 mg fluoride tablets daily for 30 months. However, these increases were not statistically significant.[140] Daily use of 1 mg fluoride tablets for three school years significantly increased the fluoride concentration in the outer 10 μ of primary teeth by 148 ppm in anterior and 80 ppm in posterior surfaces.[141] The uptake, however, occurred during the first few months and did not increase further with time.

After considering the results of analyses of many teeth collected from children using various types of topical fluoride preparations, it appears that the greatest increase of fluoride in sound enamel will occur at the beginning of a series of applications after which the rate of F deposition will slow so that each subsequent application will provide progressively less fluoride to the enamel until, finally, no additional uptake will be observed. That is, any gain in fluoride is offset by an equal loss. In the case of most mouth rinses or tablets, this seems to happen quite rapidly (perhaps within a few weeks), whereas with more concentrated preparations uptake may continue for several years. Of course, newly formed enamel defects (e.g., demineralized areas) will acquire additional fluoride regardless of the fluoride concentration of adjacent sound enamel.

Sequential APF-SnF_2 applications

Based upon the knowledge that acidulated-phosphate-fluoride applications deposit more fluoride in enamel than other commonly used topical preparations, but that stannous fluoride provides greater enamel solubility reduction, *Shannon* and co-workers[142-146] tested the effect of combined use of the agents. They found that application of acidulated-phosphate-fluoride followed by stannous fluoride *in vitro* produced a less soluble root or enamel surface than either agent used alone. Furthermore, the reaction products were more difficult to remove with flowing tap water. Reversing the order of application (i.e., SnF_2 followed by APF) was not as effective, but one study showed that mixing the two solutions prior to application appeared to provide essentially the same benefit as when acidulated-phosphate-fluoride was used first.[146] They suggested that the reason for improved solubility reduction from the APF-SnF_2 combination was the formation of both CaF_2 from acidulated-phosphate-fluoride and $Sn_3F_3PO_4$ from stannous fluoride rather than the formation of just one product if only a single agent had been used.

A study of the reactions that occurred in a neutral calcium phosphate solution (that might simulate saliva) following sequential applications of APF and SnF_2 to enamel suggested that the calcium fluoride that had formed during the treatment dissolved and promoted the formation of new apatitic mineral.[13]

Enamel pretreatment

In addition to a pumice prophylaxis, two other types of enamel pretreatment have been studied in an attempt to improve fluoride uptake from topical applications. These include mild etching of the enamel with acid and treatment with polyvalent metal ions (e.g., aluminum).

A one-minute pretreatment with 0.01 to 0.1 N phosphoric acid results in a large increase in deposited fluoride, which can be as much as five times greater than in unetched enamel.[107,147-149] As already mentioned, this is because the acid enlarges diffusion pathways, thus allowing greater fluoride penetration and reaction with the enamel that was dissolved and reprecipitated during the etch. It has been suggested that the precipitated mineral is dicalcium phosphate dihydrate ($CaHPO_4 \cdot 2H_2O$), which is transformed by the fluoride application to calcium fluoride and/or fluorapatite.[15,16]

Polyvalent metal ions increase fluoride

uptake through complexation with fluoride and reaction with enamel. In general, any polyvalent metal capable of forming strong fluoride complexes while simultaneously binding firmly to apatite crystals increases fluoride uptake.[150] Although incorporation of the metal ion into the treatment solution will increase uptake, it is more effective when applied prior to fluoride application. Pretreatment with a solution of an aluminum salt (e.g., chloride or nitrate), followed by acidulated-phosphate-fluoride or stannous fluoride, was shown to increase fluoride uptake significantly *in vitro*,[150-152] and pretreatment of rats' teeth *in vivo* with an aluminum salt solution also increased fluoride uptake.[153-155] Titanium tetrafluoride has been reported to deposit more fluoride in enamel than acidulated-phosphate-fluoride,[156] and pretreatment with titanium trichloride or zirconyl chloride followed by acidulated-phosphate-fluoride not only resulted in greater fluoride deposition but also reduced the rate of artificial caries formation.[157] A beneficial effect of metal ion pretreatment, however, has not clearly been established *in vivo*.[154,155]

Barrier coating

As discussed in an earlier section, much more fluoride diffuses into enamel during a topical application than is permanently retained. Most of it diffuses back out during the first few minutes or hours and is lost in the saliva. To prevent the outward diffusion of fluoride and increase the reaction time of absorbed fluoride, an impermeable coating material can be applied over the treated enamel.[70,158] Fig 6-14 shows the findings from a laboratory study where human enamel was treated for 4 minutes with acidulated-phosphate-fluoride, coated with a barrier material, and then immersed in an aqueous calcium phosphate solution to simulate saliva. After various times, the coating was removed and the enamel placed back in the solution for 24 hours to allow loss of unreacted fluoride. The figure shows that the barrier improved the ultimate retention of fluoride at least threefold and that the maximum benefit occurred within the first 6 hours. The presence of the barrier for longer than 6 hours did not appear to increase fluoride retention further. In an *in vivo* study, 18 months after application of acidulated-phosphate-fluoride, enamel contained 1,350 ppm F, but when a cyanoacrylate sealant was applied after the treatment, the enamel contained 3,280 ppm F.[159] Similarly, in another study, 612 ppm F was found without the sealant and 1,203 ppm F with the sealant.[160] In yet another study, however, no effect of a sealant could be found.[161]

The application of sealant or lacquer incorporating the fluoride has also been shown to increase the concentration of fluoride in enamel *in vivo*[162] and *in vitro*,[98, 163-165] and its acid resistance *in vitro*.[166-168] It has been suggested that fluoride is able to slowly diffuse from the lacquer into the enamel, thus prolonging the treatment time. However, it is likely that some of the uptake from the lacquer occurs during the time that the solvent is evaporating. In this event, the dry lacquer functions in the same fashion as the barrier coating described above. Nevertheless, the data of one study[162] suggest that some fluoride does diffuse from the coating into the enamel and therefore rapid uptake during the drying period and slow uptake by diffusion out of the lacquer may occur consecutively. A somewhat similar approach was taken by *Manly* and *Harrington*,[169] who incorporated fluoride into an oral adhesive bandage and found significant enamel fluoride uptake if the bandage was first hydrated by flowing water or calcium phosphate solutions.

Iontophoresis

Because the fluoride ion is a charged particle and therefore will move in an electric field, it has been thought that application of an electric potential to the tooth might facilitate the fluoride ion's penetration into enamel. Although a number of studies have tested this possibility, the findings have not been consistent.

Several investigators have found increased fluoride uptake when fluoride solutions are used with iontophoresis, although the effect was often of small magnitude.[170-173] Increased anticaries activity of fluoride in rats,[174] enamel solubility reduction,[175,176] and desensitizing effects[177-180] have also been reported. In contradiction to the positive findings have been a number of studies where no effect could be found.[123,181-186] It has to be concluded that increased fluoride uptake resulting from the use of iontophoresis remains unproven.

Summary

Resistance to dental caries is increased through the interaction of fluoride with dental enamel. In general, the reaction of low fluoride concentrations results in the substitution of fluoride for hydroxyl groups in the hydroxyapatite crystal lattice to form fluorapatite. Higher concentrations usually form calcium fluoride. In the oral environment, it is likely that some of the fluoride from calcium fluoride is subsequently utilized in the formation of fluorapatite.

Several different fluoride agents have been used for the treatment of enamel, each differing somewhat in its reactions with enamel. Sodium fluoride functions essentially as described above, with the concentrated solutions, including APF, reacting initially to form predominantly calcium fluoride. Stannous fluoride also forms calcium fluoride but, in addition, a coating of tin compounds, highly resistant to acid, and which limits the penetration of fluoride into the enamel. A preparation containing amine fluoride compounds, used in some areas of the world, also forms predominantly calcium fluoride.

Sodium monofluorophosphate differs from the ionic fluoride compounds above because it forms only fluorapatite, even when used at high concentrations. The mechanism for the formation of fluorapatite from monofluorophosphate is not known, but it has been suggested that it is directly incorporated into the hydroxyapatite crystal or that it decomposes at the crystal surface providing ionic fluoride for subsequent substitution of hydroxyl groups.

Much of the fluoride taken up by enamel from solutions of high fluoride concentration is not permanently retained. Some of the fluoride is absorbed by the enamel but does not react and quite readily diffuses back out, while some reacts to form relatively soluble compounds that slowly dissolve and are ultimately lost. The period of slow loss can be as long as several months or more, depending on the type and number of applications given to the teeth.

The amount of fluoride taken up by enamel depends on a number of factors. Larger amounts are acquired when the teeth are young, contain low natural fluoride levels, or have areas of porosity, (e.g., from caries activity). The formulation used for the fluoride treatment will deposit more fluoride in enamel if it has a low pH, high fluoride concentration, or contains polyvalent metal ions. Conversely, fluoride deposition will be reduced if the formulation contains large amounts of humectants, thickening agents, or abrasives that react with fluoride. Fluoride uptake will also be increased by longer treatment times, high temperature, repeated applications, acid pretreatments, and barrier coatings.

References

1. Posner, A.S.; Eanes, E.D.; Harper, R.A.; and Zipkin, I. 1963. X-ray diffraction analysis of the effect of fluoride on human bone apatite. *Arch. Oral Biol.* 8:549-70.
2. Zipkin, I.; Posner, A.S.; and Eanes, E.D. 1962. The effect of fluoride on the X-ray diffraction pattern of the apatite of human bone. *Biochem. Biophys. Acta* 59:255-58.
3. Young, R.A.; van der Lugt, W.; and Elliott, J.C. 1969. Mechanism for fluorine inhibition of diffusion in hydroxyapatite. *Nature* (Lond.) 223:729-30.
4. van der Lugt, W.; Kottnerus, I.M.; and Young, R.A. 1970. NMR determination of fluoride position in mineral hydroxyapatite. *Caries Res.* 4:89-95.
5. Mellberg, J.R.; Laakso, P.V.; and Nicholson, C.R. 1966. The acquisition and loss of fluoride by topically fluoridated human tooth enamel. *Arch. Oral Biol.* 11:1213-20.
6. McCann, H.G., and Bullock, F.A. 1955. Reactions of fluoride ion with powdered enamel and dentin. *J. Dent. Res.* 34:59-67.
7. Rolla, G., and Bowen, W.H. 1978. Surface adsorption of fluoride and ionic exchange reactions on hydroxyapatite. *Acta Odontol. Scand.* 36:219-24.
8. Spinelli, M.A.; Brudevold, A.; and Moreno, E. 1971. Mechanism of fluoride uptake by hydroxyapatite. *Arch. Oral Biol.* 16:187-203.
9. Leach, S.A. 1959. Reaction of fluoride with powdered enamel and dentin. *Brit. Dent. J.* 106:133-42.
10. McCann, H.G. 1953. Reactions of fluoride ion with hydroxyapatite. *J. Biol. Chem.* 201:247-59.
11. Ramsey, A.C.; Duff, E.J.; Patterson, L.; and Stuart, J.L. 1973. The uptake of F^- by hydroxyapatite at varying pH: theoretical considerations and experiments. *Caries Res.* 7:231-44.
12. McCann, H.G. 1968. The solubility of fluorapatite, and its relationship to that of calcium fluoride. *Arch. Oral Biol. 13:987-1001.*
13. Jeansonne, B.G., and Feagin, F.F. 1973. Reactions of enamel surfaces and neutral calcium phosphate solutions after combinations of APF and SnF_2. *J. Dent. Res.* 52:348-51.
14. Gray, J.A. and Francis, M.D. 1963. Physical chemistry of enamel dissolution. In: *Mechanisms of hard tissue destruction*, ed. R.F. Sognnaes, pp. 213-60. Washington, D.C.: AAS Pub. No. 75.
15. Chow, L.C., and Brown, W.E. 1973. Reaction of dicalcium phosphate dihydrate with fluoride. *J. Dent. Res.* 52:1220-27.
16. Wei, S.H.Y.; Tang, T.E.; and Wefel, J.S. 1974. Reactions of dicalcium phosphate dihydrate with fluoride solutions. *J. Dent. Res.* 53:1145-54.
17. Arnold, F.A.; Dean, H.T.; and Singleton, D.E. 1944. The effect on caries incidence of a single topical application of fluoride solution to the teeth of young adult males of a military population. *J. Dent. Res.* 23:155-62.
18. Rickles, N.H., and Becks, H. 1951. The effects of an acid and a neutral solution of sodium fluoride on the incidence of dental caries in young adults. *J. Dent. Res.* 30:757-65.
19. Stones, H.H.; Lawton, F.E.; Bransby, E.R.; and Hartley, H.O. 1949. The effect of topical applications of potassium fluoride and the ingestion of tablets containing sodium fluoride on the incidence of dental caries. *Brit. Dent. J.* 86:263-71.
20. Brudevold, F.; Savory, A.; Gardner, D.E.; Spinelli, M.; and Speirs, R. 1963. A study of acidulated fluoride solutions. I. *In vitro* effects on enamel. *Arch. Oral Biol.* 8:167-77.
21. Wellock, W.D., and Brudevold, F. 1963. A study of acidulated fluoride solutions. II. The caries inhibiting effect of single annual topical applications of an acidic fluoride and phosphate solution: a two year experience. *Arch. Oral Biol.* 8:179-82.
22. Pameijer, J.H.N.; Brudevold, F.; and Hunt, E.E., Jr. 1963. A study of acidulated fluoride solutions. III. The cariostatic effect of repeated topical sodium fluoride applications with and without phosphate: a pilot study. *Arch. Oral Biol.* 8:183-85.
23. Frazier, P.D., and Engen, D.W. 1966. X-ray diffraction study of the reaction of acidulated fluoride with powdered enamel. *J. Dent. Res.* 45:1144-48.
24. Wei, S.H.Y., and Forbes, W.C. 1968. X-ray diffraction analysis of the reactions between intact and powdered enamel and several fluoride solutions. *J. Dent. Res.* 47:471-77.
25. Baud, C.A., and Bang, S. 1970. Electron probe and X-ray diffraction and microanalysis of human enamel treated *in vitro* by fluoride solution. *Caries Res.* 4:1-13.
26. DeShazer, D.O., and Swartz, C.J. 1967. The formation of calcium fluoride on the surface of hydroxyapatite after treatment with acidic fluoride phosphate solutions. *Arch. Oral Biol.* 12:1071-75.
27. Mellberg, J.R.; Nicholson, C.R.; Franchi, G.J.; Englander, H.R.; and Mosley, G.W. 1977. Enamel fluoride uptake and retention from intensive APF gel applications *in vivo*. *J. Dent. Res.* 56:716-21.

28. Muhler, J.C., and van Huysen, G. 1947. Solubility of enamel protected by sodium fluoride and other compounds. *J. Dent. Res.* 26:119-27.
29. Hefferren, J.J. 1963. Qualitative and quantitative tests for stannous fluoride. *J. Pharm. Sci.* 52:1090-96.
30. Hercules, D.M., and Craig, N.L. 1978. Fluorine and tin uptake by enamel studied by X-ray photoelectron spectroscopy (ESCA). *J. Dent. Res.* 57:296-305.
31. Jordan, T.H.; Wei, S.H.Y.; Bromberger, S.H.; and King, J.C. 1971. $Sn_3F_3PO_4$: the product of the reaction between stannous fluoride and hydroxyapatite. *Arch. Oral Biol.* 16:241-46.
32. Berndt, A.F. 1972. Reaction of stannous fluoride with hydroxyapatite: the crystal structure of $Sn_3F_3PO_4$. *J. Dent. Res.* 51:53-57.
33. Nordquist, W.D.; Krutchkoff, D.J.; and Wei, S.H.Y. 1977. Influence of variable SnF_2 exposure time on *in vitro* $Sn_3F_3PO_4$ formation. *Caries Res.* 11:39-45.
34. Wei, S.H.Y., and Forbes, W.C. 1974. Electron microprobe investigations of stannous fluoride reactions with enamel surfaces. *J. Dent. Res.* 53:51-56.
35. Hoerman, K.C.; Klima, J.E.; Birks, L.S.; Nagel, D.J.; Ludwick, W.E.; and Lyon, H.W. 1966. Tin and fluoride uptake in human enamel *in situ.* Electron probe and chemical microanalysis. *J. Amer. Dent. Assoc.* 73:1301-5.
36. Collins, R.; Nebergall, W.; and Langer, H. 1961. A study of the reactions of various tin (II) compounds with calcium hydroxyapatite. *J. Am. Chem. Soc.* 83:3727-28.
37. Babcock, F.D.; King, J.C.; and Jordan, T.H. 1978. The reaction of stannous fluoride with hydroxyapatite. *J. Dent. Res.* 57:933-38.
38. Scott, D.B. 1960. Electron microscopic evidence of fluoride-enamel reaction. *J. Dent. Res.* 39:1117.
39. Cooley, W.E. 1961. Reactions of tin (II) and fluoride ions with etched enamel. *J. Dent. Res.* 40:1199-1210.
40. Muhler, J.C. 1960. Stannous fluoride enamel pigmentation: evidence of caries arrestment *J. Dent. Child.* 27:157-61.
41. Wellock, W.D.; Maitland, A.; and Brudevold, F. 1965. Caries increments, tooth discoloration, and state of oral hygiene in children given single annual applications of acid phosphate fluoride and stannous fluoride. *Arch. Oral Biol.* 10:453-60.
42. Horowitz, H.S., and Chamberlain, S.R. 1971. Pigmentation of teeth following topical applications of stannous fluoride in a non-fluoride area. *J. Publ. Hlth. Dent.* 31:32-37.
43. Fanning, E.A.; Gotjamanos, T.; Vowles, N.J.; van der Weilen, I.; and Cellier, K.M. 1968. The effects of fluoride dentifrices on the incidence and distribution of stained tooth surfaces in children. *Arch. Oral Biol.* 13:467-69.
44. Naylor, M.N., and Emslie, R.D. 1967. Clinical testing of stannous fluoride and sodium monofluorophosphate dentifrices in London school children. *Brit. Dent. J.* 123:17-25.
45. Slack, G.L.; Berman, D.S.; Martin, W.J.; and Hardie, J.M. 1967. Clinical testing of a stannous fluoride-calcium pyrophosphate dentifrice in Essex school girls. *Brit. Dent. J.* 123:26-33.
46. Horowitz, H.S., and Thompson, M. 1967. Evaluation of stannous fluoride dentifrice for use in dental public health programs. III. Supplementary findings. *J. Amer. Dent. Assoc.* 74:979-86.
47. Isaac, S., and Brudevold, F. 1957. Discoloration of teeth by metallic ions. *J. Dent. Res.* 36:753-58.
48. Shapiro, M., and Hood, J.S. 1956. Discoloration of gingiva and teeth by stannous fluoride. *J. Calif. Dent. Assoc. & Nev. Dent. Soc.* 32:174-77.
49. Snyder, J.R. 1964. Tooth enamel pigmentation tested with a new dental index during the 1961-1963 Moorhead dental study. *Northwest Dent.* 43:151.
50. Hals, E.; Torell, P.; and Morch, T. 1960. Effect of topically applied agents on enamel. V. Experiments *in vitro* with tin fluoride solutions. *Acta Odont. Scand.* 18:455-60.
51. Shannon, I.L., and Feller, R.P. 1973. Effect of extended storage on aqueous solutions of stannous fluoride. *J. Ind. Dent. Assn.* 45(4):59-64.
52. von der Fehr, F.F. 1961. The effect of fluorides on the caries resistance of enamel. *Acta Odont. Scand.* 19:431-42.
53. Shannon, I.L. 1969. Water free solutions of stannous fluoride and their incorporation into a gel for topical application. *Caries Res.* 3:339-47.
54. Shannon, I.L. 1963. Inactivation of stannous fluoride by calcium pyrophosphate. *J. So. Calif. Dent. Assn.* 31:396-99.
55. Ericsson, Y. 1961. The compatability of fluorides and common dentifrice components. pp. 79-91. Zurich: *Caries Symposium.*
56. Fischer, R.B.; Muhler, J.C.; and Wust, C.J. 1954. Effects of several fluoride reagents on the surface structure of powdered dental enamel. *J. Dent. Res.* 33:50-54.
57. Eanes, E.D. 1976. The reaction of monofluorophosphate with amorphous and apatitic calcium phosphates. *Caries Res.* 10:59-71.
58. Ingram, G.S. 1972. The reaction of mono-

fluorophosphate with apatite. *Caries Res.* 6:1-15.
59. Feller, R.P.; Shannon, I.L.; Matranga, L.F.; Osborne, H.W.; and Perez, R.S. 1976. Reduction of enamel solubility by sodium monofluorophosphate. *J. Dent. Res.* 55:510-14.
60. Ericsson, Y. 1963. The mechanism of monofluorophosphate action on hydroxyapatite and dental enamel. *Acta Odont. Scand.* 21:341-58.
61. Ingram, G.S. 1973. Some factors affecting the interaction of hydroxyapatite with sodium monofluorophosphate. *Caries Res.* 7:315-23.
62. Duff, E.J. 1973. Orthophosphates. XV. A suggested mechanism for the inhibition of dental caries by monofluorophosphate. *Caries Res.* 7:70-84.
63. Gron, P.; Brudevold, F.; and Aasenden, R. 1971. Monofluorophosphate interaction with hydroxyapatite and intact enamel. *Caries Res.* 5:202-14.
64. Ericsson, Y. 1967. Biologic splitting of PO_3F ions. *Caries Res.* 1:114-52.
65. Muhlemann, H.R.; Schmid, H.; and Konig, K.G. 1957. Enamel solubility reduction with inorganic and organic fluorides. *Helv. Odont. Acta* 1:23-33.
66. Muhlemann, H.R.; Rossinsky, K.; and Schait, A. 1967. Physikalisches, chemisches, and mikromorphologisches verhalten von schmelz noch behandlung mit anorganishen und aminfluoriden. *Schweiz. Mschr. Zahnheilk.* 77:230-48.
67. Rinderer, L.; Schait, A.; and Muhlemann, H.R. 1965. Loss of fluoride from dental enamel after topical fluoridation. *Helv. Odont. Acta* 9:148-50.
68. Shern, R.; Swing, K.W.; and Crawford, J.J. 1970. Prevention of plaque formation by organic fluorides. *J. Oral Med.* 25:93-97.
69. Schneider, P., and Muhlemann, H.R. 1974. The antiglycolytic action of amine fluorides on dental plaque. *Helv. Odont. Acta* 18 (Suppl. VIII): 63-70.
70. Mellberg, J.R.; Nicholson, C.R.; and Laakso, P.V. 1967. The effect of a barrier coating on fluoride uptake by human tooth enamel. *Arch. Oral Biol.* 12:1177-87.
71. Brudevold, F.; McCann, H.G.; Nilsson, R.; Richardson, B.; and Coklica, V. 1967. The chemistry of caries inhibition: problems and challenges in topical treatments. *J. Dent. Res.* 46:37-45.
72. Aasenden, R.; Brudevold, F.; and Richardson, B. 1968. Clearance of fluoride from the mouth after topical treatment or the use of a fluoride mouthrinse. *Arch. Oral Biol.* 13:625-36.
73. Mellberg, J.R.; Peterson, J.K.; and Nicholson, C.R. 1974. Fluoride uptake and caries inhibition from self-application of an acidulated phosphate fluoride prophylaxis paste. *Caries Res.* 8:52-60.
74. Sundvall-Hagland, I.; Brudevold, F.; Armstrong, W.D.; Gardner, D.E.; and Smith, F.A. 1959. A comparison of the increment of fluoride in enamel and the reduction in dental caries resulting from topical fluoride applications. *Arch. Oral Biol.* 1:74-79.
75. Mercer, V.N., and Muhler, J.C. 1965. The clinical demonstration of caries arrestment following topical stannous fluoride treatments. *J. Dent. Child.* 32:65-72.
76. Mericle, M.R., and Muhler, J.C. 1964. Reactions of NaF and SnF_2 with dental enamel having varying Ca:P ratios. *J. Dent. Res.* 43:1222-27.
77. Derrow, D.E.; Stookey, G.K.; and Muhler, J.C. 1961. Studies on the duration of a single application of 8% stannous fluoride in rats. *J. Dent. Res.* 40:712-13.
78. Shannon, I.L. 1965. The effect of exposing stannous fluoride treated enamel surfaces to whole saliva. *U.S. Army Air Force Tech. Rep.* SAM-TR-65-28.
79. Atkinson, H.F. 1948. The permeability of human enamel. II. An investigation employing a method of cataphoresis. *Brit. Dent. J.* 84:113-19.
80. Linden, L. 1968. Microscopic observations of fluid flow through enamel *in vitro*. *Odont. Revy* 19:1-17.
81. Adler, P.; Straub, J.; and Popovics, M. 1950. Intravital uptake of fluoride by the teeth under various conditions. *J. Dent. Res.* 29:549-50.
82. Adler, P, and Straub, J. 1950. Uptake of fluorine intravitally by intact human teeth from a topical sodium fluoride solution. *J. Experentia* 6:24.
83. Myers, H.M.; Hamilton, J.G.; and Becks, H. 1952. A tracer study of the transfer of F^{18} to teeth by topical application. *J. Dent. Res.* 31:743-50.
84. Bruun, C. 1973. Uptake and retention of fluoride by intact enamel *in vivo* after application of neutral sodium fluoride. *Scand. J. Dent. Res.* 81:92-100.
85. Mellberg, J.R., and Nicholson, C.R. 1968. *In vitro* fluoride uptake by erupted and unerupted tooth enamel. *J. Dent. Res.* 47:176.
86. Nicholson, C.R., and Mellberg, J.R. 1969. Effect of natural fluoride concentration of human tooth enamel on fluoride uptake *in vitro*. *J. Dent. Res.* 48:302-6.
87. Brudevold, F.; Hein, J.W.; Bonner, J.F.; Nevin, R.B.; Bibby, B.G.; and Hodge, H.C. 1957. Reaction of tooth surfaces with 1 ppm of fluoride as sodium fluoride. *J. Dent. Res.* 36:771-79.
88. Ericsson, Y. 1958. The distribution and reac-

tions of fluoride ions in enamel-saliva environment investigated with the radioactive fluorine isotope F 18. *Acta Odont. Scand.* 16:127-41.

89. Little, M.F.; Cooper, H.C.; and Rowley, J. 1971. Inorganic-organic interactions in human dental enamel. In International symposium on tooth enamel. Tooth enamel II. Its composition, properties, and fundamental structures. Eds. R.W. Fearnhead and M.V. Slack. Bristol: John Wright & Sons.
90. Weatherell, J.A.; Robinson, C.; and Hallsworth, A.S. 1972. Changes in the fluoride concentration of the labial enamel surface with age. *Caries Res.* 6:312-24.
91. Rogers, G.A., and Wagner, M.J. 1969. Protection of stripped enamel surfaces with topical fluoride applications. *Am. J. Orthodont.* 65:551-59.
92. Mellberg, J.R., and Loertscher, K.L. 1973. Fluoride acquisition *in vitro* by etched enamel from acidulated phosphate fluoride preparations. *J. Dent. Res.* 52:447-50.
93. Mellberg, J.R., and Shulman, L. 1974. The treatment of human teeth with fluoride for replantation and allotransplantation. *J. Dent. Res.* 53:844-46.
94. Wei, S.H.Y., and Forbes, W.C. 1969. Reactions of powdered sound dentin with several fluoride solutions. *J. Dent. Res.* 48:149-52.
95. Mühlemann, H.R. 1967. Die kariesprophylaktische wirkung der aminfluoride-10 jahre erfahrungen. *Die Quintessenz* 18: Ref 3192, Issues 5 to 8.
96. Heifetz, S.B.; Mellberg, J.R.; Winter, S.J.; and Doyle, J. 1970. *In vivo* fluoride uptake by enamel of teeth of human adults from various topical fluoride procedures. *Arch. Oral Biol.* 15:1171-81.
97. Kirkegaard, E. 1977. *In vitro* fluoride uptake in human dental enamel from various fluoride solutions. *Caries Res.* 11:16-23.
98. Arends, J., and Schuthof, J. 1975. Fluoride content in human enamel after fluoride application and washing — an *in vitro* study. *Caries Res.* 9:363-72.
99. Petersson, L.G. 1976. Fluorine gradients in outermost surface enamel after various forms of topical application of fluorides *in vivo. Odont. Revy* 27:25-50.
100. Duke, S., and Forward, G.C. 1978. Calcium fluoride and fluoridated hydroxyapatite formation in relation to the acid dissolution rate of enamel mineral. *Caries Res.* 12:12-20.
101. Mellberg, J.R. 1980. Rate of fluoride uptake by surface and subsurface sound enamel from sodium monofluorophosphate. *Caries Res.* 14:50-55.
102. Mellberg, J.R., and Loertscher, K.L. 1972. Fluoride acquisition *in vitro* by sound human tooth enamel from sodium fluoride and ammonium silicofluoride-phosphate solutions. *Arch. Oral Biol.* 17:1107-16.
103. Congleton, J.B.; Crenshaw, M.A.; and Bawden, J.W. 1978. The diffusion of fluoride from acidulated phosphate fluoride topical products. *J. Dent. Child.* 45:133-36.
104. Duckworth, R., and Braden, M. 1967. The uptake and release of fluorine-18 by human intact surface enamel *in vitro. Arch. Oral Biol.* 12:217-30.
105. Ericsson, Y. 1961. Fluorides in dentifrices. Investigations using radioactive fluorides. *Acta Odont. Scand.* 19:41-77.
106. Mellberg, J.R. 1966. Fluoride uptake by intact human tooth enamel from acidulated fluoride phosphate preparations. *J. Dent. Res.* 45:303-36.
107. Wei, S.H.Y. 1973. Fluoride uptake by enamel from topical solutions and gels: an *in vitro* study. *J. Dent. Child.* 40:299-302.
108. Mellberg, J.R., and Nicholson, C.R. 1964. *In vitro* evaluation of an acidulated phosphate fluoride prophylaxis paste. *Arch. Oral Biol.* 13:1223-34.
109. Wefel, J.S., and Wei. S.H.Y. 1979. *In vitro* evaluation of fluoride uptake from a thixotropic gel. *Ped. Dent.* 1:97-99.
110. Brewer, M.M., and Cussler, E.L. 1975. Accelerating monofluorophosphate uptake by hydroxyapatite. *Caries Res.* 9:119-26.
111. Shannon, I.L., and Gibson, W.A. 1963. Inactivation of stannous fluoride by calcium pyrophosphate. *J. So. Calif. Dent. Assn.* 31:396-99.
112. Hagen, A.R. 1972. The state of fluorine in dentifrice systems. *Acta Odont. Scand.* 30:167-86.
113. Hefferren, J.J.; Zimmerman, M.; and Koehler, H.M. 1966. Reactions of stannous fluoride with some inorganic compounds. *J. Dent. Res.* 45:1395-1402.
114. Vrbic, V.; Brudevold, F.; and McCann, H.G. 1967. Acquisition of fluoride by enamel from fluoride pumice pastes. *Helv. Odont. Acta* 11:21-26.
115. Kelly, G.E.; Stookey, G.K.; and Muhler, J.C. 1969. Laboratory studies concerning the development of a stannous fluoride-phosphate prophylactic paste. *J. Dent. Child.* 5:321-54.
116. DePaola, P.F.; and Mellberg, J.R. 1973. Caries experience and fluoride uptake in children receiving semi-annual prophylaxis with an acidulated phosphate fluoride paste. *J. Amer. Dent. Assoc.* 87:155-59.

117. Ericsson, Y. 1962. Aluminum compounds in fluoridated toothpastes and dental prophylaxis pastes. *Acta Odont. Scand.* 20:441-51.

118. Mellberg, J.R.; Nicholson, C.R.; and Trubman, A. 1973. The acquisition of fluoride by tooth enamel *in vivo* from self-applied APF gel and prophylaxis paste. *Caries Res.* 7:173-78.

119. Muhler, J.C.; Stookey, G.K.; and Bixler, D. 1965. Evaluation of the anticariogenic effect of mixtures of stannous fluoride and soluble phosphates. *J. Dent. Child.* 32:154-69.

120. Regolati, B., and Hotz, P. 1970. Effects of pyrophosphate and diphosphonate on fluoride uptake by hydroxyapatite. *Helv. Odont. Acta* 14:42-44.

121. Regolati, B., and Muhlemann, H.R. 1970. Effect of diphosphonate and fluoride on caries, fluorine content, and dissolution of rat molars. *Helv. Odont. Acta* 14:37-42.

122. Knutson, J.W.; Armstrong, W.D.; and Feldman, F.M. 1947. The effects of topically applied sodium fluoride on dental caries experience. *Publ. Hlth. Rep.* 62:425-30.

123. Ericsson, Y. 1958. The distribution and reaction of fluoride ions in enamel-saliva environment investigated with the radioactive fluorine isotope F18. *Acta Odont. Scand.* 16:127-41.

124. Rossinsky, K.; Schroeder, H.E.; and Muhlemann, H.R. 1967. Electron microscopic study of interference of salivary cuticle with topical fluoridation. *Helv. Odont. Acta* 11:163-68.

125. Bruun, C., and Stoltze, K. 1976. *In vivo* uptake of fluoride by surface enamel of cleaned and plaque covered teeth. *Scand. J. Dent. Res.* 84:268-75.

126. Joyston-Bechal, S.; Duckworth, R.; and Braden, M. 1976. The effect of artificially produced pellicle and plaque on the uptake of ^{18}F by human enamel *in vitro*. *Arch. Oral Biol.* 21:73-78.

127. Tinanoff, N.; Wei, S.H.Y.; and Parkins, F.M. 1974. Effect of a pumice prophylaxis on fluoride uptake in tooth enamel. *J. Amer. Dent. Assoc.* 88:384-89.

128. Tinanoff, N.; Wei, S.H.Y.; and Parkins, F.M. 1975. Effect of the acquired pellicle on fluoride uptake in tooth enamel *in vitro*. *Caries Res.* 9:224-30.

129. Joyston-Bechal, S.; Duckworth, R.; and Braden, M. 1973. The mechanism of uptake of ^{18}F by enamel from sodium fluoride and acidulated phosphate fluoride solutions labeled with ^{18}F. *Arch. Oral Biol.* 18:1077-89.

130. Stookey, G.K. 1973. The influence of length of topical application of stannous fluoride upon enamel fluoride content. *J. Indiana Dent. Assoc.* 52:498-501.

131. Scheinin, A. 1954. Studies on the acid solubility and fluorine content of sodium fluoride treated powdered dental enamel. Effects of concentration, temperature, time, and ultrasound. *Suomen Hammaslack* 50:53-64.

132. Barancos, R.J., and Strachan, D.S. 1966. The effect of temperature in the uptake of topical fluoride. IADR annual meeting, Abstract No. 217.

133. Putt, M.S.; Beltz, J.F.; and Muhler, J.C. 1978. Effect of temperature of SnF_2 solution on tin and fluoride uptake by bovine enamel. *J. Dent. Res.* 57:772-76.

134. Mellberg, J.R.; Englander, H.R.; and Nicholson, C.R. 1967. Acquisition of fluoride *in vivo* by deciduous enamel from daily topical sodium fluoride applications over 21 months. *Arch. Oral Biol.* 12:1139-48.

135. Mellberg, J.R., and Nicholson, C.R. 1974. Fluoride uptake *in vivo* by deciduous enamel of children from neutral fluoride and APF mouthrinses. *Caries Res.* 8:148-54.

136. Mellberg, J.R.; Nicholson, C.R.; Packer, M.W.; and Laswell, H.R. 1973. Fluoride concentrations in deciduous teeth of children using fluoride mouthrinses. *Caries Res.* 7:324-31.

137. Mellberg, J.R., and Nicholson, C.R. 1974. Weekly mouthrinsing with 3000 ppm of fluoride: the effect of concentration of fluoride in the enamel. *J. Publ. Hlth. Dent.* 34:2-7.

138. Aasenden, R.; DePaola, P.F.; and Brudevold, F. 1972. Effects of daily rinsing and ingestion of fluoride solutions upon dental caries and enamel fluoride. *Arch. Oral Biol.* 17:1705-14.

139. Ahrens, G. 1976. Effect of fluoride tablets on uptake and loss of fluoride in superficial enamel *in vivo*. *Caries Res.* 10:85-95.

140. Shern, R.J.; Driscoll, W.S.; and Korts, D.C. 1977. Enamel biopsy results of children receiving fluoride tablets. *J. Amer. Dent. Assoc.* 95:310-14.

141. Mellberg, J.R.; Nicholson, C.R.; and Law, F.E. 1972. Fluoride concentrations in deciduous tooth enamel of children chewing sodium fluoride tablets. *J. Dent. Res.* 51:551-54.

142. Shannon, I.L. 1970. Enamel solubility reduction by topical application of combinations of fluoride compounds. *J. Oral Med.* 25:12-17.

143. Shannon, I.L. 1970. *In vitro* enamel solubility reduction through sequential application of acidulated phosphofluoride and stannous fluoride. *J. Can. Dent. Assoc.* 36:308-10.

144. Shannon, I.L. 1971. Antisolubility effects of acidulated phosphofluoride and stannous fluoride in the treatment of crown and root surfaces. *Aust. Dent. J.* 16:240-42.

145. Shannon, I.L., and Wightman, J.R. 1970. Treatment of root surfaces with a combination of acidulated phosphofluoride and stannous fluoride. *J. Louisiana Dent. Assoc.* 28:14-17.
146. Shannon, I.L., and Feller, R.P. 1972. Enamel solubility reduction by mixtures of stannous fluoride and acidulated phosphofluoride. *J. Dent. Assoc. So. Afr.* 27:342-47.
147. Aasenden, R.; Brudevold, F.; and McCann, H.G. 1968. The response of intact and experimentally altered human enamel to topical fluoride. *Arch. Oral Biol.* 13:543-52.
148. Gedalia, I.; Azriel, B.; Zalkind, M.; Ersdorfer, J.E.; and Segal, B. 1971. Uptake of topically applied fluoride in enamel pretreated with phosphoric or citric acid. *J. Dent. Res.* 50:1358.
149. Brudevold, F.; Aasenden, R.; McCann, H.G.,III; and McCann, H.G. 1969. Use of an enamel biopsy method for determination of *in vivo* uptake of fluoride from topical treatments. *Caries Res.* 3:119-33.
150. McCann, H.G. 1969. The effect of fluoride complex formation on fluoride uptake and retention in human enamel. *Arch. Oral Biol.* 14:521-31.
151. Gerhardt, D.E., and Windeler, A.A. 1972. Fluoride uptake in natural tooth surfaces pretreated with aluminum nitrate. *J. Dent. Res.* 51:870.
152. Clarkson, B.N. 1976. The effect of metal ion pretreatment of enamel on fluoride uptake from acidulated phosphate fluoride. *J. Int. Assoc. Dent. Child.* 12:9-16.
153. Regolati, B.; Schait, A.; and Muhlemann, H.R. 1971. Studies on the effects of aluminum and fluoride on caries fluorine content and dissolution rate in rat molars. *J. Dent. Res.* 50:764-65.
154. Regolati, B.; Schait, A; Schmid, R.; Marthaler, T.M.; and Muhlemann, H.R. 1969. Effects of aluminum and fluoride on caries, fluorine content, and dissolution of rat molars. *Helv. Odont. Acta* 13:59-64.
155. Regolati, B.; Schait, A.; Schmid, R.; and Muhlemann, H.R. 1974. The effect of titanium, aluminum, and fluoride on rat caries. *Helv. Odont. Acta* 18:92-96.
156. Mundorff, S.A.; Little, M.F.; and Bibby, B.G. 1972. Enamel dissolution II. Action of titanium tetrafluoride. *J. Dent. Res.* 51:1567-71.
157. Clarkson, B.H. 1978. The effect of metal/fluoride complexes on fluoride uptake and caries-like lesion formation in enamel. *J. Dent. Res.* 57:784-89.
158. Richardson, B. 1967. Fixation of topically applied fluoride in enamel. *J. Dent. Res.* 46:87-91.
159. Dogan, I.L.; van Leeuwin, M.; and Kirklin, M. 1973. *In vivo* studies on the "sealing" of fluoride in teeth: two year clinical results. IADR annual meeting, Abstract No. 240.
160. Stamm, J.W. 1974. Fluoride uptake from topical sodium fluoride varnish measured by an *in vivo* enamel biopsy. *J. Can. Dent. Assoc.* 40:501-5.
161. Friedman, M.; van der Merwe, E.H.M.; Bischoff, J.I.; and Frysh, H. 1974. Sealing of fluoride on teeth *in vivo*: a preliminary report. *J. Dent. Res.* 53:722.
162. Petersson, L.G. 1975. *In vivo* fluorine uptake in human enamel following treatment with a varnish containing sodium fluoride. *Odont. Revy* 26:253.
163. Koch, G., and Peterson, L.G. 1972. Fluoride content of enamel surface treated with a varnish containing sodium fluoride. *Odont. Revy* 23:437-46.
164. Bang, S., and Kim, Y.J. 1973. Electron microprobe analysis of human tooth enamel coated *in vivo* with fluoride varnish. *Helv. Odont. Acta* 17:84-88.
165. Edenholm, H.; Johnson, G.; Koch, G.; and Petersson, L.G. 1977. Fluoride uptake and release in deciduous enamel after application of fluoride varnishes. *Swed. Dent. J.* 1:59-64.
166. Schmidt, H.F.M. 1964. Ein neus touchierungsmittel mit besonders land anhaltendem intensivem fluoridierungseffekt. *Stoma* 17:14-20.
167. Schmidt, H.F.M. 1964. In vitro untersuchungen uber die herabsetzung der loslichkeit menschlichen zahnschmelzes durch behandlung mit dem neuen touchierungsmittel fluor-lack ein vergleich mit einer 8% igen zinnfluoridlosung. *Stoma* 17:185.
168. Gulzow, H.J., and Jellinghous, M. 1973. Caries prophylaxis by local application of fluorides as solution, jelly, or lacquer. *Deutsch Zahnaerztl Z.* 28:592-97.
169. Manly, R.S., and Harrington, D.P. 1968. Release of fluoride to enamel by an adhesive bandage. *J. Am. Coll. Dent.* 35:34-44.
170. Barbakow, F.; van der Merwe, E.; Scanes, S.; and Fatti, L.P. 1973. Evaluation of an iontophoretic technique for increasing the fluoride concentration in enamel. *J. Dent. Res.* 52:616.
171. Gedalia, I.; Goldhaber, P.; and Golub, L. 1970. Fluoride uptake by enamel after immersion in 2% sodium fluoride solution with iontophoresis. *J. Dent. Res.* 49:1555.
172. Srinivasan, S.; Duic, L.; Reynolds, L.W.; and Kimmelman, B.B. 1975. Enhanced fluoride uptake by teeth through use of iontophoretic techniques. *Pharm. Ther. Dent.* 2:253-56.
173. Zadok, J.; Gedalia, I.; Weinman, J.; and Daphni, L. 1976. Fluoride uptake by root dentin after

immersion in 2% NaF solution with iontophoresis. *J. Dent. Res.* 55:310.

174. Roberts, M.W., and Henriques, B.L. 1974. Iontophoresis: a method of increasing the effects of fluoride dentifrice; a study in rats. *Aust. Dent. J.* 19:264-68.

175. Schegel, P.L.; Stowell, E.C.; and Emmerson, C.C. 1962. The influence of an electrical potential on topically applied fluorides. *J. So. Calif. Dent. Assoc.* 30:321-27.

176. Wagner, M.J., and Weil, T.M. 1966. Reductions of enamel acid solubility with electrophoretic fluoride applications. *J. Dent. Res.* 45:1563.

177. Collins, E.M. 1962. Densensitization of hypersensitive teeth. *Dental Digest* 68:360-63.

178. Jensen, A.L. 1964. Hypersensitivity controlled by iontophoresis: a double blind clinical investigation. *J. Amer. Dent. Assoc.* 68:216-25.

179. Murthy, K.S.; Tatlin, S.T.; and Singh, I. 1973. A comparative evaluation of topical application and iontophoresis of sodium fluoride for desensitization of hypersensitive dentin. *Oral Surg., Oral Med., Oral Pharm.* 36:448-58.

180. Scott, H.M., Jr. 1962. Reduction of sensitivity by electrophoresis. *J. Dent. Child.* 29:225-41.

181. Simmons, J.J. 1961. Ion densensitization of teeth. *Texas Dent. J.* 79:11-17.

182. Sandino, J.P.; Merlin, J.C.; Thomas, R.; and Vincent, R. 1973. *In vivo* study of the influence of an electrical potential on the diffusion of fluoride ions in dental enamel. *Schweiz Mschr. Zahn.* 83:587-93.

183. Pouezat, J.A. 1974. Electron microprobe analysis of fluoride in teeth treated *in vitro* by iontophoresis. *Inform. Dent.* 56:23-28.

184. Bang, S., and Pouezat, J.A. 1970. *In vitro* studies of fluoride permeability of human dental enamel: comparison of topical and iontophoretic applications. *J. Dent. Res.* 49:690.

185. Velitchkova, P. 1975. A comparative study of fluoride introduction in dental enamel by rubbing and electrophoresis. *Stomatologia* (Sofia) 1:33-36.

186. Minkov, B.; Marmari, I., Gedalia, I.; and Garfunkel, A. 1975. The effectiveness of sodium fluoride with and without iontophoresis on the reduction of hypersensitive dentin. *J. Periodont.* 46:246-49.

Chapter 7

Professionally Applied Topical Fluoride

The topical application of fluorides to erupted teeth has been investigated since the early 1940s. Based upon the assumed mechanism that fluoride will be deposited in the outer layers of enamel, making the teeth more resistant to acid dissolution, topical fluoride application by a dentist, hygienist, or other dental auxiliary has become an established caries-preventive procedure in most dental offices.

Currently, the dentist has a choice of topical fluoride agents. Additionally, the fluoride may be used in an aqueous solution, a viscous gel, a prophylaxis paste, or a dental varnish. The vehicle selected will, in part, determine the technique of application. The effect of these variables—fluoride agent, vehicle, and application technique—on the efficacy of the topical fluoride procedure will be discussed in the following sections.

The fluoride agent

A number of fluoride compounds have been studied as potential caries-preventive topical agents. These include lead fluoride,[1-3] potassium fluoride,[4,5] iron fluoride,[6] ammonium fluoride,[7] amine fluoride,[8] zirconium fluoride,[9] titanium tetrafluoride,[10,11] potassium fluorostannite,[12] sodium hexafluorozirconate,[13] sodium silicofluoride,[14] and stannous hexafluorozirconate.[15] Amine fluoride has gradually been receiving recognition as a topical caries-preventive agent. However, none of these fluoride compounds has proved superior in inhibiting dental caries nor gained acceptance over the three agents currently in use—neutral sodium fluoride, acidulated phosphate fluoride, and stannous fluoride.

Neutral sodium fluoride

Sodium fluoride (NaF) was the first topically applied fluoride compound. Studies using this agent were independently initiated in the 1940s by *Bibby*[16] and by *Knutson* and coworkers of the United States Public Health Service.[1,17-19] The concentration and application technique recommended by the Public Health Service was the technique accepted and first used by the dental profession.[20]

Technique of application

The Public Health Service recommended the use of an aqueous 2% NaF solution. If the NaF reagent is pure and uncontaminated, this solution has a pH of 7. Treatments were given in a series of four appointments. At the initial appointment, the teeth were first

Table 7-1 Effect of professionally applied neutral sodium fluoride solutions on the permanent teeth of children residing in fluoride-deficient communities

Study	Initial age (years) of subjects	No. applications per year	Duration of study (years)	Percent reduction DMFT	Percent reduction DMFS
Galagan and *Knutson*[1]	7–15	2	1	22	14
		4	1	41	34
		6	1	41	28
Galagan and *Knutson*[21]	6–16	2	1	20	13
		2	1	15	13
		3	1	27	24
Davies[22]	9–12	4	1		58
Hewat et al.[23]	13–14	4	1		18
Chrietzenberg[24]	6–12	4	1		47
Marshall-Day[25]	14–15	4	1		10
Bergman[26]	11–12	4	3		43
Cohen and *Schiffrin*[27]	6–16	4	2		43
Howell et al.[28]	8–15	4*	2	24	36
McLaren and *Brown*[29]	6–11	4*	1		39
			2		18
Nevitt et al.[30]	9–14	4	1.3		23
Harris[31]	6–11	4	5	33	
Law et al.[32]	7–13	4	1	35	36
Torell and Ericsson[33]	10	2	2		20
Averill et al.[34]	7–11	2	2	16	11
Cons et al.[35]	6–11	4*	3	17	11
Szwejda[36]	6–10	4*§	1	14	17
			2	19	21
			3	17	19
			1	48	42
			2	36	32
			3	38	41
Mercer and *Muhler*[37]	6–15	2	1	6	9
			2	29	27
Iizuka et al.[38]	6–11	4	2	36	45

*Treated only during the first study year.
§Two different application techniques employed.

cleaned with an aqueous pumice slurry. The teeth were then isolated with cotton rolls and dried with compressed air. Teeth were either isolated by quadrant or by half-mouth (right and left sides). Using cotton-tipped applicator sticks, the 2% NaF solution was painted on the air-dried teeth so that all surfaces were visibly wet. Then, with the teeth still isolated, the solution was allowed to dry for 3 to 4 minutes. This procedure was repeated for each of the isolated segments until all of the teeth were treated. A second, third, and fourth fluoride application, each *not* preceded by a prophylaxis, was scheduled at intervals of approximately one week. The four-visit procedure was recommended for ages 3, 7, 10, and 13 years, coinciding with the eruption of different groups of primary and permanent teeth. Thus, most of the teeth would be treated soon after their eruption, maximizing the protection afforded by the topical application.

Clinical efficacy

The most appropriate method for evaluating a potential anticaries agent is to determine its effect on caries incidence in the human mouth, that is, in controlled clinical trials. During the past 40 years, numerous trials have evaluated the caries protection afforded by the professional application of topical NaF. Because of the large number of studies, it is not possible to cite all of them; however, a representative list is presented in Table 7-1.[1,21-38]

For the studies listed in Table 7-1, and in other tables in this chapter, results are presented as the *percentage* reduction in new decayed, missing, or filled teeth (DMFT) or surfaces (DMFS) in the fluoride-treated group compared to a control group. While this is the accepted procedure, one should be aware that the use of the *percentage* difference, instead of the *absolute* difference in the caries increment between the two groups, can be misleading. For instance, a 50% reduction when the caries increment in the control group averages 2 DMFS per child a year means an average saving of one surface per child. However, when the caries increment in the control group is 1.2 DMFS per child, the same percentage reduction means only 0.6 surface saved per child. Although a 50% reduction is very respectable, in the latter example, the actual number of surfaces saved may have little clinical impact.

The studies presented in Table 7-1 evaluated professionally applied topical applications of NaF to the permanent teeth of children residing in fluoride-deficient communities.[1,21-38] While there is a wide range of reductions, from 9 to 58% for DMFS, approximately two-thirds of the studies reported reductions of over 20%. The average reduction for DMF surfaces for the 19 studies listed in Table 7-1 is 29%.

Clinical considerations

Topical applications of NaF began to be used by the dental profession at large in the late 1940s and early 1950s. The four-visit regimen at specific ages, as recommended by the United States Public Health Service, was not convenient for most private offices in which patients were normally recalled at 6- or 12-month intervals. Probably for this reason, the use of NaF has largely been superseded by other fluoride compounds, which are recommended for application on a schedule that is more convenient for office routine.

Stannous fluoride

Largely through the efforts of *Muhler* and his associates[39] at Indiana University, stannous fluoride (SnF_2) became the second topical fluoride agent to gain wide acceptance.

Stannous fluoride was selected from a large

number of fluoride salts that were tested for their effect on reducing enamel solubility. In laboratory experiments, the presence of the stannous ion with fluoride produced an enamel surface that was less acid soluble than surfaces treated with other fluoride compounds, including NaF. Although later experiments by *Mühlemann* and co-workers[40] showed that under certain experimental conditions NaF may be superior to SnF_2 in reducing enamel solubility, and *Brudevold* and *McCann*[41] questioned the entire concept of enamel solubility-reduction experiments, there is considerable evidence supporting the caries-inhibiting properties of SnF_2.

Technique of application

Stannous fluoride has been used at 8 and 10% concentrations in solutions equivalent to 2 and 2.5% fluoride. Although the 10% solution is usually used for adults and the 8% for children, there is no evidence of an actual clinical difference between the two.

Solutions of SnF_2 are not stable. Soon after mixing, they become cloudy due to the formation of tin hydroxide.[42] Since the stannous ion is believed to contribute to the anticaries benefits of SnF_2, aged solutions are considered to be clinically less effective. *Muhler* et al.[39] recommended that a fresh solution of SnF_2 be prepared for each patient.* While this recommendation has always been followed, there has been no clinical trial evaluating the efficacy of a fresh SnF_2 solution compared to an aged one. *Dunn* and *Shannon*[43] believe that aged solutions should maintain clinical effectiveness, but support their theory only with laboratory evidence of enamel solubility reduction.

Stannous fluoride is recommended for administration at 6- or 12-month intervals. When a patient is highly caries susceptible, the applications may even be more frequent. The treatment consists of two steps, in which the teeth are first thoroughly cleaned and then a freshly prepared aqueous solution of SnF_2 is applied.[44] Each tooth surface is cleaned with flour of pumice or other dental cleaning agent for 5 to 10 seconds, and unwaxed dental floss is passed between the interproximal areas. (Unwaxed floss has been recommended and continues to be used because it is believed that waxed floss may coat the tooth surface and adversely affect fluoride uptake. Laboratory studies, however, have shown that use of waxed floss does not substantially alter fluoride acquisition by enamel.[45]) A quadrant or half-mouth is isolated with cotton rolls and the SnF_2 is applied with cotton-tipped applicators. The solution is applied continuously, keeping the teeth moist, for 4 minutes. After treatment, the patient may expectorate but is instructed not to eat, drink, or rinse for at least 30 minutes. This instruction is made empirically since it may result in the teeth having a slightly longer fluoride contact. However, the importance of this instruction has yet to be proven.

It has been suggested that it is not necessary to apply SnF_2 for as long as 4 minutes, but that 30 or even 15 seconds is adequate. *Mercer* and *Muhler*[46] found similar caries inhibition using 4-minute and 30-second treatment times, and *Scola* and *Ostrom*[47] found even greater protection from 15 seconds than from 4 minutes. Contrary to these reports, *Horowitz* and *Heifetz*,[48] treating children in a fluoridated community, found that 30-second applications were less effective than 4-minute applications. Practitioners who use topical applications of SnF_2 in their preventive programs should continue to use a 4-minute treatment as originally recommended for this procedure.

*8% solution: 0.8 gm SnF_2 added to water to make 10 ml. 10% solution: 1.0 gm SnF_2 added to water to make 10 ml.

Table 7-2 Effect of professionally applied stannous fluoride solutions* on the permanent teeth of children residing in fluoride-deficient communities

Study	Initial age (years) of subjects	No. applications per year	Duration of study (years)	Percent reduction DMFT	DMFS
Jordan et al.[49]	12–13	1	2	38	38
Law et al.[32]	7–13	1	1	19	24
Mercer and *Muhler*[50]	6–14	1	1	50	51
		2	1	53	53
Peterson and *Williamson*[51]	9–13	1	2	26	24
Salter et al.[52]	6–7	1	1	65	56
		2	1	29	30
Harris[53]	7–12	2	3	23	
Mercer and *Muhler*[46]	5–15	2	1	38(81)§	39(78)
			2	44(68)	47(69)
Grissom et al.[54]	6–11	2	2		16
Wellock et al.[55]	8–12	1	1	+9	0
Torell and *Ericsson*[33]	10	1	2		4
Hass[56]	6–12	1	1	30	21
Horowitz and *Lucye*[128]	8–11	1	2	+3	+8
Cartwright et al.[57]	6–19	2	2	37	
Cons et al.[35]	6–11	1	3	8	8
Mercer and *Muhler*[37]	6–15	1	1	57	57
			2	55	57
Iizuka et al.[38]	6–11	1	2	13	23

*Only studies using an 8% SnF_2 concentration are listed.
§Two independent examiners.

Clinical efficacy

Table 7-2 presents the results of the topical application of 8% SnF_2 applied either once or twice a year to the permanent teeth of children residing in fluoride-deficient communities. In trials conducted by *Muhler* or his co-workers, caries reductions of approximately 40% or more were reported, and when 2% NaF and 8% SnF_2 were evaluated concurrently, SnF_2 demonstrated superior reductions.[58-62] However, the caries reductions obtained by other investigators using SnF_2 were generally less than those reported by the Indiana group. The average reduction (DMFS) for the studies listed in Table 7-2 is 32%. This figure is consistent with *Buonocore* and *Bibby's*[63] figure of 36%, which they obtained by averaging the results of 14 studies using topical SnF_2.

Variation between the results of independent clinical trials is not unexpected. Such factors as the age, initial caries experience, and number of subjects; the therapeutic agent employed, its concentration, and the frequency and method of application; the diagnostic criteria employed in the identification of caries, whether radiographs were used, and the duration of the study are all variables that cannot always be standardized and that will influence the outcome of a clinical trial. The consistently higher findings of the Indiana group of investigators, however, may be attributed to the claim that topical applications of SnF_2 can produce an arrestment of early carious lesions.[64-66] Arrestment of a lesion can lead to a reversal in clinical diagnosis. That is, a surface diagnosed as carious at an initial examination would be considered sound at a subsequent examination. A large number of reversals in the SnF_2-treated group would favor that group by elevating the percentage reduction. As discussed in Chapter 1, lesions have been known to clinically reverse. It is not clear, however, to what extent SnF_2 is active in reversing clinical lesions. A complicating factor, identified from laboratory studies on extracted teeth, is the ability of the tin moiety in SnF_2 solutions to alter the radiographic interpretation of "white spot" lesions by increasing the radiodensity of the demineralized enamel.[67,68] If a similar alteration occurs clinically, a carious lesion may be masked radiographically, rather than reversed.

Clinical considerations

The recommendation that SnF_2 be applied every 6 or 12 months is more suited for most dental office routines in which patients are usually recalled at these intervals. Because of the adaptability of SnF_2 treatments to office routine, many dentists switched from NaF to SnF_2 when the latter became available in the 1950s.

Stannous fluoride, however, has some disadvantages. The recommendation that it be prepared fresh for each patient is inconvenient. It has an astringent taste that many children find difficult to accept, and nausea appears to be more frequent with SnF_2 than with NaF. This may be partially due to the higher concentration of fluoride in the 8% SnF_2 solution. Pigmentation of teeth following topical application of SnF_2 has been reported. A brown discoloration can occur in "white spot" lesions, in plaque, and around the margins of some restorations.[55,64,69-71] The discoloration is the result of the deposition of tin phosphates that, with time, transform to colored compounds (probably tin sulfides), which is esthetically undesirable.[72,73]

Acidulated phosphate fluoride

In the 1960s, a new topical fluoride preparation, *acidulated phosphate fluoride* (APF) was introduced by *Brudevold* and his co-workers[74] at Forsyth Dental Center. The development of APF was based on the known information that slightly demineralized enamel acquired more fluoride than uneffected enamel. It was hypothesized that the addition of phosphate to acidified sodium fluoride would inhibit the enamel dissolution associated with the solution's low pH, but would still allow an increased fluoride uptake. The APF solution developed by these investigators was acidulated with orthophosphoric acid and buffered to a pH of approximately 3. Clinical testing of this preparation demonstrated that it was effective in reducing caries incidence.

Although *Muhler* and co-workers[75] prepared and clinically tested an APF solution using SnF_2, this preparation was never marketed. Currently available acidulated phosphate fluoride preparations all contain NaF as the active ingredient. The general formulation has 1.23% of fluoride as NaF, buffered to a pH of 3-4 in a 0.1 M phosphoric acid.

Technique of application

Acidulated phosphate fluoride solutions are available in aqueous solutions and gels. Fluoride preparations in gel form will be discussed later in this chapter. The preferred method of application using *aqueous* preparations of APF is the *paint-on* technique already described for SnF_2, with the exception that because APF is stable, it need not be freshly prepared for each patient. Acidulated phosphate fluoride is also recom-

Table 7-3 Effect of professionally applied acidulated phosphate fluoride solutions on the permanent teeth of children residing in fluoride-deficient communities

Study	Agent	Initial age (years) of subjects	No. applications per year	Duration of study (years)	Percent reduction DMFT	Percent reduction DMFS
Wellock and *Brudevold*[76]	1.2% F (NaF + HF)	8–11	1	1	55	71
	0.1 M H_3PO_4		1	2	67	70
	pH approximately 3					
Wellock et al.[55]	1.2% F (NaF + HF)	8–12	1	1	44	46
	0.1 M H_3PO_4		1	2	44	52
	pH approximately 3					
Muhler et al.[75]	8% SnF_2 + NaH_2PO_4, pH approximately 3	6–13	2	1	66	67
	3.6% NaF + K_2HPO_4, pH approximately 6	6–13	2	1	51	52
Averill et al.[34]	2% NaF + NaH_2PO_4, H_3PO_4, pH approximately 4.5	7–11	2	2	12	+2
Cartwright et al.[57]	1.2% F (NaF + HF)	6–9	2	2	49	
	0.1 M H_3PO_4					
	pH approximately 3					
Horowitz[77,78]	1.2% F (NaF + HF)	10–12	1	1	17	22
	0.1 M H_3PO_4		1	2	26	33
	pH approximately 3		1	3	27	30
Horowitz and *Doyle*[79]	1.2% F (NaF + HF)		2	1	28	27
	0.1 M H_3PO_4		2	2	26	33
	pH approximately 3		2	3	40	43
DePaola et al.[80]	1% NaF reduced to	6–8	3	1	23	21
	0.25% after first year;		3	2	6	11
	0.1 M H_3PO_4		3	3	1	13
	pH approximately 4					
Jordan et al.[81]	1.2% F (NaF + HF)	6–12	1	1	26	35
	0.1 M H_3PO_4					
	pH approximately 3					
Ingraham and *Williams*[82]	1.2% F (NaF + HF)	6–10	1	2	18	11
	0.1 M H_3PO_4					
	pH approximately 3					
Cons et al.[35]	1.2% F (NaF + HF)	6–11	1	3	16	+1
	0.1 M H_3PO_4					
	pH approximately 3					
Szwejda[36]	1.2% F (NaF + HF)	6–10	1	2	20	27
	0.1 M H_3PO_4		1	3	15	20
	pH approximately 3					
Iizuka et al.[38]	2% NaF	6–11	1	2	44	44
	0.15 M H_3PO_4					
	pH approximately 3.5					
Vrbic et al.[83]	4% NaF	10–12	1	3	16	23
	0.1 M H_3PO_4		2	3	29	31
	pH approximately 4.5					
Zahran[84]	2% NaF	7–9	2	1	3	8
	0.15 M H_3PO_4		2	2	18	18
	pH approximately 3		2	3	8	17
			2	4	2	5
Downer et al.[85]	1.2% F (NaF + HF)	14–15	2	3	34*	31*
	0.1 M H_3PO_4					
	pH approximately 3					

*Includes a prophylaxis with an APF paste and daily supervised brushing with an MPF dentifrice.

mended for application at 6- or 12-month intervals.

Clinical efficacy

Table 7-3 lists clinical studies using *aqueous* solutions of APF applied to the permanent teeth of children residing in fluoride-deficient communities. As with NaF and SnF_2, a wide range of effectiveness has been reported. Averaging the results of the studies listed in Table 7-3, a reduction of 28% is obtained.

Clinical considerations

Because APF is recommended for use in a treatment regimen and with a frequency identical to that recommended for SnF_2, the use of this agent easily accommodates most dental office schedules. Acidulated phosphate fluoride has the advantage over SnF_2 of being stable and of not producing staining of the enamel. Aqueous solutions are generally not flavored, however, and the taste is poorly tolerated by some children.

Amine fluoride

As used in dentistry, the amine fluorides represent a loose classification of compounds in which inorganic fluoride (e.g., HF) is reacted with the amine portion of an organic compound. The amine fluorides, therefore, differ from other organic fluoride compounds, such as the fluorinated hydrocarbons, in which the fluoride is attached directly to a carbon atom.

In 1957, *Mühlemann* and co-workers,[40] of the University of Zurich, first studied the effects of amine fluorides on enamel solubility *in vitro*. They found that, under the conditions of their study, certain organic fluorides were superior to inorganic fluorides in reducing enamel solubility. They attributed the improved effect to a combination of chemical protection afforded by the fluoride and physicochemical protection due to the organic portion of the molecule.

In addition to their ability to reduce enamel solubility, the amine fluorides have other properties that enhance their potential as cariostatic agents. Some of them are surface active, that is, they have an affinity for enamel and thus will hold the fluoride for a longer time against the tooth. They also have antibacterial properties. Their antibacterial effects appear to be greater than those that can be accounted for by the presence of fluoride alone and have been attributed to the organic portion of the molecule. Reduced plaque formation and antiglycolytic activity have both been reported with these compounds,[86-92] although not all studies have been positive.[93,94]

Laboratory experiments have shown amine fluoride preparations to be effective agents for reducing enamel solubility, increasing enamel fluoride, reducing plaque deposits, and preventing caries in experimental animals.[95-102] For the prevention of dental caries in humans, amine fluorides have been tested in dentifrices,[103-107] mouthrinses,[106,107] and topical gels, where they have been either brushed on the teeth or applied with a tray.[8,108] While the caries inhibiting potential of amine fluoride preparations appears to be good, despite their surfactant and antibacterial properties, it is not known if they are superior to the other currently available fluoride agents. Much of the research on amine fluorides has been conducted in Europe, especially by *Mühlemann* and coworkers. Interest by American researchers in the clinical application of amine fluorides has remained low.

The fluoride vehicle

Topical fluorides have been applied to the teeth as aqueous solutions or gels and have been incorporated into prophylaxis pastes and varnishes. The results of numerous clinical studies indicate that the vehicle in which the fluoride is incorporated can influence the level of clinical effectiveness.

Aqueous solutions

Aqueous solutions were the first, and for many years the principal vehicle in which professionally applied topical fluorides were available. All of the studies cited in Tables 7-1, 7-2, and 7-3 were performed using aqueous solutions of NaF, SnF_2, or APF. Obviously, the aqueous form of the fluoride is effective in reducing dental caries. However, application of aqueous fluorides using the two-step prophylaxis and topical fluoride method is a time-consuming procedure. Since the operator is either a dentist or dental hygienist whose time is compensated at a relatively high rate, professional topical fluoride application is very costly relative to the benefits derived.[109] For this reason, other vehicles for fluoride were sought that could be more expeditiously applied in a program of professional topical fluoride application.

Fluoride gels

Acidulated phosphate fluoride is available commercially as a gel. Gels are produced by the addition of an alkyl cellulose to the fluoride preparation, which increases its viscosity. These products have essentially the same formulation as the aqueous solution but with the addition of the gelling agent. Although neutral NaF can also be prepared as a gel, the authors are not aware of any product currently marketed in this form recommended for professional topical fluoride application. It has been reported that water-free gels of SnF_2 can be prepared and are effective in reducing enamel solubility in laboratory experiments.[110,111] However, a SnF_2 gel was never tested clinically in a professional program of topical fluoride application.

Fluoride gels have the advantage of being used in trays so that the entire mouth can be treated in a single application. The tray method is easier and less time-consuming than the paint-on technique used for aqueous solutions. Because of the convenience of the tray application, many dental offices now use an APF gel for professional topical fluoride treatments.

Table 7-4 lists studies using an APF gel-tray technique in which a professional application was usually performed once or twice a year. Most of these studies are positive, indicating that this method is effective in reducing dental caries. Nevertheless, the caries reductions reported using an APF gel-tray technique have been somewhat less than those reported from an APF aqueous solution paint-on technique (see Table 7-3). It is not known whether this difference is due to the different physical consistencies of the fluoride preparations or to the different application techniques. Alternatively, the reason may be that in most of the gel-tray studies, the gel was applied once, rather than twice a year. Some believe that the lack of a custom fit when commercial disposable trays are used may be a factor.

Fluoride-containing prophylaxis pastes

Prophylaxis pastes with fluoride were developed to allow the practitioner the opportunity to provide both the cleaning and the fluoride application in one step. While the ease and time saving of a single procedure is attractive, this approach has not proved to be an effective cariostatic method.

Table 7-4 Effect of acidulated fluoride gels applied topically with trays

Study	Initial age (years) of subjects	No. applications per year	Duration of study (years)	Percent reduction DMFT	DMFS
Horowitz [77,78]	10–12	1	1	12	14
Horowitz and *Doyle* [79]		1	2	12	22
		1	3	16	24
Horowitz and *Kau* [112]		*	5		21
Bryan and *Williams* [113]	8–12	1	1	45	28
Bryan and *Williams* [114]		**	2	45	37
Ingraham and *Williams* [82]	6–10	1	2	52	41
Swejda et al.[115]	7	1	1	+.3	+.5
Cons et al.[35]	6–11	1	4	25	18
Szwejda [116]	7–8	1	2	3	4
Shern et al.[8]	6–13	5§	2	+.5	
Mainwaring and *Naylor* [117]	11–15	2	3		14

*No additional applications; examined 2 years after discontinuation of treatment.
**No additional applications; examined 1 year after discontinuation of treatment.
§Five treatments applied on consecutive days during first year only.

One problem associated with fluoride-containing prophylaxis pastes is their formulation. There is a greater difference between the ingredients of different manufacturers' prophylaxis pastes than between different fluoride gels or aqueous solutions. Formulation problems with fluoride prophylaxis pastes include selection of a compatible abrasive, the presence of humectants, and the effect of viscosity. Use of incompatible abrasives (e.g., pumice), high concentrations of humectants (e.g., glycerol), or a high viscosity greatly reduces or inhibits fluoride uptake by enamel.[118]

Clinical trials of fluoride-containing prophylaxis pastes are listed in Table 7-5. Some of the first fluoride-containing prophylaxis pastes used either NaF or SnF_2 with lava pumice or silex as the abrasive. While clinical tests with these pastes were frequently positive, the pastes were never marketed. The first marketed fluoride-containing prophylaxis paste contained SnF_2 as the active ingredient and zirconium silicate as the abrasive. Since this product has recently been withdrawn from the market, its effectiveness is moot. Other marketed products contain either NaF, APF, or monofluorophosphate (used in dentifrice formulations). Few clinical studies of these marketed products have been reported. In two independent studies in which APF was applied twice a year by hygienists, one study reported a caries reduction while the other did not.[126,127] Fluoride is taken up by enamel following treatment with a fluoride-containing prophylaxis paste.[126,129] However, the increase appears to be transient[127,130] so that infrequent applications, once or twice a year, may not produce a significant long-term reduction in enamel solubility.

Table 7-5 Effect of professionally applied fluoride-containing prophylaxis pastes

Study	Initial age (years) of subjects	Agent and abrasive	No. applications per year	Duration of study (years)	Percent reduction DMFT	DMFS
Bibby et al.[119]	6–15	4% NaF, pumice	2	1		25
Peterson et al.[120]	10–13	17.5% SnF_2 silex, silicone	2	2	35 (39)*	42 (34)*
Scola and *Ostrom* [121,47]	17–24	17.5% SnF_2, pumice	1	1	12	12
			1	2	26	12
Bixler and *Muhler* [122,123]	5–18	8.9% SnF_2, pumice	2	1	31	35
			2	2	30	34
			2	3	33	35
Horowitz and *Lucye* [128]	8–10	8.9% SnF_2, pumice	1	2	+8	+6
Szwejda [36]	6–10	SnF_2**	1	2	13	17
			1	3	17	19
			1	2	9	20
			1	3	19	20
Szwejda [124]	6–10	1.9% NaF, 0.8% HF, H_3PO_4, sodium metaphosphate	1	1	12	
				2	0	
				3	1	8
Peterson et al.[125]	10–13	2.1% F ($KF \cdot H_2O$), H_3PO_4, pumice	1	2	14 (12)*	16 (15)*
DePaola and *Mellberg* [126]	10–13	APF: 0.4% F, ammonium fluorosilicate, SiO_2	2	2	17	21
Barenie et al.[127]	9–14	APF: 0.4% F, ammonium fluorosilicate, SiO_2	2	2	+7(+8)*	+5(+8)*

*Two independent examiners.
**No other description of the paste ingredients.

Fluoride varnishes

After topical fluoride application, there is a substantial leaching of absorbed fluoride from surface enamel.[131-133] To prevent this immediate loss, fluoride has been incorporated into varnishes that have the ability to adhere to enamel for long periods and, it is hypothesized, to slowly release the fluoride to the teeth. The retentive and possible slow release effects of these products increase the exposure time of the teeth to the fluoride by several days, without increasing chair time, and presumably allow fluoride to be more permanently bound to the teeth.

A NaF-containing varnish (Duraphat®—2.2% F) and an organic fluoride-containing varnish (Fluor Protector®—0.7% F) are available commercially in some countries, though not in the United States. The varnishes are applied to cotton roll-isolated teeth using a cotton-tipped applicator after the teeth have first received a prophylaxis and interproximal flossing. The varnishes harden in approximately 2 minutes and the time for application is approximately 5 or 6 minutes.

Teeth treated with fluoride varnishes will acquire a high concentration of fluoride in the outer enamel.[134-136] However, in one study, after extracted primary teeth were coated with fluoride varnishes for 24 hours and then stored in synthetic saliva for one week, a large loss of fluoride was reported.[136] After the 24-hour application of Duraphat® or Fluor Protector®, the fluoride content in the outer layer (2-5μ) of enamel rose from below 1,000 ppm to over 5,000 and 7,000 ppm respectively. Following a week's storage in synthetic saliva, the fluoride concentration of Duraphat®-treated enamel was approximately 3,500 ppm and that of Fluor Protector®-treated enamel was approximately 5,500 ppm.

Arends and *Schuthof*[137] have shown that both commercial fluoride varnishes will inhibit enamel decalcification and *in vitro* "white spot" formation. Other investigators have clinically tested the varnishes.[138-144] *Koch* and *Petersson*[140] found a dramatic 75% reduction in new caries in a one-year study in which children received two topical applications of fluoride varnish. While other clinical studies have also been positive, the reductions have been less dramatic[141-144] or the study design was not ideal.[138,139] Currently, the clinical evidence does not indicate that fluoride in this type of a vehicle is superior to fluoride in aqueous solutions.

Methods of application

The two most common professionally applied topical fluoride methods are the *paint-on technique* and the *tray technique*. While a spray application has been tried, it was never generally recommended.[145] Both the paint-on and the tray techniques involve a two-step procedure in which the teeth are first cleaned with pumice or other dental prophylaxis paste and the proximal surfaces of the teeth are flossed, and then the topical fluoride agent is applied.

Paint-on technique

All accessible surfaces of the teeth first receive a prophylaxis using a rotating rubber cup and dental prophylaxis paste. Since a pumice prophylaxis abraids a layer of fluoride-rich surface enamel,[146-149] a less abrasive paste, such as a silicon dioxide one, should be used.[130] A fluoride-containing prophylaxis paste is recommended for this step, since it may replace some of the enamel fluoride lost from the surface by abrasion. The rubber cup should be splayed while it is rotating so that the paste will contact as much of the proximal surfaces as possible. Next, unwaxed floss is passed between each interdental area removing plaque from each adjacent proximal surface before proceeding to the next area. Care should be taken to advance the floss in the hand so that a clean section engages each new tooth surface.

The patient is instructed to rinse the mouth, and the teeth are isolated using cotton rolls. Saliva absorbers may also be used to cover the parotid duct openings, and a saliva ejector should be placed beneath the tongue for maximum saliva control (Fig. 7-1). Either a quadrant at a time or half of the mouth (left or right) may be isolated and treated (Fig. 7–2a and b). The isolated teeth are then dried with compressed air and the fluoride is applied with cotton-tipped applicators. When using a paint-on technique, the fluoride is usually employed as an aqueous solution. The solution is continuously reapplied keeping the isolated teeth moist for 4 minutes. During this time, unwaxed dental floss, which has been soaked in the fluoride solution, is passed interproximally. The same procedure is then repeated for each quadrant or the other half of the mouth depending upon the method of isolation employed.

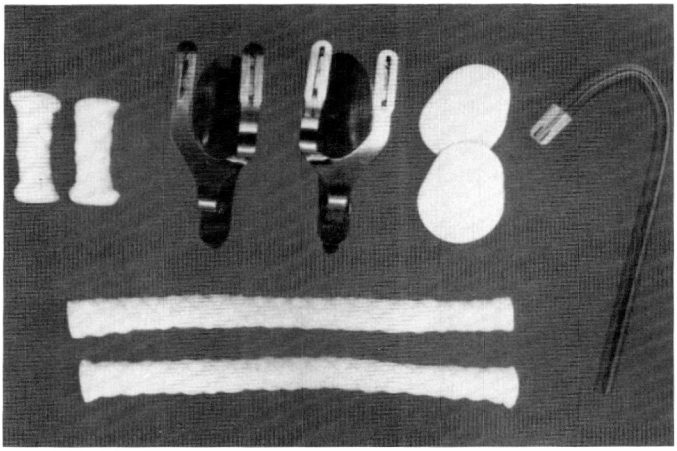

Fig. 7-1 Long and/or short cotton rolls, saliva absorbers, and a saliva ejector may all be used to keep the teeth dry during a topical fluoride application.

After treatment, the patient may expectorate, but is instructed not to rinse, eat, or drink for one-half hour.

Tray technique

With the introduction of APF, topical fluorides began to be marketed as gels. Fluoride gels can be applied in trays, and numerous types of trays, ranging from wax or paper to rubber with foam inserts, are commercially available (Fig. 7-3).

The teeth are first thoroughly cleaned as described for the paint-on technique. The patient is allowed to rinse and the teeth are dried with compressed air. Then a ribbon of fluoride gel is placed in each of two trays, which are inserted over the maxillary and mandibular teeth, and a saliva ejector is inserted. By using two trays simultaneously, the whole mouth can be treated in one application (Fig. 7-4). The trays are left in place for 4 minutes. During this time any excess that oozes from the trays may be aspirated by the saliva ejector or expectorated into a paper napkin that the patient holds.

After removal of the trays, the patient may expectorate but is instructed not to rinse, eat, or drink for 30 minutes.

Need for prophylaxis step

Application of topical fluoride is time-consuming. Whether a dentist performs the treatment or it is done by an auxiliary who is paid at a lower rate, the professional time involved makes it a costly procedure with a low cost-effectiveness ratio.[109] The prophylaxis and interproximal flossing takes approximately 15 minutes; the topical fluoride application takes 16 minutes (paint-on technique by quadrant), 8 minutes (paint-on technique by half-mouth), or 4 minutes (gel-tray technique). Thus, no matter which technique is employed, one professional can treat only two or three patients an hour.

While fluoride application times of less than one minute have been studied, they have not been generally recommended.[48,124] The time-consuming step in the procedure, however, is the prophylaxis step. For instance, if a gel-tray application technique was employed, nearly three-fourths of the treatment time would have been expended in cleaning the teeth.

Recently, the need for the prophylaxis step has been questioned. The rationale for the prophylaxis is that it removes materia alba, plaque, and other natural coatings from the

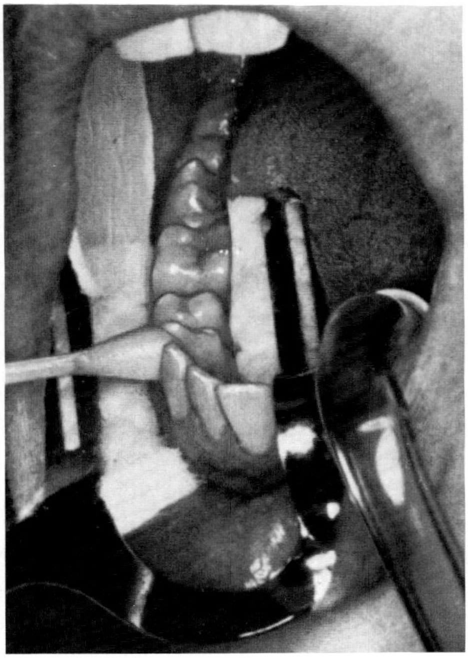

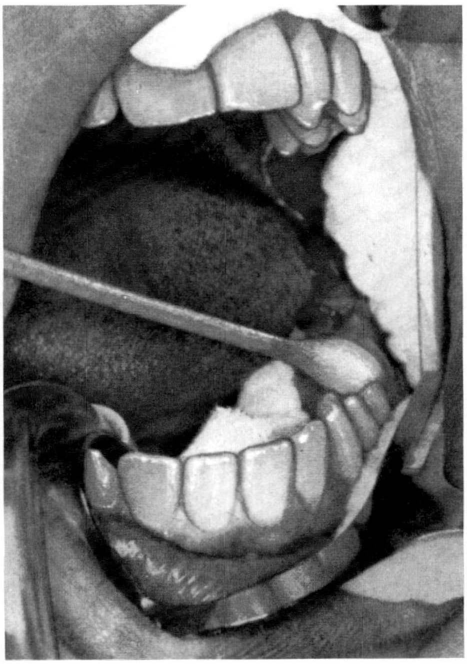

Figs. 7-2a and b Quadrant (a) [above] and half-mouth (b) isolation during topical fluoride application using the paint-on technique.

tooth surface that could act as a barrier to fluoride uptake.[20] In an *in vivo* study on schoolchildren, however, *Tinanoff* and coworkers[150] found no difference in fluoride uptake when an APF gel was applied by tray to permanent incisors that had been cleaned only with a toothbrush and water compared to incisors that had received a pumice prophylaxis. In another study, the same investigators, using blocks of human enamel, found that while the presence of organic pellicle could reduce the amount of fluoride uptake by surface enamel from an APF aqueous solution, cleaning the surface with either a toothbrush and water or pumice would result in similar levels of fluoride acquisition.[151] Of special interest is the study by *Bruun* and *Stoltze*,[152] who applied both neutral NaF and amine fluoride to plaque-covered and cleaned premolars in 12- to 14-year-old children. These investigators found that amine fluoride was deposited in the outer enamel, regardless of whether the surface first had been cleaned. Additionally, their results indicated that the presence of plaque may actually enhance the uptake of fluoride from NaF.

The results of these recent studies suggest that it may be possible to further streamline the technique of topical fluoride application by eliminating the preparatory prophylaxis step. Such a change would improve the cost-effectiveness of professionally applied topical fluoride programs. However, before this change could be recommended, it would be necessary to conduct clinical trials to determine whether caries reductions (as opposed to fluoride uptake) using the modified method are comparable to the more traditional, but professionally more time-consuming, two-step prophylaxis-application approach. These studies are already in progress.

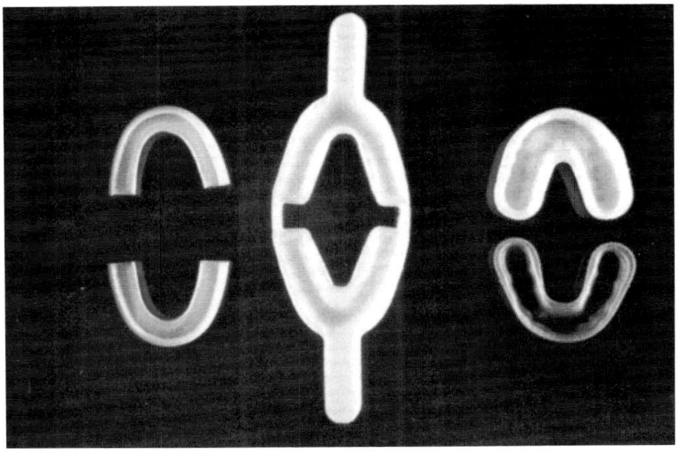

Fig. 7-3 Examples of commercially available disposable trays used with the gel-tray method of topical fluoride application.

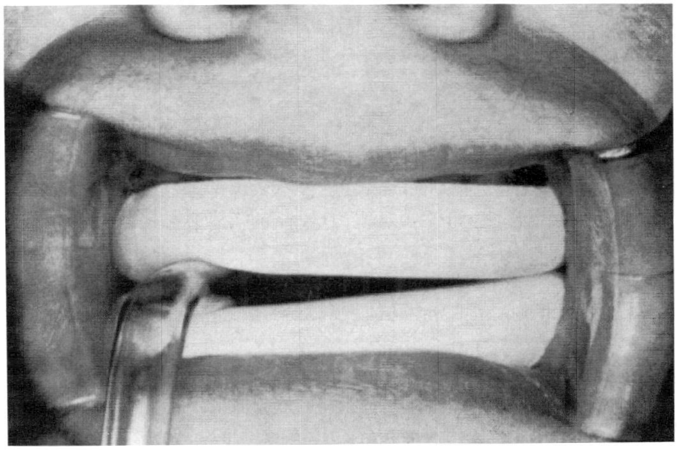

Fig. 7-4 Gel-tray topical fluoride application. The entire mouth is treated with a single 4-minute treatment.

Effectiveness of professionally applied topical fluoride in different clinical situations

The many clinical trials listed in Tables 7-1 through 7-5 were all conducted in fluoride-deficient communities and evaluated the effectiveness of professionally administered topical fluoride, specifically on the permanent teeth of children. There are other clinical circumstances in which the efficacy of topical fluoride treatments must be known. These are discussed in the following sections.

Effectiveness in optimally fluoridated communities

Compared to the large number of trials conducted in fluoride-deficient communities, the number of clinical studies in which the effect of professionally applied topical fluoride has been assessed in residents of optimally fluo-

Table 7-6 Effect of professionally applied topical fluoride on the permanent teeth of children residing in optimally fluoridated communities

Study	Fluoride agent	Initial age (years) of subjects	No. applications per year	Duration of study (years)	Percent reduction DMFT	Percent reduction DMFS
Downs and *Pelton*[153]	2% NaF	6–18	4	1	0	0
Galagan and *Vermillion*[154]	2% NaF	7–16	4	1	9	0
Muhler[155,156]	8% SnF_2	6–17	2	1	35	31
				2	46	35
				2.5	54	49
Horowitz and *Heifetz*[157,48]	8% SnF_2	7–9	1	1	17	10
				2	20	13
				3	21	21
Szwejda[124]	10% SnF_2	8–9	1	3	14	20
	1.23% APF solution		1	3	19	23
	APF gel		1	3	9	4
	APF prophylaxis paste		1	3	1	+2

ridated communities is exceedingly small. Of the studies listed in Table 7-6, in which NaF, SnF_2, and APF were tested on the permanent teeth of children, only the report by *Muhler* using SnF_2 obtained the degree of caries reduction generally observed in fluoride-deficient communities.[155,156] However, even the results of this study are equivocal. Since the community in which the study was conducted had been fluoridated for only 6 years when the study began, many of the 6- to 17-year-old subjects had not received lifelong benefits of waterborne fluoride.

In assessing the potential benefit from the use of topical fluoride applications in fluoridated areas, it must be recognized that in fluoridated communities the caries activity is already low. Thus, while a 30 to 40% caries reduction in a fluoride-deficient community may mean an annual reduction of one or more new carious surfaces per person, in a fluoridated community, the same percentage reduction may mean a decrease in the annual caries increment of less than one-half a surface. While this reduction may be *statistically* significant, it is not necessarily *clinically* significant; in fact, the cost of the preventive program could conceivably be more than the cost of restoring the teeth had the development of caries not been prevented.

Based upon the limited evidence available, the *routine* use of professionally administered topical fluoride to children who are lifelong residents of an optimally fluoridated community cannot be recommended. Dentists who practice in fluoridated communities must decide on an individual basis which patients could benefit from this procedure. Children who previously resided in a fluoride-deficient community and who, therefore, have had only limited benefits from community water fluoridation should be considered candidates for professionally applied topical fluoride. Children with an uncharacteristically high caries activity for the fluoridated community in which they reside should also receive professional topical fluoride applications.

Table 7-7 Effect of professionally applied topical fluoride on the primary teeth of children residing in fluoride-deficient or optimally fluoridated communities

Study	Fluoride agent	Initial age (years) of subjects	No. applications per year	Duration of study (years)	Percent reduction DEFT	Percent reduction DEFS
Fluoride-deficient communities						
Jordan et al.[158]	2% NaF	6–12	1	1	5	+3
			2	1	15	10
			3	1	40	17
Ast[159]	2% NaF	2–7	4	1		22
Jordan[160]	2% NaF	4–6	1	3	34	
Wittich[161]	2% NaF	3–6	2	2		22
Sundvall-Hagland et al.[162]	2% NaF	3–5	4*	1		34
				2		23
				3		12
Compton et al.[163]	8% SnF_2	2–4	1	1		28
Salter et al.[52]	8% SnF_2	6–7	1	1	45	42
Burgess et al.[164]	8% SnF_2	2–4	1	1		15
				2		25
Optimally fluoridated communities						
McDonald and *Muhler*[165]	2% NaF	3–12	4	1	21	12
	4% SnF_2	3–12	4	1	57	37
Schutze et al.[166]	APF prophylaxis paste	3–5	2	2		+16

*Treated first year only.

Effectiveness in the primary dentition

Studies in which topical fluorides have been professionally applied to the primary dentition are listed in Table 7-7. While the results of the studies conducted in fluoride-deficient communities generally are positive, the caries reductions reported for the primary teeth are not as great as those usually observed in the permanent dentition.

Only one study was conducted in which topical fluoride solutions were professionally applied to the primary teeth of children residing in a fluoridated community. In that study, *McDonald* and *Muhler*[165] reported superior results from SnF_2 applications compared to applications of NaF.

Because it is difficult to adequately isolate the primary dentition of young (preschool) children when performing a topical fluoride treatment, it has become common practice in some dental offices to omit the application of a fluoride solution and instead to administer a prophylaxis using a fluoride-containing prophylaxis paste. Only one study has evaluated the effectiveness of this procedure.[166] This study, conducted in a fluoridated community, failed to find an effect from biannual treatments.

Effectiveness in adults

Table 7-8 lists studies of professionally applied topical fluoride to the dentition of adults. Of the nine studies, two failed to demonstrate caries reductions; the others

Table 7-8 Effect of professionally applied topical fluoride on the teeth of adults residing in fluoride-deficient or optimally fluoridated communities

Study	Fluoride agent	Initial age (years) of subjects	No. applications per year	Duration of study (years)	Percent reduction DMFT	DMFS
Fluoride-deficient communities						
Arnold et al.[167]	1% NaF	17–23	1	1	0	0
Klinkenberg and *Bibby*[2]	1% NaF	18–40	5	1	47	45
Rickles and *Becks*[168]	2% NaF	22–34	2	2	19	37
Kutler and *Ireland*[169]	2% NaF	20–42	4	1	0	0
Carter et al.[170]	2% NaF	19–39	4	1	12	
Muhler[171]	10% SnF_2	17–39	1	1	24	16
Harris et al.[172]	10% SnF_2	30.1*	1	1		15(7)**
Scola and *Ostrom*[47]	SnF_2 multiple therapy***	17–24	1	2	50	48
Optimally fluoridated communities						
Muhler et al.[66]	SnF_2 multiple therapy***	dental students	2	2.5	68	64

*Mean age.
**Two independent examiners.
***Includes prophylaxis with SnF_2-containing prophylaxis paste, topical application of 10% SnF_2 solution, and use of SnF_2-containing dentifrice.

reported reductions of 7 to 64%. Thus, topical fluoride applications to the permanent teeth of adults can be beneficial. However, it must be remembered that the incidence of new carious lesions is greatest during the first few years after eruption. Compared to teeth in a younger population, noncarious teeth (or surfaces) in adults are less likely to decay. Therefore, the potential benefit of topical fluoride applications in adults is less than in children because of the decreased caries susceptibility of the remaining caries-free surfaces. Nevertheless, since many adults do develop carious lesions, the caries history of the individual adult patient should be evaluated to determine whether he or she should receive a professionally applied topical fluoride application.

Root surface carious lesions

Caries of the roots of the teeth is a dental condition almost unique to adults.[173-176] Portions of the roots can be exposed to cariogenic challenges in the oral cavity as a result of apical migration of the gingival attachment or from periodontal surgery. Since root surface lesions are similar to enamel lesions, differing mainly in the types of microorganisms that may be present, topical fluoride applications to root surfaces should provide a cariostatic benefit. While it has been shown that the amount of fluoride acquired by root surfaces is greater than that taken up by the enamel,[177] and that the acid solubility of root surfaces can be reduced by fluoride treatments,[178] there has been no clinical trial in which professionally applied topical fluoride has been specifically evaluated for its ability to prevent root surface lesions in adults.

Root surface hypersensitivity

Hypersensitivity of exposed root surfaces is another dental problem common to adults. Once the thin layer of covering cementum on the exposed root is lost, the unprotected dentin reacts to tactile, chemical, and thermal irritants within the oral cavity.

Despite the fact that root hypersensitivity affects most adults at some time and can be quite painful, there is no treatment that has been universally accepted as effective. A variety of materials have been applied topically as desensitizing agents to the exposed portion of the root. The rationale of treatment appears to be either to render the odontoblastic processes or nerve fibrils present in the dentin incapable of transmitting impulses, or to physically occlude the dentinal tubules, possibly through a process of mineralization. Desensitization has been attempted using such diverse materials as glycerin, formaldehyde, phenol, silver nitrate, strontium chloride, potassium nitrate, calcium hydroxide, dicalcium acid phosphate, calcium sucrose phosphate-calcium orthophosphate complex, and dental resins.[179-182] Topically applied fluoride compounds are also used for root desensitization. They are either self-applied, usually in a dentifrice[183-189] (see Chapter 8), or they are applied professionally in the dental office.[190-195]

Professional applications to reduce root hypersensitivity have included the use of a 33.3% NaF paste,[195] a 2% NaF solution,[190,192-194] and a 10% NaF solution.[191]

The method of topical application of these different fluoride preparations is similar in that they are applied to the exposed root surfaces of the isolated teeth for several minutes and the application is repeated at frequent intervals for several weeks. In the case of the 2% NaF solution, the hypersensitive teeth are isolated and carefully dried. Since air drying may be painful, drying is achieved by wiping the teeth with dry cotton pellets. A piece of cotton, soaked in the NaF solution (room temperature) is placed against the exposed cervical dentin for 3 minutes. During this time, additional NaF solution is applied to the cotton to keep it wet. Applications are performed twice a week for 4 to 6 weeks.

In 1960, iontophoresis of fluoride was introduced for the treatment of cervical hypersensitivity.[196,197] *Iontophoresis,* or *electrophoresis,* as used in health care, refers to the movement of charged particles (ions) into the body by means of an electric current. In the treatment of hypersensitive dentin, the negatively charged fluoride ion is electrically induced into the tooth by placing one pole from a battery or commercial desensitizer on an NaF-bathed tooth (usually using NaF-soaked cotton), while the other electrode is held in the patient's hand or attached to the patient's arm. *Minkov* and associates[190] compared the effects on cervical hypersensitivity of a topical application of 2% NaF solution with and without the use of iontophoresis. They found that both treatments reduced hypersensitivity and that there was no difference in the effectiveness of the two methods. *Gangarosa* and *Park,*[193] however, claimed that *Minkov* et al. applied the wrong electrode to the teeth. Also using a 2% NaF solution, *Gangarosa* and *Park* found that good immediate reductions in sensitivity could be obtained when the cathode, or negative pole, of the commercial desensitizer was applied to the teeth, compared to moderate reductions when the positive anode, which had been used by *Minkov's* group, was applied. While *Gangarosa* and *Park* did not treat teeth for comparison using an NaF solution without iontophoresis, they did demonstrate that iontophoresis with sodium chloride was ineffective in reducing root hypersensitivity.

Whatever method is chosen for treating cervical hypersensitivity in the office, it is recommended that patients continue self-treatment at home. This can be done by having the patient routinely use a dentifrice containing strontium chloride, which is especially marketed for patients with cervical hypersensitivity,[198-200] or by the use of a monofluorophosphate-containing dentifrice, which has also been shown to be effective in such cases.[183,185,186] At least one clinician recommends home use of an APF gel (1.23% fluoride) in custom-fitted polyvinyl trays applied at a frequency of one or more times a week for several months.[189]

While the mechanism whereby fluoride reduces dentin hypersensitivity is not understood, recent evidence suggests that stimuli may be either mechanically blocked by precipitated fluoride compounds in the dentin tubules, or biochemically blocked by labile fluoride in the organic dentin matrix.[201]

Effect of multiple topical fluoride preparations

The value of multiple topical fluoride preparations used simultaneously in the same patient was first evaluated by *Muhler* and his associates. They tested the daily use of a SnF_2-containing dentifrice together with biannual topical fluoride treatments using a SnF_2 solution preceded by a prophylaxis with a SnF_2 prophylaxis paste.[47,66,85,117,120-123,128,202,203] The studies were conducted in both optimally fluoridated and fluoride-deficient communities. In general, as seen in Table 7-9, the multiple therapy produced superior caries reductions compared to what would have been expected from the use of any one fluoride preparation alone. The clinical trial of *Scola* and *Ostrom,*[47,121] in which naval personnel were treated with multiple SnF_2 therapy, supported the findings of *Muhler's* group, while the investigations of *Peterson* and co-workers[120] and *Horowitz* and *Lucye*[128] did not. Other investigators used different fluoride compounds in multiple topical fluoride preparation programs with varying degrees of success.[85,117,202]

Since most children normally brush at home with a fluoridated dentifrice, it is important to know whether additional protection can be obtained from professionally applied topical fluoride applications. Although not conclusive, the results of the studies listed in Table 7-9 support the hypothesis that the two regimens used in the same patient can provide a greater protection than can be obtained from the use of either technique alone.

The efficacy of fluoride-containing prophylaxis pastes was discussed in a previous section. It was recommended that these pastes should not be used in place of the conventional two-step prophylaxis-topical fluoride procedure, but that they could replace fluoride-free pastes during this procedure or whenever a prophylaxis is performed. While it is desirable to know whether use of a fluoride-containing prophylaxis paste prior to a topical fluoride application will increase the expected caries reduction, the studies listed in Table 7-9 do not provide this information. With one exception, the design of these studies did not include a treatment group that received a topical fluoride application in which the preliminary prophylaxis was performed with a fluoride-free paste. In the one investigation that allowed comparison, none of the treatment groups derived any benefit from the fluoride therapy.[128]

A unique method using multiple fluoride preparations was employed by *Lindhe* and *Axelsson.*[204] They gave professional prophylaxes every 2 weeks to 7- to 14-year-old children using a sodium monofluorophosphate prophylaxis paste and supervised toothbrushing once a month with a 0.2% NaF solution. After one year, there were 98% fewer carious lesions in the fluoride-treated group compared to a control group of children. This procedure, which obviously is an attempt to combine fluoride therapy and plaque control, required an exceptional amount of professional time and, therefore, may not be very practical. However, the dramatic reduction demonstrates that intensive

Table 7-9 Effect of professionally applied multiple fluoride therapy on the permanent teeth of individuals residing in fluoride-deficient or optimally fluoridated communities

Study	Fluoride treatments*	Initial age (years) of subjects	No. applications per year	Duration of study (years)	Percent reduction DMFT	Percent reduction DMFS
Fluoride-deficient communities						
Bixler and *Muhler*[122,123]	P**	5–18	2	1	31 (39)+	35 (34)
	P + D				31 (27)	37 (32)
	P + T				46 (40)	48 (42)
	P + T + D				73 (55)	75 (58)
	P	5–18	2	2	24 (36)	31 (37)
	P + D				29 (25)	37 (32)
	P + T				35 (46)	39 (43)
	P + T + D				66 (50)	70 (55)
	P	5–18	2	3	29 (36)	29 (38)
	P + D				35 (33)	39 (36)
	P + T				39 (58)	40 (56)
	P + T + D				63 (49)	67 (50)
Horowitz and *Lucye*[128]	P**	8–11	1	2	+8	+6
	T				+2	+8
	P + T				+3	1
Peterson et al.[120]	P**	10–13	1	2	28	34
	P + T				29	32
	P		2	2	35	42
Scola and *Ostrom*[121,47]	P**	17–24	1	1	12	12
	P + D				29	48
	P + T				47	43
	P + T + D				51	45
	P	17–24	1	2	26	12
	P + D				47	42
	P + T				34	27
	P + T + D				50	48
Beiswanger et al.[202]	T + D***	7–14	1	1	49 (45)§	48 (57)
				2	22 (24)	19 (24)
Downer et al.[85]	P + T + D****	11–12	2	3	34	31
Mainwaring and *Naylor*[117]	D_1*****	11–12	2	3		16
	D_2					17
	T					13
	D_1 + T					28
Optimally fluoridated communities						
Gish and *Muhler*[203]	P**	6–14	2	1	29 (45)+	40 (42)
	P + T				68 (58)	75 (58)
	P + T + D				62 (76)	69 (73)
Muhler et al.[66]	P + T + D**	dental students	2	2.5	68	64

+ Two independent examiners. §Reductions compared to use of APF topical zone.
* P = Fluoride containing prophylaxis paste. T = Professional topical fluoride application. D = Fluoide-containing dentifrice.
** SnF_2 active ingredient in P, T, and D. *** SnF_2 active ingredient in D; APF active ingredient in T (solution).
**** Sodium monofluorophosphate active ingredient in D; APF active ingredient in P and T (solution).
***** Sodium monofluorophosphate active ingredient in D_1 and D_2; APF active ingredient in T used as gel with tray.

therapy can produce highly favorable results.

Fluoride treatment of avulsed teeth

An emergency situation faced by dentists is the traumatic avulsion of an anterior tooth. If the tooth can be located, it is recommended that it be replanted as soon as possible after the accident. Replanted teeth, however, do not have a good prognosis and most of them are eventually lost because of external resorption of the root.
Studies conducted on laboratory animals have shown that the immersion of extracted teeth in fluoride solutions will greatly inhibit root resorption following replantation.[205,206] The immersion treatment significantly increases the amount of fluoride in the cementum,[177,207] and it has been proposed that this makes the root surface more resistant to resorption. Additionally, following replantation, some of the fluoride is released to the adjacent alveolar bone and may inhibit osteoclastic activity in the surrounding bone.[207]
It has been suggested that avulsed teeth be treated by immersion in a fluoride solution prior to their replantation. To date, however, no clinical study utilizing this technique has been reported.

Fluoride-containing dental materials and devices

Restorative materials, cements, and varnishes

Decay along the margins of restorations is called *recurrent caries.*[208] These lesions are not literally the reappearance of the same lesion for which the tooth was restored, but usually are new lesions that initiated at either the uncut enamel surface adjacent to the restoration or along the cut walls of the cavity preparation.[209,210]
Laswell[211] examined the status of restorations in naval recruits and found that recurrent caries was associated with 9.2% of existing amalgam restorations, 8% of resin restorations, and only 3.8% of silicate restorations. This finding confirmed the impression of practicing dentists that teeth restored with silicate were less susceptible to recurrent caries than those restored with other materials. Fluoride is incorporated into silicate powder during the manufacturing process and can be present in concentrations as high as 130,000 ppm. This fluoride slowly leaches out of the restoration and is taken up by the adjacent tooth enamel. *Hallsworth* and *Weatherell*[212] found a fluoride content of approximately 3,000 ppm in incisor enamel that was in direct contact with a silicate cement restoration, compared to a fluoride concentration of less than 100 ppm in inner enamel elsewhere in the tooth. Several laboratory studies have confirmed that transfer of fluoride occurs between silicate cement and enamel and that, as a consequence, the enamel is less susceptible to acid dissolution.[213-217] The alteration of solubility is believed to be the mechanism that makes the cavosurface margins of silicate cement restorations less susceptible to recurrent caries.[218,219]
Dental researchers have deliberately added fluoride to other dental restorative materials, to luting cements, and to cavity varnishes in order to impart a cariostatic property to these materials similar to that achieved by the silicate cements. Silver amalgam containing stannous fluoride or calcium fluoride has been prepared and evaluated by *in vitro* methodology for enamel solubility reduction and fluoride uptake.[220,221] Similar studies have also been performed with zinc phosphate cements to which stannous fluoride or sodium fluoride was added;[222-224] with cavity varnishes and liners to which calcium monofluorophosphate ($CaPO_3F$), potassium

fluorozirconate (K_2ZrF_6), sodium fluoride, or amine fluorides have been added;[225-227] and with composite resins, silicophosphate cements, and polycarboxylate cements.[214-216,228,229]

For all of the dental materials listed above, laboratory studies have demonstrated their ability to impart fluoride to enamel or to reduce enamel solubility. While these findings indicate the potential value of adding fluoride to dental materials, almost no study has actually clinically tested fluoride-enriched dental materials for their ability to prevent recurrent caries.[230] Additionally, the incorporation of fluoride into amalgam and dental cements, with the possible exception of the carboxylates, adversely affects the physical properties of the materials for oral use. Because of the dearth of clinical evidence of caries protection and the unknown effects of added fluoride on clinical performance, materials to which fluoride has been deliberately added must be considered experimental at this time.

Sealants are effective in preventing occlusal caries as long as they adhere to the tooth surface. Retention of sealants, however, is not indefinite and, if a lost sealant is not replaced, caries can develop in the vulnerable pits and fissures.

Dental researchers have investigated the use of fluoride with the sealant technique in order to provide caries protection to occlusal surfaces after sealants have been lost. Topical fluoride application and occlusal sealant placement have been provided concomitantly.[231] However, it is generally agreed that a topical fluoride treatment should not be performed on occlusal surfaces either *immediately* before acid conditioning or between the acid conditioning step and sealant placement.[232-236] Topical fluorides react with conditioned enamel to form globular reaction products (possibly amorphous calcium fluoride), which significantly decrease the bond strength between the sealant and enamel surface.[237]

In an attempt to circumvent the adverse effects of topical fluorides on sealant retention, fluorides have been added to either the acid etchant[238] or to the sealant itself.[239,240] Addition of sodium fluoride to the phosphoric acid conditioning solution resulted in a reduced bond strength between the sealant and etched enamel surface and, therefore, this procedure is contraindicated.[238] On the other hand, the addition of sodium fluoride to several different sealant systems produced a significant increase in the fluoride content of the enamel against which the sealants were placed without significantly affecting the bond strength between the resin and enamel surface, impairing the resins' physical properties, or increasing microleakage at the sealant-enamel interface.[239] In a laboratory study, a fluoride-containing polyurethane resin, known to release fluoride to the enamel, was effective in arresting carious lesions in rat molars, although no comparison was made of the effects of the polyurethane system without fluoride additions.[240]

Of the several methods in which fluoride therapy and sealant therapy have been combined, the addition of fluoride to the sealant itself appears to offer the most promising results.

Dental devices

Both dental floss and dental prophylaxis cups have been impregnated with fluorides as additional methods for imparting fluoride to the teeth.[241-244]

Fluoride-impregnated dental floss

Chaet and *Wei*[241] evaluated the fluoride uptake of extracted human molar teeth from multiple contact with dry nonwaxed dental floss that had been previously treated with an APF solution. Approximately three times as much fluoride was analyzed in the surfaces treated with the fluoride-impregnated dental floss as in those treated with plain dental floss. Using dental assistants and dental students as subjects, these same investigators evaluated the effect of the fluoride-impregnated floss on the colonization of *Streptococcus mutans* on interproximal surfaces. While the number of *in vivo* interproximal areas harboring *Streptococcus mutans* was significantly reduced by the use of the fluoride-impregnated dental floss, adherence to the twice-daily flossing regimen was poor. Since the subjects had a dental background that should have enhanced motivation and the period of the trial was short, it seems unlikely that the use of dental floss, with or without fluoride, will ever be a significant method of reducing dental decay in the general population.

Fluoride-impregnated prophylaxis cup

The temperature of the enamel surface is raised during a prophylaxis because of the friction between the prophylaxis cup and the tooth. High temperatures enhance fluoride uptake from topical fluoride solutions.[245-247] It was, therefore, reasoned that if a fluoride-impregnated prophylaxis cup was developed, fluoride would be released from the prophylaxis cup under optimal conditions and be deposited in the outer layer of the enamel. Laboratory studies have confirmed that prophylaxis cups made from a blend of thermoplastic resins and impregnated with sodium fluoride and stannous fluoride will increase the fluoride content of enamel and will increase the resistance of the treated surfaces to acid dissolution.[242-244] However, the amount of fluoride deposited in enamel when a fluoride-containing prophylaxis paste is used was generally found to be similar whether a conventional or fluoride-impregnated prophylaxis cup was used.[242,243] Therefore, there appears to be no advantage to use of a fluoride-impregnated prophylaxis cup if a fluoride-containing prophylaxis paste is already being used.

Summary

Professionally applied topical fluoride treatments have been evaluated for approximately 40 years. The topical fluoride compounds that have been most thoroughly studied are neutral NaF, acidulated phosphate fluoride (APF), and SnF_2. These compounds appear to exhibit a similar range of clinical effectiveness when applied to the permanent teeth of children residing in fluoride-deficient communities. Amine fluorides are also effective as topical fluoride agents; however, it is not known whether these compounds are superior to the inorganic fluorides already in use.

In the development of professional topical fluoride therapy, different vehicles for the topical agents and different methods of application have been evaluated. Fluoride has been used in aqueous solution, in a gel, and in dental prophylaxis pastes. The most consistent results have been obtained when the fluoride was used in aqueous solution. Conversely, the results of studies employing fluoride-containing prophylaxis pastes suggest that this method of fluoride therapy should not be the sole means of application when performing topical fluoride treatment. A two-step topical fluoride technique is recommended whereby the teeth are first cleaned and then the topical fluoride is applied. The incorporation of the fluoride into a viscous gel allows a convenient and time-saving tray application. While the need for the preliminary cleaning step has been recently questioned, there is, at this time, no clinical evidence that would prompt a recommendation that it be eliminated.

Topical fluoride applications are effective in the primary dentition; however, the caries reductions are generally not as great as those reported for the permanent teeth. Topical treatments are also effective in adults, although the need to prevent enamel lesions may be less, since the teeth of older patients are presumably less susceptible to decay. Theoretically, topical fluoride treatments should protect against root caries in adult patients with exposed root surfaces. In adults with hypersensitive roots, topical fluoride therapy has proved effective in controlling the hypersensitivity.

The *routine* use of professional topical fluoride applications cannot be recommended for patients who are lifelong residents of an optimally fluoridated community. However, individual patients with a high caries activity, despite a history of communal water fluoride contact, and transients, who previously resided in a fluoride-deficient community, are candidates for professional topical fluoride therapy.

Fluoride compounds have been added to various dental materials in order to prevent recurrent caries. The fluoride from these materials will usually be acquired by the adjacent tooth enamel with a concomitant reduction in enamel solubility. It is, therefore, expected that they would be effective in reducing the incidence of recurrent caries in restored teeth. However, because clinical tests of these agents are scant, they cannot be unreservedly recommended.

References

1. Galagan, D.J., and Knutson, J.W. 1947. The effect of topically applied fluorides on dental caries experience. V. Report of findings with two, four, and six applications of sodium fluoride and lead fluoride. *Pub. Health Rep.* 62:1477-83.
2. Klinkenberg, E., and Bibby, B.G. 1950. The effect of topical applications of fluorides on dental caries in young adults. *J. Dent. Res.* 29:4-7.
3. Knutson, J.W., and Scholz, G.C. 1950. The effect of topically applied fluorides on dental caries experience. *N.Y.J. Dent.* 20:72-78.
4. Cheyne, V.D. 1942. Human dental caries and topically applied fluorine: a preliminary report. *J Amer. Dent. Assoc.* 29:804-7.
5. Stones, H.H.; Lawton, F.E.; Bransby, E.R.; and Hartley, H.O. 1949. The effect of topical applications of potassium fluoride and of the ingestion of tablets containing sodium fluoride on the incidence of dental caries. *Brit. Dent. J.* 86:263-71.
6. Fjaestad-Seger, M.; Norstedt-Larsson, K.; and Torell, P. 1962. Forsak med enkla metodor for klinisk fluorapplikation. *Sverig. Tandlak. Forb. Tindu.* 53:169-73.
7. Caslavska, V.; Brudevold, F.; Vrbic, V.; and Moreno, E.C. 1971. Response of human enamel to topical application of ammonium fluoride. *Arch. Oral Biol.* 16:1173-80.
8. Shern, R.J.; Duany, L.F.; Senning, R.S.; and Zinner, D.D. 1976. Clinical study of an amine fluoride gel and acidulated phosphate fluoride gel. *Community Dent. Oral Epidemiol.* 4:133-36.
9. Hals, E.; Torell, P.; and Morch, T. 1960. Effect of topically applied agents on enamel. IV. The effect of zirconium fluoride solutions topically applied *in vitro*. *Acta Odontol. Scand* 18:521-26.
10. Shrestha, B.M.; Mundorff, S.A.; and Bibby, B.G. 1972. Enamel dissolution: I. Effects of various agents and titanium tetrafluoride. *J. Dent. Res.* 51:1561-66.
11. Reed, A.J.; and Bibby, B.G. 1976. Preliminary report on effect of topical applications of titanium tetrafluoride on dental caries. *J. Dent. Res.* 55:357-58.
12. Gish, C.W.; Muhler, J.C.; and Howell, C.L. 1959. The effect of topically applied potassium fluorostannite on the dental caries experience in children. III. Results at the end of three years. *J. Dent. Res.* 38:881-82.
13. Moller, I.J.; Schaltz, G.; and Altermann, S. 1969. A clinical trial on the caries-inhibiting effect of sodium hexafluorostannate. *Caries Res.* 3:315-25.
14. Peterson, J.K.; and Jordan, W.A. 1957. Relative caries inhibiting value of topically applied sodium silicofluoride and sodium fluoride: final report on a two year study at Mound, Minnesota. *J. Dent. Res.* 36:124-28.
15. Muhler, J.C.; Bixler, D.; and Stookey, G.K. 1968. The clinical effectiveness of stannous hexafluorozirconate as an anticariogenic agent. *J. Amer. Dent. Assoc.* 76:558-63.
16. Bibby, B.G. 1944. The use of fluorine in the prevention of dental caries. II. Effect of sodium fluoride applications. *J. Amer. Dent. Assoc.* 31:317-21.
17. Knutson, J.W.; and Armstrong, W.D. 1943. The effect of topically applied sodium fluoride on dental caries experience. *Pub. Health Rep.* 58:1701-15.
18. Knutson, J.W.; and Armstrong, W.D. 1945. The

effect of topically applied sodium fluoride on dental caries experience. II. Report of findings for second study year. *Pub. Health Rep.* 60:1085-90.

19. Knutson, J.W.; and Armstrong, W.D. 1946. The effect of topically applied sodium fluoride on dental caries experience. III. Report of findings for the third study year. *Pub. Health Rep.* 61:1683-89.
20. Knutson, J.W. 1948. Sodium fluoride solutions: technic for application to the teeth. *J. Amer. Dent. Assoc.* 36:37-39.
21. Galagan, D.J.; and Knutson, J.W. 1948. Effect of topically applied fluoride on dental caries experience. VI. Experiments with sodium fluoride and calcium chloride. Widely spaced applications. Use of different solution concentrations. *Pub. Health Rep.* 63:1215-21.
22. Davies, G.N. 1950. Dental caries control and the general practitioner. *N. Z. Dent. J.* 46:25-31.
23. Hewat, R.E.T.; Eastcott, D.F.; and Leslie, G.H. 1951. Control of dental caries by topical application of sodium fluoride. (Second experimental study in Wellington.) *N. Z. Dent. J.* 47:123-33.
24. Chrietzberg, J.E. 1951. Toothbrushing as a substitute for quick cleansing in the topical fluoride technic. *J. Amer. Dent. Assoc.* 42:435-38.
25. Marshall-Day, C.D. 1951. Effect of topical sodium fluoride on dental caries during adolescence. *J. Dent. Res.* 30:514.
26. Bergman, G. 1953. Topical application of sodium fluoride using school children as subjects. *Acta Odontol. Scand.* 11 (Suppl. 12):53-112.
27. Cohen, A.; and Schiffrin, L. 1953. Dental caries in handicapped children after topical sodium fluoride. *Oral Surg., Oral Med., Oral Path.* 6:562-66.
28. Howell, C.H.; Gish, C.W.; Smiley, R.D.; and Muhler, J.C. 1955. Effect of topically applied stannous fluoride on dental caries experience in children. *J. Amer. Dent. Assoc.* 50:14-17.
29. McLaren, H.R.; and Brown, H.K. 1955. A study of the use of a topically applied stannous fluoride solution in the prevention of dental caries. *Can. J. Pub. Health* 46:387-95.
30. Nevitt, G.A.; Witter, D.H.; and Bowman, W.D. 1958. Topical applications of sodium fluoride and stannous fluoride. *Pub. Health Rep.* 73:847-50.
31. Harris, R. 1959. Observations on the effect of topical sodium fluoride on caries incidence in children. *Aust. Dent. J.* 4:257-60.
32. Law, F.E.; Jeffreys, M.H.; and Sheary, H.C. 1961. Topical applications of fluoride solutions in dental caries control. *Pub. Health Rep.* 76:287-90.
33. Torell, P.; and Ericsson, Y. 1965. Two year clinical tests with different methods of local caries-preventive fluorine application in Swedish school children. *Acta Odontol. Scand.* 23:287-322.
34. Averill, H.M.; Averill, J.E.; and Ritz, A.G. 1967. A two-year comparison of three topical fluoride agents. *J. Amer. Dent. Assoc.* 74:996-1001.
35. Cons, N.C.; Janerich, D.T.; and Senning, R.S. 1970. Albany topical fluoride study. *J. Amer. Dent. Assoc.* 80:777-81.
36. Szwejda, L.F. 1971. Fluorides in community programs: results after four years of study of various agents topically applied by two technics. *J. Public Health Dent.* 31:166-76.
37. Mercer, V.H.; and Muhler, J.C. 1972. Comparison of single topical applications of sodium fluoride and stannous fluoride. *J. Dent. Res.* 51:1325-30.
38. Iizuka, Y.; Higaki, M.; Ikeda, M.; Hogaki, M.; Haga, K.; Ito, K.; Sekine, H.; and Kubota, M. 1972. Comparison of three topical fluoride agents. II. A two-year experience. *Bull. Kanagawa Dent. Col.* 1:22-27.
39. Muhler, J.C.; Nebergall, W.H.; and Day, H.G. 1954. Studies on stannous fluoride and other fluorides in relation to the solubility of enamel in acid and the prevention of experimental dental caries. *J. Dent. Res.* 33:33-49.
40. Mühlemann, H.R.; Schmid, H.; and Konig, K.G. 1957. Enamel solubility reduction studies with inorganic and organic fluorides. *Helv. Odont. Acta* 1:23-33.
41. Brudevold, F.; and McCann, H.G.1968. Enamel solubility tests and their significance in regard to dental caries. *Ann. N. Y. Acad. Sci.* 153:20-51.
42. Hefferren, J.J. 1963. Qualitative and quantitative tests for stannous fluoride. *J. Pharm. Sci.* 52:1090-96.
43. Dunn, B.W.; and Shannon, I.L. 1967. The topical application of stannous fluoride in the United States Air Force. *J. Oral Ther. & Pharm.* 4:32-48.
44. Dudding, N.J.; and Muhler, J.C. 1962. Technique of application of stannous fluoride in a compatible prophylactic paste and as a topical agent. *J. Dent. Child.* 29:219-24.
45. Thornton, C.B.; and Stewart, G.P. 1978. Effect of waxed versus unwaxed floss on fluoride uptake by enamel. *J. Dent. Child.* 45:203-6.
46. Mercer, V.; and Muhler, J.C. 1964. The effect of a 30-second topical SnF_2 treatment on dental caries reductions in children. *J. Oral Ther. & Pharm.* 1:141-46.
47. Scola, F.P.; and Ostrom, C.A. 1968. Clinical

evaluation of stannous fluoride when used as a constituent of a compatible prophylactic paste, as a topical solution, and in a dentifrice in Naval personnel. II. Report of findings after two years. *J. Amer. Dent. Assoc.* 77:594-97.

48. Horowitz, H.S.; and Heifetz, S.B. 1969. Evaluation of topical applications of stannous fluoride to teeth of children born and reared in a fluoridated community: final report. *J. Dent. Child.* 36:355-61.
49. Jordan, W.A.; Snyder, J.R.; and Wilson, V. 1959. Study of a single application of 8% stannous fluoride. *J. Dent. Child.* 26:355-59.
50. Mercer, V.H.; and Muhler, J.C. 1961. Comparison of a single application of stannous fluoride with a single application of sodium fluoride or two applications of stannous fluoride. *J. Dent. Child.* 28:84-86.
51. Peterson, J.K.; and Williamson, L. 1962. Effectiveness of topical application of eight percent stannous fluoride. *Pub. Health Rep.* 77:39-40.
52. Salter, W.A.T.; McCombie, F.; and Hole, L.W. 1962. The anticariogenic effects of one and two applications of stannous fluoride on the deciduous and permanent teeth of children age six and seven. *J. Canad. Dent. Assoc.* 28:363-71.
53. Harris, R. 1963. Observations on the effect of eight percent stannous fluoride on dental caries in children. *Aust. Dent. J.* 8:335-40.
54. Grissom, D.K.; Dudenbostel, R.E.; Cassel, W.J., Jr.; and Murray, R.T. 1964. A comparative study of systemic sodium fluoride and topical stannous fluoride applications in preventive dentistry. *J. Dent. Child.* 31:314-22.
55. Wellock, W.D.; Maitland, A.; and Brudevold, F. 1965. Caries increments, tooth discoloration, and state of oral hygiene in children given single annual applications of acid phosphate-fluoride and stannous fluoride. *Arch. Oral Biol.* 10:453-60.
56. Hass, R.L. 1965. Effectiveness of a single application of stannous fluoride after toothbrushing. *J. Amer. Dent. Assoc.* 71:1391-95.
57. Cartwright, H.V.; Lindahl, R.L.; and Bawden, J.W. 1968. Clinical findings on the effectiveness of stannous fluoride and acid phosphate fluoride as caries reducing agents in children. *J. Dent. Child.* 35:36-40.
58. Gish, C.W.; Howell, C.L.; and Muhler, J.C. 1957. A new approach to the topical application of fluorides for the reduction of dental caries in children. A preliminary report. *J. Dent. Res.* 36:784-86.
59. Gish, C.W.; Howell, C.L.; and Muhler, J.C. 1957. A new approach to the topical application of fluorides in children, with results at the end of two years. *J. Dent. Child.* 24:194-96.
60. Gish, C.W.; Muhler, J.C.; and Howell, C.L. 1958. Stannous fluoride versus sodium fluoride—a progress report. *J. Dent. Child.* 25:177-79.
61. Gish, C.W.; Muhler, J.C.; and Howell, C.L. 1959. A new approach to the topical application of fluorides in children with results at end of four years. *J. Dent. Child.* 26:300-3.
62. Gish, C.W.; Muhler, J.C.; and Howell, C.L. 1962. A new approach to the topical application of fluorides for the reduction of dental caries in children: results at the end of five years. *J. Dent. Child.* 29:65-71.
63. Buonocore, M.G.; and Bibby, B.G. 1964. Fluoride dentifrices, topical fluorides, and fluoridation. In *Pharmacotherapeutics of oral disease,* eds. A.H. Kutscher, E.V. Zegarelli, and G.A. Hyman, pp. 222-31. New York: McGraw.
64. Muhler, J.C. 1960. Stannous fluoride enamel pigmentation: evidence of caries arrestment. *J. Dent. Child.* 27:157-61.
65. Mercer, V.H.; and Muhler, J.C. 1965. The clinical demonstration of caries arrestment following topical stannous fluoride treatments. *J. Dent. Child.* 32:65-72.
66. Muhler, J.C.; Spear, L.B., Jr.; Bixler, D.; and Stookey, G.K. 1967. The arrestment of incipient dental caries in adults after the use of three different forms of SnF_2 therapy: results after 30 months. *J. Amer. Dent. Assoc.* 75:1402-6.
67. Lobene, R.R.; Zulgar-Nain, B.J.; and Hein, J.W. 1966. Masking of enamel caries by topically applied stannous fluoride: a source of error in clinical diagnosis. *J. Oral Ther.* 3:35-43.
68. Glass, R.L. 1967. Radiographic evidence of tin uptake by human tooth structure. *Arch. Oral Biol.* 12:401-6.
69. Hyde, E.J.; and Muhler, J.C. 1963. Pigmentation of teeth treated with stannous fluoride and its association with caries incidence and oral hygiene. *J. Canad. Dent. Assoc.* 29:514-20.
70. Horowitz, H.S.; and Chamberlin, S.R. 1971. Pigmentation of teeth following topical applications of stannous fluoride in a non-fluoridated area. *J. Public Health Dent.* 31:32-37.
71. Muhler, J.C. 1957. Effect on gingiva and occurrence of pigmentation on teeth following the topical application of stannous fluoride or stannous chlorofluoride. *J. Periodontol.* 28:281-86.
72. Isaac, S.; and Brudevold, F. 1957. Discoloration of teeth by metallic ions. *J. Dent. Res.* 36:753-58.
73. Shapiro, M.; and Hood, J.L. 1956. Discoloration of gingiva and teeth by stannous fluoride. *J. Calif. Dent. Assoc. & Nevada Dent. Soc.* 32:174-77.

74. Brudevold, F.; Savory, A.; Gardner, D.E.; Spinelli, M.; and Speirs, R. 1963. A study of acidulated fluoride solutions. I. *In vitro* effects on enamel. *Arch. Oral Biol.* 8:167-77.

75. Muhler, J.C.; Stookey, G.K.; and Bixler, D. 1965. Evaluation of the anticariogenic effect of mixtures of stannous fluoride and soluble phosphates. *J. Dent. Child.* 32:154-69.

76. Wellock, W.D.; and Brudevold, F. 1963. A study of acidulated fluoride solutions. II. The caries inhibiting effect of single annual topical applications of an acidic fluoride and phosphate solution. A two-year experience. *Arch. Oral Biol.* 8:179-82.

77. Horowitz, H.S. 1968. The effect on dental caries of topically applied acidulated phosphate-fluoride: results after one year. *J. Oral Ther. & Phar.* 4:286-91.

78. Horowitz, H.S. 1969. Effect on dental caries of topically applied acidulated phosphate-fluoride: results after two years. *J. Amer. Dent. Assoc.* 78:568-72.

79. Horowitz, H.S.; and Doyle, J. 1971. The effect on dental caries of topically applied acidulated phosphate-fluoride: results after three years. *J. Amer. Dent. Assoc.* 82:359-65.

80. DePaola, P.F.; Wellock, W.D.; Maitland, A.; and Brudevold, F. 1968. The relationship of cariostasis, oral hygiene, and past caries experience in children receiving three sprays annually with acidulated phosphate-fluoride: three year results. *J. Amer. Dent. Assoc.* 77:91-94.

81. Jordan, W.A.; Pugnier, V.A.; and McKee, D.P. 1969. Evaluating acidulated phosphate fluoride solution as a caries inhibitor. *Northwest Dent.* 48:207-10.

82. Ingraham, R.Q.; and Williams, J.E. 1970. An evaluation of the utility of application and cariostatic effectiveness of phosphate-fluoride in solution and gel states. *J. Tenn. Dent. Assoc.* 50:5-12.

83. Vrbic, V.; Kosmelj, B.; and Ravnik, C. 1974. A three-year study among Yugoslavian school children on caries reduction after topical application of 4 percent NaF-PO_4. *Community Dent. Oral Epidemiol.* 2:163-65.

84. Zahran, M. 1976. Effect of topically applied acidulated phosphate fluoride on dental caries. *Community Dent. Oral Epidemiol.* 4:240-43.

85. Downer, M.C.; Holloway, P.J.; and Davies, T.G.H. 1976. Clinical testing of a topical fluoride caries preventive programme. *Brit. Dent. J.* 141:242-50.

86. Shern, R.; Swing, K.W.; and Crawford, J.J. 1970. Prevention of plaque formation by organic fluorides. *J. Oral Med.* 25:93-97.

87. Kavanagh, B.J.; Murphy, C.V.; Dolan, M.M.; and Yankell, S.L. 1974. *In vitro* plaque prevention with fluorides: comparison of teeth with nichrome wires. *J. Periodontol.* 45:314-15.

88. Dolan, M.M.; Kavanagh, B.J.; and Yankell, S.L. 1972. Artificial plaque formation with organic fluorides. *J. Periodontol.* 43:561-63.

89. Dolan, M.M.; Murphy, C.V.; Kavanagh, B.; and Yankell, S.L. 1973. Effects of fluorides in the *in vitro* plaque model system from human salivary sediment. *J. Dent. Res.* 52:1323-26.

90. Luscher, B.; Regolati, B.; and Mühlemann, H.R. 1974. Effect of amine fluorides on plaque and caries (*in vitro* and animal investigations). *Helv. Odont. Acta.* 18 (Suppl. 8):71-78.

91. Shern, R.J.; Rundell, B.B.; and Defever, C.J. 1974. Effects of an amine fluoride mouthrinse on the formation and microbial content of plaque. *Helv. Odont. Acta.* 18 (Suppl. 8):57-62.

92. Schneider, P.H.; and Mühleman, H.R. 1974. The antiglycolytic action of amine fluorides on dental plaque. *Helv. Odont. Acta.* 18 (Suppl. 8):63-70.

93. Ringelberg, M.L.; and Webster, D.B. 1977. Effects of an amine fluoride mouthrinse and dentifrice on the gingival health and the extent of plaque of school children. *J. Periodontol.* 48:350-53.

94. Stoller, N.H.; Cohen, D.W.; and Yankell, S.L. 1977. Clinical evaluations of an amine fluoride mouthrinse on gingival inflammation and plaque accumulation. *J. Periodontol.* 48:650-53.

95. Mühlemann, H.R.; and Schmid, H. 1958. Anticaries dentifrices under laboratory conditions. *J. Dent. Belg.* 49:353-72.

96. Riethe, P. 1968. Various forms of application of amine fluoride compounds in animal experiments. *Dtsch. Zahnaerztl Z.* 23:20-25.

97. Mühlemann, H.R.; Schait, A.; and Konig, K.G. 1968. Fluorine uptake of enamel and animal caries inhibition of topical sodium fluoride and amine fluorides at low fluoride concentrations. *Helv. Odont. Acta* 12:61-66.

98. Rinderer, L.; Schait, A.; and Mühlemann, H.R. 1965. Loss of fluoride from dental enamel after topical fluoridation. *Helv. Odont. Acta.* 9:148-50.

99. Balmelli, O.P.; Regulati, B.; and Mühlemann, H.R. 1974. Inhibition of streptococcal deposits on rat molars by amine fluoride. *Helv. Odont. Acta* 18 (Suppl. 8):71-78.

100. Konig, K.G.; Marthaler, T.M.; and Mühlemann, H.R. 1958. Anticaries effect of inorganic fluorides and some organic fluorides in albino rats. *Helv. Odont. Acta* 1:33-37.

101. Mühlemann, H.R.; Meyer, R.W.; Konig, K.G.; and Marthaler, T.M. 1961. The cariostatic effect of

some antibacterial compounds in animal experimentation. *Helv. Odont. Acta* 5:18-22.

102. Shern, R.J.; Amsbaugh, S.M.; and Reynolds, R. 1977. Effects of daily rinses using sodium fluoride and organic fluorides on rat caries. *J. Dent. Res.* 56:1063-66.

103. Marthaler, T.M. 1968. Caries inhibition after seven years of unsupervised use of an amine fluoride dentifrice. *Brit. Dent. J.* 124:510-15.

104. Marthaler, T.M. 1974. Caries inhibition by an amine fluoride dentifrice. Results after six years in children with low caries activity. *Helv. Odont. Acta* 18 (Suppl. 8):35-44.

105. Patz, J.; and Mavjoks, R. 1970. Die kariesprophylaktische wirkung einer amin fluoridhaltigen zahn paste bei jugendlichen nach dreijahrigem unuberwachtem gebrauch. *Dtsch. Zahnaerztl Z.* 25:617-25.

106. Ringleberg, M.L.; Webster, D.B.,Jr.; and Dixon, D.O. 1978. Effects of an amine fluoride dentifrice and mouthrinse on the dental caries of school children after 18 months. *J. Prev. Dent.* 5 (4):26-30.

107. Ringelberg, M.L.; Webster, D.B.; Dixon, D.O.; and LeZotte, D.C. 1979. The caries preventive effect of amine fluorides and inorganic fluorides in a mouthrinse or dentifrice after 30 months of use *J. Amer. Dent. Assoc.* 98:202-8.

108. Marthaler, T.M.; Konig, K.G.; and Mühlemann, H.R 1970. The effect of a fluoride gel used for supervised toothbrushing 15 or 30 times per year. *Helv. Odont. Acta* 14:67-77.

109. Heifetz, S.B. 1978. Cost-effectiveness of topically applied fluorides. In *The relative efficiency of methods of caries prevention in dental public health,* ed. B.A. Burt, pp. 69-104. Ann Arbor: Univ. of Michigan.

110. Shannon, I.L. 1969. Water-free solutions of stannous fluoride and their incorporation into a gel for topical application. *Caries Res.* 3:339–47.

111. Cowan, R.D.; and Shannon, I.L. 1972. Protective effectiveness of a stannous fluoride gel. *Aust. Dent. J.* 17:293-96.

112. Horowitz, H.S.; and Kau, M.C.W. 1974. Retained anticaries protection from topically applied acidulated phosphate-fluoride: 30- and 36-month post-treatment effects. *J. Prev. Dent.* 1 (1):22-27.

113. Bryan, E.T.; and Williams, J.E. 1968. The cariostatic effectiveness of a phosphate-fluoride gel administered annually to school children. I. The results of the first year. *J. Public Health Dent.* 28:182-85.

114. Bryan, E.T.; and Williams, J.E. 1970. The cariostatic effectiveness of a phosphate-fluoride gel administered annually to school children: final results. *J. Public Health Dent.* 30:13-16.

115. Szwejda, L.F.; Tossy, C.V.; and Below, D.M. 1967. Fluorides in community programs: results from a fluoride gel applied topically. *J. Public Health Dent.* 27:192-94.

116. Szwejda, L.F. 1971. Fluorides in community programs: results after two years from a fluoride gel applied topically. *J. Public Health Dent.* 31:241-42.

117. Mainwaring, P.J.; and Naylor, M.N. 1978. A three-year clinical study to determine the separate and combined caries-inhibiting effects of sodium monofluorophosphate toothpaste and an acidulated phosphate-fluoride gel. *Caries Res.* 12:202-12.

118. Mellberg, J.; and Nicholson, C.R. 1968. *In vitro* evaluation of an acidulated phosphate fluoride prophylaxis paste. *Arch. Oral Biol.* 13:1223-34.

119. Bibby, B.G.; Zander, H.; McKelleget, M.; and Labunsky, B. 1946. Preliminary reports on the effect on dental caries of the use of sodium fluoride in a prophylactic cleaning mixture and in a mouthwash. *J. Dent. Res.* 25:207-11.

120. Peterson, J.K.; Jordan, W.A.; and Snyder, J.R. 1963. Effectiveness of stannous fluoride-silex-silicone prophylaxis paste. Two-year report. Moorehead, Minnesota. *Northwest Dent.* 42:276-78.

121. Scola, F.P.; and Ostrom, C.A. 1966. Clinical evaluation of stannous fluoride when used as a constituent of a compatible prophylactic paste, as a topical solution, and in a dentifrice in Naval personnel. I. Report of findings after first year. *J. Amer. Dent. Assoc.* 73:1306-11.

122. Bixler, D.; and Muhler, J.C. 1964. Effect on dental caries in children in a non-fluoride area of combined use of three agents containing stannous fluoride: a prophylactic paste, a solution, and a dentifrice. *J. Amer. Dent. Assoc.* 68:792-800.

123. Bixler, D.; and Muhler, J.C. 1966. Effect on dental caries in children in a non-fluoride area of combined use of three agents containing stannous fluoride: a prophylactic paste, a solution, and a dentifrice. II. Results at the end of 24 and 36 months. *J. Amer. Dent. Assoc.* 72:392-96.

124. Szwejda, L.F. 1972. Fluorides in community programs: a study for four years of the cariostatic effects of prophylactic pastes, rinses, and applications of various fluorides. *J. Public Health Dent.* 32:110-18.

125. Peterson, J.K.; Horowitz, H.S.; Jordan, W.A.; and Pugnier, V. 1969. Effectiveness of an acidulated phosphate fluoride-pumice prophylactic paste: a two-year report. *J. Dent. Res.*

48:346–50.
126. DePaola, P.F.; and Mellberg, J.R. 1973. Caries experience and fluoride uptake in children receiving semi-annual prophylaxes with an acidulated phosphate fluoride paste. *J. Amer. Dent. Assoc.* 87:155-59.
127. Barenie, J.T.; Ripa, L.W.; Trummel, C.; Mellberg, J.R.; and Nicholson, C.R. 1976. Effect of professionally applied biannual applications of phosphate-fluoride prophylaxis paste on dental caries and fluoride uptake: results after two years. *J. Dent. Child.* 43:340-44.
128. Horowitz, H.S.; and Lucye, H. 1966. A clinical study of stannous fluoride in a prophylaxis paste and as a solution. *J. Oral Ther. & Pharm.* 3:17-25.
129. Heifetz, S.B.; Mellberg, J.R.; Winter, S.J.; and Doyle, J. 1970. *In vivo* fluoride uptake by enamel of teeth of human adults from various topical fluoride procedures. *Arch. Oral Biol.* 15:1171-81.
130. Mellberg, J.R.; Nicholson, C.R.; Ripa, L.W.; and Barenie, J. 1976. Fluoride deposition in human enamel *in vivo* from professionally applied fluoride prophylaxis paste. *J. Dent. Res.* 55:976-79.
131. Brudevold, F.; McCann, H.G.; Nilsson, R.; Richardson, B.; and Coklica, V. 1967. The chemistry of caries inhibition problems and challenges in topical treatments. *J. Dent. Res.* 46 (Suppl. to No. 1):37-45.
132. Spinelli, M.A.; Brudevold, F.; and Moreno, E. 1971. Mechanism of fluoride uptake by hydroxyapatite. *Arch. Oral Biol.* 16:187-203.
133. Arends, J.; and Schuthof, J. 1975. Fluoride content in human enamel after fluoride application and washing—an *in vitro* study. *Caries Res.* 9:363-72.
134. Koch, G.; and Petersson, L.G. 1972. Fluoride content of enamel surface treated with a varnish containing sodium fluoride. *Odontol. Revy* 23:437-46.
135. Petersson, L.G. 1975. *In vivo* fluoride uptake in human enamel following treatment with a varnish containing sodium fluoride. *Odontol. Revy* 26:253-66.
136. Edenholm, H.; Johnson, G.; Koch, G.; and Petersson, L.G. 1977. Fluoride uptake and release in deciduous enamel after application of fluoride varnishes. An *in vitro* pilot study. *Swed. Dent. J.* 1:59-64.
137. Arends, J.; and Schuthof, J.A.D. 1977. Influence of F-releasing varnishes on the acid resistance of enamel. *Quintessence Int.* 8 (11):85-89.
138. Murray, J.J.; Winter, G.B.; and Hurst, C.P. 1977. Duraphat fluoride varnish: a two-year clinical trial in five-year-old children. *Brit. Dent. J.* 143:11-17.
139. Wegner, H. 1976. The clinical effect of application of fluoride varnish. *Caries Res.* 10:318-20.
140. Koch, G.; and Petersson, L.G. 1975. Caries preventive effect of a fluoride-containing varnish (Duraphat) after one year's study. *Community Dent. Oral Epidemiol.* 3:262-66.
141. Hetzer, G.; and Irmisch, B. 1973. Kariesprotektion durch fluor-lack (Duraphat)—Klinische ergebnisse und erfahrungen. *Dtsch. Stomatol.* 23:917-22.
142. Heuser, H.; and Schmidt, H.F. 1968. Zahnkariesprophylaxe durch tiefenimpragnierung des zahnschmelzes mit fluor-lack. *Stoma* 21:91-100.
143. Maiwald, H.J.; and Geiger, L. 1973. Lokal application von fluorschutzlack zur karies prophylaxe in kollektiven. *Dtsch. Stomatol.* 23:56-63.
144. Maiwald, H.J. 1974. Lokalapplikation von fluorschutzlack zur kariespravention in kollektiven nach dreijahriger kontrollzeit. *Stomatol. DDR.* 24:123-25.
145. DePaola, P.F. 1967. Combined use of a sodium fluoride prophylaxis paste and a spray containing acidulated sodium fluoride solution. *J. Amer. Dent. Assoc.* 75:1407-11.
146. Vrbic, V.; Brudevold, F.; and McCann, H.G. 1967. Acquisition of fluoride by enamel from fluoride pumice pastes. *Helv. Odont. Acta* 11:21-26.
147. Koch, G.; Petersson, L.G.; and Johnson, G. 1975. Abrasion och fluorinlagring vid puts av emalj. *Svensk Tandlakare Tidskrift* 68:1-7.
148. Zuniga, M.A.; and Caldwell, R.C. 1969. The effect of fluoride-containing prophylaxis pastes on normal and "white spot" enamel. *J. Dent. Child.* 36:345-49.
149. Stookey, G.K. 1978. *In vitro* estimates of enamel and dentin abrasion associated with a prophylaxis. *J. Dent. Res.* 57:36.
150. Tinanoff, N.; Wei, S.H.Y.; and Parkins, F.M. 1974. Effect of a pumice prophylaxis on fluoride uptake in tooth enamel. *J. Amer. Dent. Assoc.* 88:384-89.
151. Tinanoff, N.; Wei, S.H.Y.; and Parkins, F.M. 1975. Effect of the acquired pellicle on fluoride uptake in tooth enamel *in vitro*. *Caries Res.* 9:224-30.
152. Bruun, C.; and Stoltze, K. 1976. *In vivo* uptake of fluoride by surface enamel of cleaned and plaque-covered teeth. *Scand. J. Dent. Res.* 84:268-75.
153. Downs, R.A.; and Pelton, W.J. 1950. The effect of topically applied fluorides in dental caries experience on children residing in fluoride areas. *J. Colorado Dent. Assoc.* 29:7-10.
154. Galagan, D.J.; and Vermillion, J.R. 1955. Effect

of topical fluorides on teeth matured on fluoride-bearing water. *Pub. Health Rep.* 70: 1114–15.

155. Muhler, J.C. 1960. The effectiveness of stannous fluoride in children residing in an optimal communal fluoride area. *J. Dent. Child.* 27:51-54.
156. Muhler, J.C. 1960. The anticariogenic effectiveness of a single application of stannous fluoride in children residing in an optimal communal fluoride area. II. Results at the end of 30 months. *J. Amer. Dent. Assoc.* 61:431-38.
157. Horowitz, H.S.; and Heifetz, S.B. 1967. Evaluation of topical applications of stannous fluoride to teeth of children born and reared in a fluoridated community: interim report. *J. Dent. Child.* 34:290-95.
158. Jordan, W.A.; Wood, O.B.; Allison, J.A.; and Irwin, V.D. 1946. The effects of various numbers of topical applications of sodium fluoride. *J. Amer. Dent. Assoc.* 33:1385-91.
159. Ast, D.B. 1950. Sodium fluoride dental caries prophylaxis. *N. Y. State Dent. J.* 16:441-48.
160. Jordan, W.A. 1950. A three-year study on the effects of a 2 percent topical sodium fluoride on deciduous molars. *Northwest Dent.* 29:265-67.
161. Wittich, H.C. 1950. The effect of topical application of sodium fluoride upon deciduous teeth. *Northwest Dent.* 29:113-14.
162. Sundvall-Hagland, I.; Brudevold, F.; Armstrong, W.D.; Gardner, D.E.; and Smith, F.A. 1959. A comparison of the increment of fluoride in enamel and the reduction in dental caries resulting from topical fluoride applications. *Arch. Oral Biol.* 1:74-79.
163. Compton, F.H.; Burgess, R.C.; Mondrow, T.G.; Grainger, R.M.; and Nikiforuk, G. 1959. The Riverside preschool dental project. *J. Canad. Dent. Assoc.* 25:478-88.
164. Burgess, R.; Mondrow, W.; Nikiforuk, G.; and Compton, F. 1961. Topical stannous fluoride for preschool children. *J. Dent. Res.* 40:712 (Abstract).
165. McDonald, R.E.; and Muhler, J.C. 1957. The superiority of topical applications of stannous fluoride on primary teeth. *J. Dent. Child.* 24:84–86.
166. Schutze, H.J. Jr.; Forrester, D.J.; and Balis, S.B. 1974. Evaluation of a fluoride prophylaxis paste in a fluoridated community. *J. Canad. Dent. Assoc.* 40:675-83.
167. Arnold, F.A. Jr.; Dean, H.T.; and Singleton, D.E. Jr. 1944. The effect on caries incidence of a single topical application of a fluoride solution to the teeth of young adult males of a military population. *J. Dent. Res.* 23:155-62.
168. Rickles, N.H.; and Becks, H. 1951. The effects of an acid and a neutral solution of sodium fluoride on the incidence of dental caries in young adults. *J. Dent. Res.* 30:757-65.
169. Kutler, B.; and Ireland, R.L. 1953. The effect of sodium fluoride application on the dental caries experience in adults. *J. Dent. Res.* 32:458-62.
170. Carter, W.J.; Jay, P.; Shklair, I.L.; and Daniel, L.H. 1955. The effect of topical fluoride on dental caries experience in adult females of a military population. *J. Dent. Res.* 34:73-76.
171. Muhler, J.C. 1958. The effect of a single topical application of stannous fluoride on the incidence of dental caries in adults. *J. Dent. Res.* 37:415-16.
172. Harris, N.O.; Hester, W.R.; Muhler, J.C.; and Allen, J.F. 1964. Stannous fluoride topically applied in aqueous solution in caries prevention in a military population. SAM-TDR-64-26, U. S. Air Force School of Aerospace Medicine, Brooks Air Force Base, Texas.
173. Hazen, S.P.; Chilton, N.W.; and Mumma, R.D., Jr. 1973. The problem of root caries. I. Literature review and clinical description. *J. Amer. Dent. Assoc.* 86:137-44.
174. Jordan, H.V.; and Sumney, D.L. 1973. Root surface caries: review of the literature and significance of the problem. *J. Periodontol.* 44:158-63.
175. Sumney, D.L.; Jordan, H.V.; and Englander, H.R. 1973. The prevalence of root surface caries in selected populations. *J. Periodontol.* 44:500-4.
176. Westbrook, J.L.; Miller, A.S.; Chilton, N.W.; Williams, F.L.; and Mumma, R.D., Jr. 1974. Root surface caries: a clinical, histopathologic, and microradiographic investigation. *Caries Res.* 8:249-55.
177. Mellberg, J.R.; and Shulman, L. 1974. The treatment of human teeth with fluoride for replantation and allotransplantation. *J. Dent. Res.* 53:844-46.
178. Shannon, I.L.; Buchanan, W.E., Jr.; and Mahan, C.J. 1976. *In vitro* treatment of human root surfaces with fluorides. *J. Public Health Dent.* 36:201-6.
179. Harris, R.; and Curtin, J.H. 1976. Dentine hypersensitivity. *Aust. Dent. J.* 21:165-69.
180. Hodosh, M. 1974. A superior desensitizer—potassium nitrate. *J. Amer. Dent. Assoc.* 88:831-32.
181. Green, B.L.; Green, M.L.; and McFall, W.T.,Jr. 1977. Calcium hydroxide and potassium nitrate as desensitizing agents for hypersensitive root surfaces. *J. Periodontol.* 48:667-72.
182. Dayton, R.E.; DeMarco, T.J.; and Swedlow, D. 1974. Treatment of hypersensitive root surfaces

with dental adhesive materials. *J. Periodontol.* 45:873-78.
183. Bolden, T.E.; Volpe, A.R.; and King, W.J. 1968. The desensitizing effect of a sodium monofluorophosphate dentifrice. *Periodontics* 6:112-14.
184. Hazen, S.P.; Volpe, A.R.; and King, W.J. 1968. Comparative desensitizing effect of dentifrices containing sodium monofluorophosphate, stannous fluoride, and formalin. *Periodontics* 6:230–32.
185. Kanouse, M.C.; and Ash, M.M., Jr. 1969. The effectiveness of a sodium monofluorophosphate dentifrice on dental hypersensitivity. *J. Periodontol.* 40:38-40.
186. Shapiro, W.B.; Kaslick, R.S.; Chasens, A.I.; and Weinstein, D. 1970. Controlled clinical comparison between a strontium chloride and a sodium monofluorophosphate toothpaste in diminishing root hypersensitivity. *J. Periodontol* 41:523-25.
187. Zinner, D.D.; Duany, L.F.; and Lutz, H.J. 1977. A new desensitizing dentifrice: preliminary report. *J. Amer. Dent. Assoc.* 95:982-85.
188. Schaeffer, M.L.; Bixler, D.; and Yu, P.L. 1971. The effectiveness of iontophoresis in reducing cervical hypersensitivity. *J. Periodontol.* 42:695–700.
189. Sall, H.D. 1974. Technic for treating cervical sensitivity. *Dent. Surv.* 50 (11):60, 62, 64-65.
190. Minkov, B.; Marmari, I.; Gedalia, I.; and Garfunkel, A. 1975. The effectiveness of sodium fluoride treatment with and without iontophoresis on the reduction of hypersensitive dentin. *J. Periodontol.* 46:246-49.
191. Simon, W.J., and Hilborn, L.B. 1977. Hypersensitive dentin. *Dent. Assist.*/Sept./46:16–17
192. Gedalia, I.; Brayer, L.; Kalter, N.; Richter, M.; and Stabholz, A. 1978. The effect of fluoride and strontium application on dentin: *in vivo* and *in vitro* studies. *J. Periodontol.* 49:269–72.
193. Gangarosa, L.P.; and Park, N. 1978. Practical considerations in iontophoresis of fluoride for desensitizing dentin. *J. Prosthet. Dent.* 39:173-78.
194. Gangarosa, L.P.; Hever, G.A.; Park, N.; Hayes, B.B.; Little, C.K.; Baker, G.W.; and Smith, M.A. 1978. Desensitizing hypersensitive dentin by iontophoresis with fluoride. *N. Y. State Dent. J.* 44:92-94.
195. Murthy, K.S.; Talim, S.T.; and Singh, I. 1973. A comparative evaluation of topical application and iontophoresis of sodium fluoride for desensitization of hypersensitive dentin. *Oral Surg.* 36:448-58.
196. Siemon, W.H. 1960. A new approach in solving the problem of hypersensitivity and postoperative distress in dentine and cementum. *J. Conn. State Dent. Assoc.* 34:5-10.
197. Manning, M.M. 1961. New approach to desensitization of cervical dentin. *Dent. Surv.* 37:731-34.
198. Ross, M.R. 1961. Hypersensitive teeth: effect of strontium chloride in a compatible dentifrice. *J. Periodontol.* 32:49-53.
199. Skurnik, H. 1963. Control of dental hypersensitivity. Preliminary report on a strontium-containing dentifrice. *J. Periodontol.* 34:183-85.
200. Blitzer, B. 1967. A consideration of the possible causes of dental hypersensitivity: treatment by a strontium-ion dentifrice. *Periodontics* 5:318-21.
201. Tal, M.; Oron, M.; Gedalia, I.; and Ehrlich, J. 1976. X-ray diffraction and scanning electron microscope investigations of fluoride-treated dentine in man. *Arch. Oral Biol.* 21:285-90.
202. Beiswanger, B.B.; Billings, R.J.; Sturzenberger, O.P.; and Bollmer, B.W. 1978. Effect of an SnF_2–$Ca_2P_2O_7$ dentifrice and APF topical applications. *J. Dent. Child.* 45:137-41.
203. Gish, C.W., and Muhler, J.C. 1965. Effect on dental caries in children in a natural fluoride area of combined use of three agents containing stannous fluoride: a prophylactic paste, a solution, and a dentifrice. *J. Amer. Dent. Assoc.* 70:914-20.
204. Lindhe, J., and Axelsson, P. 1973. The effect of controlled oral hygiene and topical fluoride application on caries and gingivitis in Swedish school children. *Community Dent. Oral Epidemiol.* 1:9-16.
205. Shulman, L.B.; Kalis, P.; and Goldhaber, P. 1968. Fluoride inhibition of tooth-replant root resorption in Cebus monkeys. *J. Oral Ther. & Pharm.* 4:331-37.
206. Bjorvatn, K., and Massler, M. 1971. Effect of fluorides on root resorption in replanted rat molars. *Acta Odontol. Scand.* 29:17-29.
207. Shulman, L.B.; Gedalia, I.; and Feingold, R.M. 1973. Fluoride concentration in root surfaces and alveolar bone of fluoride-immersed monkey incisors three weeks after replantation. *J. Dent. Res.* 52:1314-16.
208. Silverstone, L.M. 1978. Operative measures for caries prevention. *Caries Res.* 12 (Suppl. 1):103-12.
209. Hals, E.; and Nernaes, A. 1971. Histopathology of *in vitro* caries developing around silver amalgam fillings. *Caries Res.* 5:58-77.
210. Kidd, E.A.M. 1977. The histopathology of artificial lesions created *in vitro* in relation to unfilled and filled cavities. *Caries Res.* 11:173–77.
211. Laswell, H.R. 1966. A prevalence study of secondary caries occurring in a young adult male

population. MSD thesis, Indiana University, School of Dentistry, Indianapolis.

212. Hallsworth, A.S., and Weatherell, J.A. 1969. The microdistribution, uptake, and loss of fluoride in human enamel. *Caries Res.* 3:109-18.

213. Phillips, R.W.; and Swartz, M.L. 1957. Effect of certain restorative materials on solubility of enamel. *J. Amer. Dent. Assoc.* 54:623-36.

214. Norman, R.D.; Phillips, R.W.; and Swartz, M.L. 1960. Fluoride uptake by enamel from certain dental materials. *J. Dent. Res.* 39:11-16.

215. Norman, R.D.; Platt, J.R.; Phillips, R.W.; and Swartz, M.L. 1961. Additional studies on fluoride uptake by enamel from certain dental materials. *J. Dent. Res.* 40:529-37.

216. Forsten, L.; Ryomaa, I.; Antilla, A.; and Keinonen, J. 1976. Fluoride uptake from restorative dental materials by human enamel. *Scand. J. Dent. Res.* 84:391-95.

217. Tveit, A.B.; and Hals, E. 1978. Penetration of ions from silicate cement restorations into Copalite-covered cavity walls. *Acta Odontol. Scand.* 36:15-24.

218. Halse, A.; and Hals, E. 1976. Electron probe microanalysis of secondary carious lesions adjacent to silicate fillings. *Calcif. Tissue Res.* 21:183-93.

219. Hals, E. 1976. Root caries: distribution and uptake of elements in lesions adjacent to silicate or amalgam restorations. *Scand. J. Dent. Res.* 84:367-71.

220. Jerman, A.C. 1970. Silver amalgam restorative material with stannous fluoride. *J. Amer. Dent. Assoc.* 80:787-91.

221. Innes, D.B.K., and Youdelis, W.V. 1966. Calcium fluoride in amalgam for caries prevention. *J. Dent. Res.* 45:94-98.

222. Wei, S.H.Y.; and Sierk, D.L. 1971. Fluoride uptake by enamel from zinc phosphate cement containing stannous fluoride. *J. Amer. Dent. Assoc.* 83:621-24.

223. Gursin, A.V. 1965. A study of the effect of stannous fluoride incorporated in dental cement. *J. Oral Ther. & Pharm.* 1:630-36.

224. Yamano, C. 1968. Effect of NaF-phosphate cement on enamel of human tooth. *J. Osaka Univ. Dent. Sch.* 13:123-37. (Cited in *Oral Research Abst.* 4:29, 1969.)

225. Soremark, R.; Hedin, M.; and Rojmyr, R. 1969. Studies on incorporation of fluoride in a cavity liner (varnish). *Odont. Revy.* 20:189-99.

226. Birkeland, J.M., and Tronstad, L. 1976. Fluoride in an experimental cavity varnish. *Scand. J. Dent. Res.* 84:200-3.

227. Nordbo, H., and Eriksen, H.M. 1976. Permeability and fluoride release of lining materials containing amine fluorides. *Scand. J. Dent. Res.* 84:386-90.

228. Forsten, L. 1976. Fluoride release from a fluoride-containing amalgam and two luting cements. *Scand. J. Dent. Res.* 84:348-50.

229. Greenland, L.; Hargreaves, J.A.; Smith, D.C.; and Beagrie, G.S. 1974. Fluoride uptake by enamel from polycarboxylate cement (Abstract #918). *J. Dent. Res.* 53 (special issue: February): 284.

230. Minoguchi, G.; Tani, Y.; and Tamai, S. 1967. Abhandlung uber die zinnfluoride ethaltenden silberamalgame und uber die rolle, die sie als vorbeugende mittel gegen die zahnkaries spielen. *Fachbl. Stomatol.* (Univ. Kyoto) 7:1-23.

231. Pugnier, V.A. 1972. Cyanoacrylate resins in caries prevention: a two-year study. *J. Amer. Dent. Assoc.* 84:829-31.

232. Gwinnett, A.J. 1973. The sequence of topical fluoride and occlusal sealant applications. *J. Am. Soc. Prev. Dent.* 3 (4):54-57.

233. Kochavi, D.; Gedalia, I.; and Anaise, J. 1975. Effect of conditioning with fluoride and phosphoric acid on enamel surfaces as evaluated by scanning electron microscopy and fluoride incorporation. *J. Dent. Res.* 54:304-9.

234. Low, T.; von Fraunhofer, J.A.; and Winter, G.B. 1975. The bonding of a polymeric fissure sealant to topical fluoride-treated teeth. *J. Oral Rehabil.* 2:303-7.

235. Lee, H.; Stoffey, D.; Orlowski, J.; Swartz, M.L.; Ocumpaugh, D.; and Neville, K. 1972. Sealing of developmental pits and fissures. III. Effects of fluoride on adhesion of rigid and flexible sealers. *J. Dent. Res.* 51:191-201.

236. Low, T.; von Fraunhofer, J.A.; and Winter, G.B. 1977. Influence of the topical application of fluoride on the *in vitro* adhesion of fissure sealants. *J. Dent. Res.* 56:17-20.

237. Skehkoleslam, Z.; Buonocore, M.G.; and Gwinnett, A.J. 1972. Effect of fluorides on the bonding of resins to phosphoric acid-etched bovine enamel. *Arch. Oral Biol.* 17:1037-45.

238. Wright, F.A.C., and Beck, D.J. 1973. Prevention of pit and fissure caries. III. Fluoride and resin-enamel bonding. *N. Z. Dent. J.* 69:77-84.

239. Swartz, M.L.; Phillips, R.W.; Norman, R.D.; Elliason, S.; Rhodes, B.F.; and Clark, H.E. 1976. Addition of fluoride to pit and fissure sealants—a feasibility study. *J. Dent. Res.* 55:757-71.

240. Lee, H.; and Ocumpaugh, D. 1973. Sealing of developmental pits and fissures. VI. Arrestment of caries with a fluoride-containing polyurethane system. *Biomater Med. Devices Artif. Organs* 1:349-58.

241. Chaet, R., and Wei, S.H.Y. 1977. The effect of

fluoride impregnated dental floss on enamel fluoride uptake *in vitro* and Streptococcus Mutans colonization *in vivo J. Dent. Child.* 44:122-26.

242. Stookey, G.K., and Schemehorn, B.R. 1976. Studies evaluating a fluoride-containing prophylactic cup. *Dental Hyg.* 50:253-57.

243. Stookey, G.K., and Stahlman, D.B. 1976. Enhanced fluoride uptake in enamel with a fluoride-impregnated prophylactic cup. *J. Dent. Res.* 55:333-41.

244. Shannon, I.L.; and Kutsko, G.T. 1977. Evaluation of fluoride-impregnated prophylaxis cups. *J. Oreg. Dent. Assoc.* 47:13-15.

245. Mellberg, J.R., and Loertscher, K.L. 1972. Fluoride acquisition *in vitro* by sound human tooth enamel from sodium fluoride and ammonium silicofluoride-phosphate solutions. *Arch. Oral Biol.* 17:1107-16.

246. Barrancos, R.J.; and Strachan, D.S. 1966. The effect of temperature on the uptake of topical fluorides (Abstract #217). *I.A.D.R. Program and Abstracts of Papers*, March: p. 92.

247. Putt, M.S.; Beltz, J.F.; and Muhler, J.C. 1978. Effect of temperature of stannous fluoride solution on tin and fluoride uptake by bovine enamel. *J. Dent. Res.* 57:772-76.

Chapter 8

Fluoride dentifrices

An important aspect of any preventive program is the maintenance of good oral hygiene, and a major part of a successful oral hygiene program is thorough and frequent toothbrushing. In industrial countries, toothbrushing is considered a normal, socially desirable habit and is practiced by a major part of the population.

As a result of the finding that topical application of fluoride is effective in inhibiting dental caries, fluoride was introduced into dentifrice formulations. Because of their wide use, dentifrices constitute a practical means of providing fluoride therapy to a large number of people. With the exception of fluoridated drinking water, fluoride dentifrices are the most widely used form of fluoride.

The development of fluoride dentifrices began prior to 1945,[1] and since then more clinical trials have been conducted to test the efficacy of fluoride dentifrices than of any other form of fluoride therapy. The conclusion of these studies is that fluoride dentifrices are an effective means of providing partial protection against dental caries.

The early fluoride dentifrices contained sodium fluoride, but now several other agents, which were selected to capitalize on one or more specific characteristics of the agent, are also used. For example, stannous fluoride provides especially good enamel solubility reduction in laboratory tests; sodium monofluorophosphate forms only the desirable fluorapatite with enamel and is particularly stable with dentifrice abrasives; amine fluoride has surfactant and antibacterial properties.

Functions of fluoride dentifrices

Dentifrices have been classified as cosmetic or therapeutic, based on whether they contain a drug for the treatment or prevention of a dental disease. It must be realized, however, that cosmetic dentifrices have therapeutic effects and therapeutic dentifrices have cosmetic effects.[2] For example, cosmetic dentifrices remove plaque, the precursor of caries and gingival disease, and therapeutic dentifrices prevent the formation of mouth odor and tooth stains from food, beverages, and tobacco. In addition, the flavor components of the dentifrice provide pleasant, lingering breath odor and encourage frequent use.

Therapeutic functions

Physicomechanical functions

It is axiomatic that "a clean tooth does not decay," and indeed it has been shown that a combination of professional prophylaxis every two weeks, oral hygiene instruction,

Table 8-1 New carious surfaces in subjects brushing immediately after eating compared to a control group using their usual brushing procedure

	N	Control	Test	Percent difference
First year	308	0.87	0.32	63
Second year	150	0.53	0.25	53

Data from *Fosdick*.[6]

and conscientious toothbrushing almost completely eliminates new caries formation.[3] Although toothbrushing is very important in maintaining oral cleanliness and aiding in the prevention of oral disease through removal of bacterial plaque, it is not able to remove all plaque. The usual brushing, even when accompanied by flossing, leaves a significant amount of plaque in proximal areas, around the necks of the teeth, and in the occlusal fissures. However, it is possible that the physicomechanical action of the toothbrush and dentifrice may reduce the cariogenicity of the remaining plaque by a rinsing or flushing action that removes fermentable materials, disrupts the delicate balance of environmental conditions necessary for acid formation, and prevents the formation of thicker, more cariogenic plaques.

In spite of these possible benefits of toothbrushing, clinical caries studies with nonfluoride-containing dentifrices have given equivocal results.[4] One reason for this may be the timing of toothbrushing relative to the ingestion of cariogenic foods. The importance of timing can be seen when the pH activity of the plaque is considered.

When fermentable carbohydrates are applied to a dental plaque, the pH falls within minutes to very low levels. *Stephan* and *Miller*[5] measured the pH fall in 3 to 4-day-old plaques after a 2-minute rinse with 10% glucose and found that the pH fell to below 5.0 within 5 minutes and remained depressed for about 45 minutes (see Fig. 1-4, Chapter 1). If the critical pH below which enamel demineralization occurs is about 5.5, the duration of dangerous pH conditions in this case was approximately 30 minutes. Toothbrushing would have to be performed well within 30 minutes after ingestion of the first cariogenic food or drink to be effective in preventing decay. When the teeth were brushed before the glucose rinse was used, the amount of acid produced by the residual plaque was small and the pH did not go below about 6.0.

When university students were instructed to brush their teeth within 10 minutes after each ingestion of food or sweets, or when brushing was not possible, to rinse their mouths thoroughly with water, *Fosdick*[6] found a highly impressive caries inhibition. Compared to a control group that continued their usual oral hygiene habits (which did not include brushing immediately after eating), the test group developed 50 to 60% fewer new carious surfaces (Table 8-1).

Because toothbrushing within minutes after ingestion of food and sweets is impractical, and we know that the pH fall in plaque remaining after toothbrushing is minimal and not likely to reach the critical pH of enamel solubility, it has been suggested that the teeth be brushed before eating.[7] If a fluoride-containing dentifrice is used, it will deposit fluoride in the residual plaque thus providing it when most needed for the possible inhibition of acid formation and enamel dissolution.

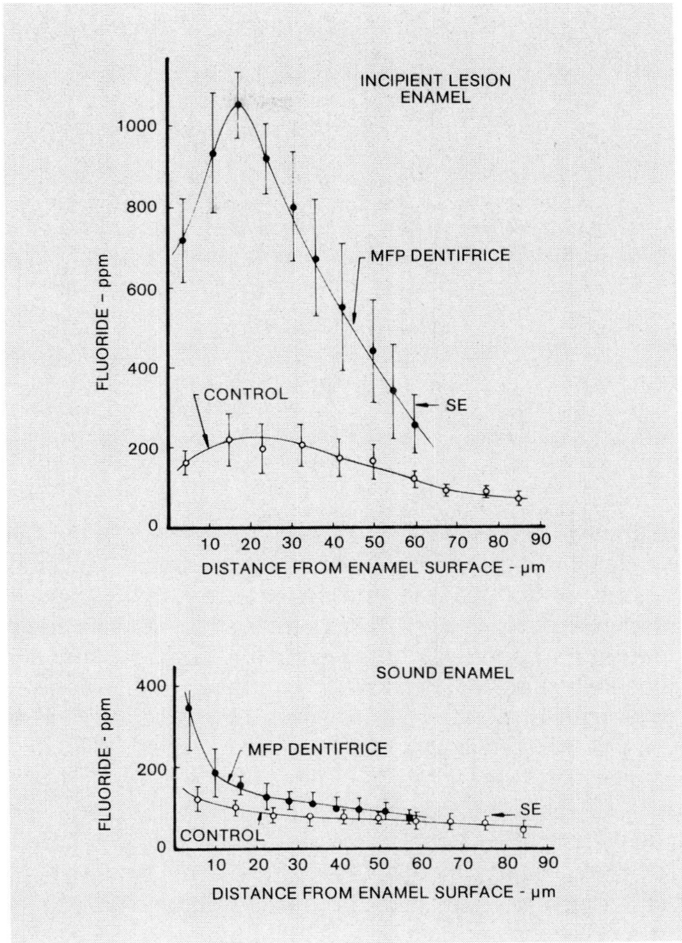

Fig. 8-1 Fluoride concentrations in sound enamel (lower) and enamel with artificial incipient lesions (upper) implanted in a denture and treated by brushing *in vivo* three times per day for 2 weeks with a sodium monofluorophosphate dentifrice.

Chemical functions

The chemical functions of fluoride dentifrices are based on the potential anticaries mechanisms of fluoride. These are more fully presented in Chapter 2 and include reactions mediated through the deposition of fluoride into enamel and plaque.

Deposition of fluoride into enamel as fluorapatite increases the acid resistance of the enamel. Although it is important that this occur in sound enamel so that it can withstand the acid of a caries attack, fluoride from dentifrices is deposited in the largest amounts in the porous enamel of incipient lesions, that is, the sites where it is needed most. Figure 8-1 shows the amount of fluoride deposited in artificial lesions (white spots) in human enamel carried for 2 weeks in a dental prosthesis and brushed three times per day with a dentifrice containing sodium monofluorophosphate. The fluoride profile reflects the morphology of an incipient lesion having a relatively sound outer layer and a highly porous, partially demineralized area below the surface. Sound enamel

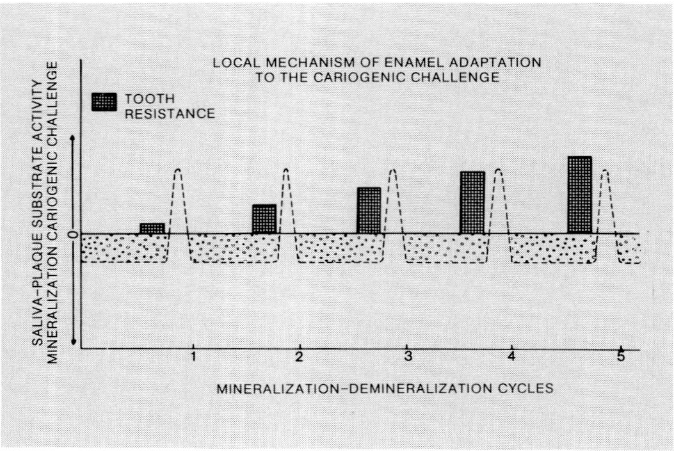

Fig. 8-2 The reactions leading to enamel adaptation are diagramatically illustrated. The fluid in contact with the tooth surface becomes unsaturated due to the low pH generated by the microbial plaque and supersaturated when salivary flow neutralizes the acid. During the unsaturation phase tooth mineral dissolves, while during the supersaturation phase minerals precipitate within the microspaces of the partially demineralized enamel. Many cycles of unsaturation and supersaturation lead to enamel adaption because the most soluble mineral dissolves and is replaced by less soluble, if proper ionic components are present in the fluid environment.
(Courtesy of T. *Koulourides*.)

similarly treated acquired only a small amount of fluoride near the surface from the relatively short 2-week treatment period.

Plaque can serve as a reservoir for fluoride that may react with enamel at a slower rate or when the conditions are more favorable. During the remission stage of the caries attack (i.e., when the pH rises above the critical level), the presence of fluoride in the liquid acid phase contacting the enamel will result in its being incorporated into the lesion as fluorapatite, thus increasing its resistance to subsequent acid attacks. Contact of fluoride in plaque with lesions in a resting or arrested state may also result in fluorapatite formation. It is not known to what extent the pellicle, other organic material, and surface mineral deposits will inhibit the uptake and penetration of fluoride.

The effect of fluoride exposure during or subsequent to caries attack has been suggested by *Koulourides*[8] to result in the situation shown diagrammatically in Figure 8-2. With each caries attack, the resistance increases and the extent of damage decreases until ultimately the resistance is great enough so that the enamel can withstand the attack. If this occurs before there is irreparable damage, the tooth will not develop an open lesion and can be thought of as fully protected from caries.

In addition to increasing the fluoride levels in sound or incipient lesion enamel, fluoride in plaque may also lessen the degree of enamel demineralization by lowering the pH at which enamel will dissolve. In essence, this should reduce the number of times the enamel will be exposed to acid below the critical pH and also the period of time during each attack when the pH is low enough to allow demineralization to occur.

Finally, the presence of fluoride in plaque may reduce the amount of acid formed due to its antienzymatic or antimetabolic effects on plaque bacteria.

Dentifrice composition

Although powders and liquids are available, the most common form of modern dentifrice is the paste. The paste consists of a solid abrasive suspended in a liquid phase containing detergent, humectant, binding agent, flavor, color, preservative, and a fluoride source (Table 8-2).

Table 8-2 Components in typical dentifrice formulations

Component	Range in formulation (%)
Abrasive	40-50
Humectant	20-40
Detergent	1-2
Binding agent	0.5-2
Flavor, color, etc.	1-4
Fluoride	0.1
Water	20-30

Abrasives

The function of the abrasive is to serve as a cleaning and polishing agent for the teeth. Without some kind of abrasive in the dentifrice, most people develop a stain or pigmented pellicle,[9-12] which, fortunately, can be removed within a short time by an abrasive-containing dentifrice.

The most important factors in selecting a particular abrasive for a fluoride-containing dentifrice are its degree of abrasivity to dental hard tissue and its compatability with fluoride. Abrasivity must be sufficient to remove and prevent the buildup of stain, but mild enough so that the enamel or exposed root surfaces are not harmed.

The abrasivity of a material is determined by its hardness, particle size, and shape. If the particle is too hard and sharp or is too large, it may wear away tooth structure. Damage may occur in exposed root surfaces, which are softer than enamel. Because of the difference in hardness between enamel and dentin, the relative abrasion of enamel and root dentin is not the same for all abrasives. A large but relatively soft or dull abrasive may remove much root dentin, but have little effect on enamel. Alternatively, a hard and sharp material of small particle size may remove less dentin but more enamel.[13,14] Often, a combination of abrasives is used to optimize cleaning and polishing effects within the bounds of safety to the hard tissue.

Of major importance to fluoride-containing dentifrices is the compatibility of the abrasive with the fluoride source. Abrasives vary widely in fluoride compatibility, and all calcium-containing abrasives have the potential to inactivate fluoride, especially if their preparation is not carefully controlled. Inactivation can occur through reactions forming calcium fluoride or fluorapatite, by adsorption to the abrasive surface, or by complexing with soluble ions.

The compatibility of calcium-containing abrasives has been improved by modification of their chemical and physical forms. For example, heat treatment of dicalcium phosphate to produce calcium pyrophosphate increased its compatibility sufficiently to allow its use in stannous fluoride and sodium fluoride dentifrices.

Fluoride compatibility with abrasives is also greatly enhanced when sodium monofluorophosphate is used as the fluoride source. Although sodium monofluorophosphate cannot be used indiscriminately with any calcium-containing abrasive, proper selection of abrasive grade and other dentifrice formation components can result in stable formulations. The compatibility of several abrasive fluoride combinations in dentifrices is shown in Figure 8-3.

The most common abrasives used in dentifrices are the following:

Insoluble sodium metaphosphate, $(NaPO_3)_x$. This compound is compatible with fluoride as it does not contain calcium or fluoride complexing ions. It is moderately abrasive.

Calcium pyrophosphate, $Ca_2P_2O_7$. This is one of the most inert calcium phosphate abrasives used in sodium fluoride, stannous fluoride, and sodium monofluorophosphate dentifrices. It is moderately abrasive.

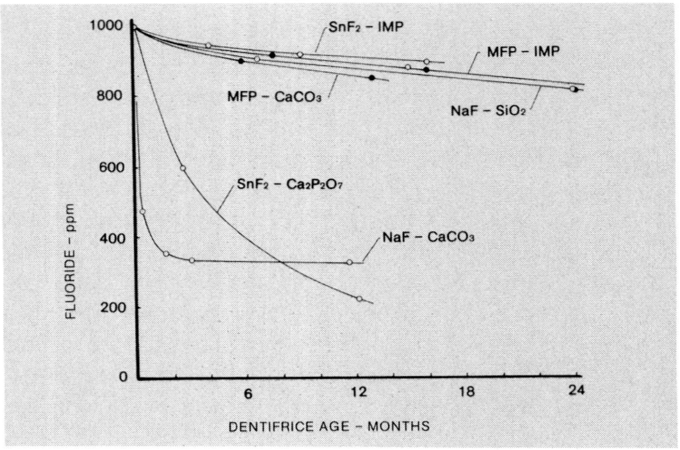

Fig. 8-3 Total soluble fluoride in dentifrices prepared with various fluoride salts and abrasives.
(Data from *Noren* and *Harse*[15] [$CaCO_3$ dentifrices] and *Kestenbaum* and *Roberts*[16].)

Dicalcium phosphate dihydrate, $CaHPO_4 \cdot 2H_2O$. This abrasive is not compatible with sodium or stannous fluoride, but is compatible with sodium monofluorophosphate in a properly formulated dentifrice. It is mildly abrasive. This compound requires a stabilizer (magnesium and pyrophosphate salts) to prevent formation of hydroxyapatite and hardening of the dentifrice in the tubes.

Dicalcium phosphate anhydrous, $CaHPO_4$. Anhydrous dical is not compatible with sodium or stannous fluoride, but can be used with sodium monofluorophosphate. It is one of the more highly abrasive materials used in dentifrices in limited amounts.

Calcium carbonate (chalk), $CaCO_3$. This material is not compatible with sodium or stannous fluoride or at an acid pH, but is compatible with sodium monofluorophosphate.[15,16] Its abrasivity varies widely depending on the source.

Alumina trihydrate, $Al_2O_3 \cdot 3H_2O$. This abrasive appears to be compatible with sodium monofluorophosphate as suggested by the positive results of a clinical trial.[17] It is moderately abrasive. The anhydrous form (calcined alumina) is more abrasive, but is not used as the principal abrasive in dentifrices.

Silica, SiO_2. Dentifrice silica abrasives consist of a family of synthetically formed materials, including precipitated silicas and xerogel silicas, which differ in method of manufacture but which have similar properties. Both are compatible with fluoride and are used in clear gel formulations because their index of refraction can be matched by the liquid phase of the dentifrice. As used in dentifrice formulations, abrasivity is moderate. Natural silicas are much more abrasive and are not used in dentifrices.

Sodium bicarbonate, $NaHCO_3$. This salt is compatible with fluoride, but has not usually been used in fluoride dentifrices. It is mildly abrasive.

Plastic particles. Polymethylmethacrylate particles are used as the abrasive in a Swedish dentifrice ("Bofors").[18,19] The plastic is compatible with all types of fluoride used in dentifrices. It has very low abrasivity, which may result in the presence of stained pellicle in some subjects.

Humectants

Humectants are compounds that are used to prevent moisture loss from the dentifrice formulation in general, and in particular from around the outlet of the tube where drying and caking would occur in their absence. The most commonly used humectants are glycerol, sorbitol, and propylene glycol. Glycerol and sorbitol have a sweet taste and thereby add to the flavor system.

Although humectants have been shown to reduce the amount of fluoride taken up by enamel in laboratory studies, this effect may be lessened by dilution with saliva. The effect of humectants on fluoride uptake by plaque—and subsequently the underlying enamel—has not been studied.

Detergents

Detergents are surface-active cleaning agents that lower surface tension, penetrate and loosen deposits, suspend debris, and aid in dispersing the dentifrice and its fluoride component throughout the mouth. The two major detergents used in dentifrices are sodium lauryl sulfate and sodium coco-monoglyceride sulfonate. Both of these compounds are compatible with fluoride.

Binding agents

The binding, or thickening, agent in the dentifrice holds the abrasive in suspension. In general, all binding agents are hydrophyllic colloids that appear to dissolve in water but actually disperse and swell to form viscous liquid phases. Commonly used binding agents are sodium alginate, Irish moss extract, cellulose derivatives (e.g., methyl cellulose and carboxymethyl cellulose), and inorganic claylike materials such as colloidal magnesium aluminum silicate.

Fluoride source

Sodium fluoride, sodium monofluorophosphate, and stannous fluoride are the three major sources of fluoride used in dentifrices. Amine fluoride is also used in some European areas. Some other fluorides (e.g., potassium fluoride[20-22] and aluminum fluoride[23]) have also been clinically tested but are not of major significance.

The standard fluoride concentration in all major dentifrices in the United States is 0.1% (1,000 ppm). This is equivalent to 0.22% NaF, 0.76% Na_2PO_3F, and 0.4% SnF_2. In Europe, some dentifrices may contain up to 1,500 ppm F.

Miscellaneous components

Flavors, sweeteners, and coloring agents are used in dentifrices to improve their taste and visual acceptability. Preservatives are added to protect the humectant and binder from bacterial and mold growth, and some abrasives from chemical changes. Corrosion inhibitors are sometimes added to prevent reaction with the dentifrice tube. Stannous fluoride dentifrices may contain stannous pyrophosphate to provide a reservoir of free stannous ions.

Laboratory evaluation

The aim of most laboratory evaluations of fluoride dentifrices—beyond safety tests (including abrasivity), which are not discussed here—is to determine whether the fluoride in the formulation is available in such a form that it can fulfill its intended purpose of inhibiting the formation of dental caries. Because of the increased understanding of the anticaries mechanisms of fluoride, the great cost of clinical trials, and the inability of a single trial to predict effects under different conditions of use or in different groups, evaluation of fluoride dentifrices by laboratory tests has received greater acceptance in recent years. Except for radically different formulations, laboratory confirmation of fluoride availability, showing that it is equal to or better than that in previously proven formulations, is considered by many to be sufficient to guarantee similar clinical efficacy. Availability is determined in a number of ways, but the most common include measuring the total soluble fluoride, ionic fluoride, enamel solubility reduction, fluoride uptake, and caries inhibition in animals.

Soluble fluoride

A reduction in fluoride availability can occur by the formation of insoluble precipitates or by adsorption to the abrasive. This is quite easily determined by measuring the amount of soluble fluoride in the dentifrice. Total soluble fluoride is usually taken as the amount of fluoride in the supernatant of a mixture of a standard amount of dentifrice (e.g., 5 g) in a standard amount of water (e.g., 100 ml). The amounts must be standardized because large amounts of water might dissolve previously insoluble fluoride precipitates.

Ionic fluoride (F^-) may be measured in the soluble fraction with a specific ion electrode. This is often done when sodium monofluorophosphate is the fluoride source in the dentifrice. Some ionic fluoride is usually present as an impurity in monofluorophosphate when the dentifrice is manufactured, but it may also arise from decomposition of monofluorophosphate during dentifrice aging.

Enamel solubility reduction

Availability of fluoride in a dentifrice formulation can be measured by its ability to react with enamel. The amount of reaction can be estimated by the degree to which the formulation can reduce enamel solubility in acid.[24] This test goes one step further than the measurement of total soluble fluoride because it takes into consideration the possible low availability of soluble fluoride complexes and the inhibition of enamel reaction by other components of the formulation.

The enamel solubility reduction test will give high values with stannous fluoride formulations because of the stannous ions that form relatively insoluble precipitates on the surface. Other enamel-reactive metals may also produce insoluble products, which will result in high values. Even the formation of calcium fluoride from sodium fluoride will affect the degree of enamel solubility reduction obtained. Because these precipitates differ in solubility and amount and are not directly related to the anticaries activity of the formulation, it is not valid to compare enamel solubility reduction values from one type of dentifrice formulation to another. The enamel solubility reduction test is primarily used to evaluate fluoride availability within a series of formulations prepared with a specific type of fluoride. This test is particularly useful to determine if a new dentifrice formulation has affected the availability of the fluoride.

Enamel solubility reduction tests are conducted using both powdered and intact enamel. When intact enamel is used, the test frequently consists of a measurement of the amount of enamel dissolved by an acid buffer within a specific time period. The difference between the amount of enamel dissolved before and after a dentifrice treatment is used to calculate the percent enamel solubility reduction.[25]

Fluoride uptake

A more direct measure of fluoride bioavailability than enamel solubility reduction is determination of the amount of fluoride acquired by enamel from a dentifrice treatment.[26] Both powdered and intact enamel are also used in this test. Powdered enamel offers greater reproducibility, whereas intact enamel is closer to the real situation. Because much of the fluoride acquired by enamel is in a loosely bound state, the treated enamel must be given a thorough wash after treatment to insure that only firmly bound fluoride remains. With intact enamel, a wash time of 24 hours is usually sufficient.[27]

The most common method of conducting fluoride uptake studies with intact enamel consists of treating blocks of known surface areas with a slurry of the dentifrice, washing the treated blocks to remove unreacted fluoride, and then dissolving thin layers (e.g., 5-10μ thick) by immersion in acid. The thickness of each layer can be calculated from analysis of calcium in the dissolved layer and the known surface area. When several layers are removed from a block, the penetration of fluoride into the enamel can be determined. Because fluoride concentrations decrease rapidly with enamel depth, comparisons between groups must be made at the same depth.

Animal tests

Perhaps the best test of fluoride bioavailability other than human clinical trials is a test of caries inhibition in an animal model. The only practical animals for caries studies are rodents, namely rats and hamsters. However, because of differences in the dentition and saliva of rodents, these tests are not truly reliable predictors of results with humans and must be used as indicators, as are other laboratory tests.

The animals are started on the caries test at weaning, about 21 to 22 days of age. They are infected with cariogenic microorganisms and fed a high sucrose diet (e.g., 60% sucrose). Once or twice per day, the teeth of the animals are treated with a slurry of the dentifrice using a cotton swab or plastic syringe. After 3 weeks or more, the animals are sacrificed, the jaws removed, and the molar teeth examined for caries. The molars are frequently sectioned through the fissures to better reveal fissure caries. Figure 8-4 shows sound and carious molars of hamsters that had been in a caries test.

Clinical evaluation

The ultimate measure of the anticaries efficacy of a fluoride dentifrice is a clinical trial with groups of human subjects. The standard clinical trial consists of a comparison of the increments of new caries found in groups using either a test or placebo dentifrice. Approximately 200 subjects are assigned in random fashion to each group and then given a test or placebo dentifrice in double blind fashion. Instead of a placebo dentifrice, a positive control dentifrice is sometimes used. The positive control is a dentifrice previously shown to be effective. Because of ethical considerations of withholding an effective anticaries preparation from the control group, the positive control will undoubtedly be used more frequently in the future. Toothbrushing is conducted either under supervision or at home for at least 1 but preferably 2 or 3 years. Dental examinations are given at yearly intervals without the examiner knowing the group identity of the subjects. The caries status of every tooth surface is recorded and the results expressed as DMFT (decayed, missing, or filled teeth) or DMFS (decayed, missing, or filled surfaces). Guidelines for conducting clinical trials have been given in two excellent publications.[28,29]

In spite of great care in designing and conducting clinical trials, the result of a single trial cannot be used as a measure of the true efficacy of the dentifrice under all condi-

Fig. 8-4a and b Sound and carious molars of hamsters.
(Courtesy of John *Facq*)

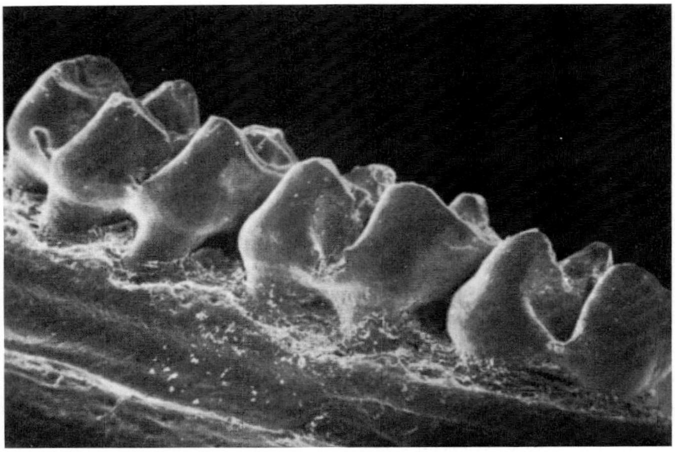

Figure 8-4a Sound hamster molars.

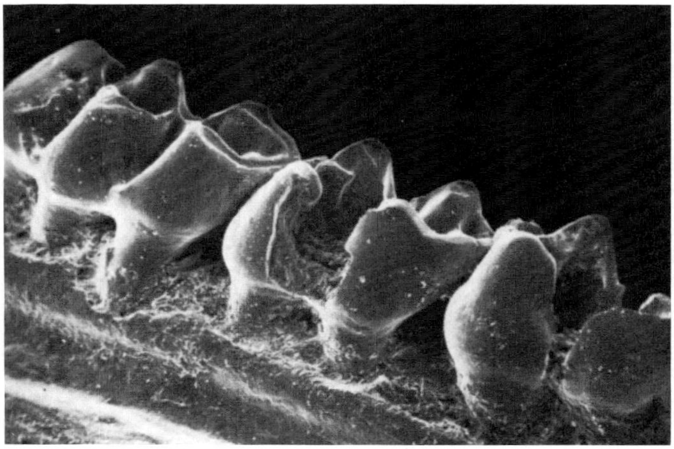

Figure 8-4b Carious hamster molars.

tions of use, by every subject, or in all areas. Although clinical trials obviously are capable of providing a more realistic estimate of anticaries efficacy than laboratory experiments, they also are subject to many problems and errors that can mask the true efficacy of the product. The subjective nature of caries scoring and the particular conditions of a clinical trial can result in quite different findings for the same product. Conditions that may affect the clinical outcome include the age of the subjects, their geographic location, caries susceptibility, differences in dietary habits, previous fluoride exposure, amount of dental care received, amount of toothbrushing supervision, dental examination methods, the skill of the examiner, and even the method used to report the results.

A recent problem in conducting clinical trials is that the caries experience of subjects in general in some areas seems to be declining.[30] This may be because of more widespread use of fluoride dentifrices, fluoridated drinking water, more dental care, and better oral hygiene habits. Under these conditions, the lesions that still form are inherently the most difficult to prevent. Therefore, to obtain the same percent caries reduction as in an area with a high caries rate, the treatment will have to be more effective.

Most clinical trial results are reported as the percent difference in new caries formation (DMFS) between the treatment and control groups. Percentage figures have the advantage that they are easily understood; however, they can also be misleading. For example, if the placebo group developed only a small number of new lesions, say an average of 1.0 new DMFS during a 2-year study, a 50% reduction by the active agent would amount to 0.25 fewer DMFS per year. However, if the placebo group developed 4.0 new DMFS during the study, a difference of 0.25 DMFS per year would be only a 12.5% caries reduction.

The percent reduction figures are point estimates of the true caries reduction for the tested dentifrice. It has been suggested that the use of interval estimates rather than point estimates for clinical trial results would be more meaningful.[31,22] Interval estimates, that is, the range in which the true caries reduction would fall, take into consideration the statistical variation (uncertainty) within a clinical trial. For example, *DePaola*[32] calculated that the point estimate of one clinical trial was 36% reduction, whereas the 95% confidence interval was 13% to 59%; that is, the true caries reduction could lie anywhere between 13% and 59%.

In spite of the problems with the use of percentage figures for reporting the results of clinical trials, they remain the most widely used reporting method and allow at least a crude comparison of the results from different trials. Therefore, the tables of clinical trials given in subsequent sections include point estimates of percent caries inhibition as rough indicators of the clinical efficacy of fluoride-containing dentifrices.

Sodium fluoride dentifrices

Because of the success of the topical application of sodium fluoride in preventing caries formation, dentifrices containing this agent were formulated and tested. However, results from early clinical trials failed to show significant caries inhibition.[33,34] The reason for these disappointing results was that probably one or more of the components of the dentifrice formulation was incompatible with sodium fluoride. The component most likely to inactivate fluoride is the abrasive. Since the early studies were conducted, the formulation of fluoride dentifrices has become more sophisticated, and compatible, clinically effective systems have been developed. A chronological summary of clinical trials of sodium fluoride dentifrices is given in Table 8-3.

Torell and *Ericsson*[35] tested a sodium fluoride dentifrice containing sodium bicarbonate, a chemically compatible abrasive, and found an 18% inhibition of new decay over a 2-year period. Sodium fluoride with insoluble sodium metaphosphate or plastic abrasives resulted in caries inhibition ranging from 9 to 48% in several studies.[18,19,37,40] More recently, dentifrices with calcium pyrophosphate ($Ca_2P_2O_7$) as the abrasive have been tested and found to be effective,[39,41-45] with caries inhibition ranging from 11 to 38%.

Because of the laboratory and clinical effectiveness shown by acidulated-phosphate-fluoride (APF) topical applications, a dentifrice was formulated that contained sodium fluoride, sodium phosphate, and used insoluble sodium metaphosphate as the abrasive at a pH of approximately 5. Although two clinical trials showed a caries inhibition of about 20%,[37,38] there was no indication that the dentifrice was superior to other sodium fluoride dentifrices.

The large variation in results from different clinical trials shown in the tables cannot be ascribed solely to differences between the dentifrices tested, but undoubtedly reflect

Table 8-3 Clinical trials of dentifrices containing sodium fluoride

Investigators	Study location	Principal abrasive*	Initial age (years) of subjects	Duration of study (years)	Percent caries reduction (DMFS)
Muhler et al.[33]	U.S.A.	$Ca_2P_2O_7$	6-16	1	10
Kyes et al.[36]	U.S.A	IMP	17-24	2	0
Torell & Ericsson[35]	Sweden	$NaHCO_3$	10-11	2	18
Brudevold & Chilton[37]	U.S.A.	DCPD	8-17	2	6
		IMP**	8-17	2	19
Peterson & Williamson[38]	U.S.A.	IMP**	9-15	3	20
Zacherl[39]	Canada	$Ca_2P_2O_7$	7-14	1.7	28
Koch[18,19]	Sweden	Plastic	8-10	3	40
		Plastic	11-12	3	48
Slack et al.[40]	England	IMP**	11-12	3	9
Zacherl[41]	Canada	$Ca_2P_2O_7$	7-13	1.7	28
		$Ca_2P_2O_7$**	7-13	1.7	14***
Weisenstein & Zacherl[42]	U.S.A.	$Ca_2P_2O_7$	5-15	1.8	11-38
Reed[43]	U.S.A.	$Ca_2P_2O_7$	5-14	2	20
Stookey & Beiswanger[44]	U.S.A.	$Ca_2P_2O_7$	8-15	2.3	25
Reed & King[45]	U.S.A.	$Ca_2P_2O_7$	8-13	2	30

*DCPD = dicalcium phosphate dihydrate; IMP = insoluble sodium metaphosphate.
**Utilized APF type system in the dentifrice.
***Area with fluoridated drinking water.

differences in the study populations, extent of supervision, examination procedures, etc., as discussed earlier. Figure 8-5 shows a frequency distribution of the results of clinical trials of sodium fluoride, stannous fluoride, and sodium monofluorophosphate dentifrices. Sixty-two percent of the trials utilizing sodium fluoride dentifrice provided from 11 to 30% caries inhibition.

Stannous fluoride dentifrices

Successful clinical studies of the use of topically applied stannous fluoride led to its use in dentifrices. Most of the early work with stannous fluoride dentifrices was conducted in the early 1950s by *Muhler* and his associates at Indiana University in conjunction with the manufacturer of the commercial product, Crest.

The abrasive selected for use in Crest was calcium pyrophosphate, which provided better fluoride stability than other abrasives conventionally used in dentifrices at that time. Although the fluoride stability profile as measured by total soluble fluoride is not as good as many other fluoride-abrasive combinations developed since Muhler's initial studies (see Fig. 8-3), the results from a single clinical trial with dentifrice aged for 10 months at 80° F before testing indicated that anticaries efficacy still remained.[46]

Because the stannous ion precipitates quite rapidly from solution by hydrolysis and oxidation, it was thought that the stannous ions

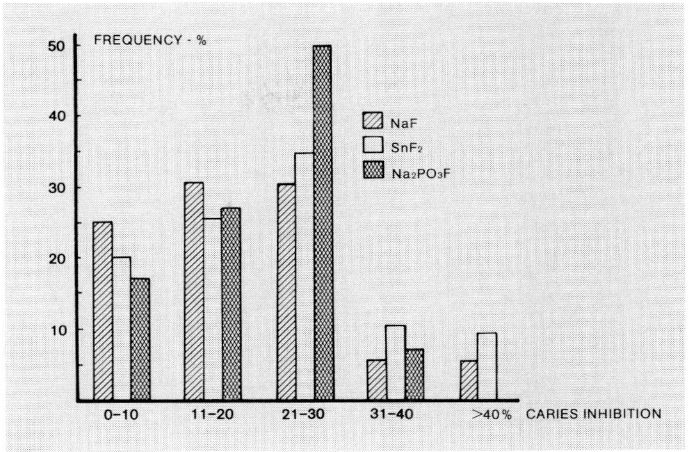

Fig. 8-5 Clinical trials of fluoride dentifrices grouped according to the caries inhibition found (% fewer DMFS).

must be stabilized. Although 1% stannous pyrophosphate is added to maintain soluble stannous ions, there is no clinical evidence to indicate that the stannous ion contributes to the efficacy of the dentifrice in inhibiting caries.

Table 8-4 lists clinical trials conducted with stannous fluoride dentifrices. Of the 47 treatment groups listed in the table, 34 used a dentifrice containing calcium pyrophosphate as the abrasive. There is a large variation in the results of the studies, but most were positive, with 61% of the trials reporting caries inhibition in the range of 11 to 30% (see Fig. 8-5).

In order to obtain greater stannous fluoride stability in a dentifrice formulation, a number of products were tested that contained insoluble sodium metaphosphate as the abrasive. Table 8-4 lists 12 studies of this type, five of which compared calcium pyrophosphate and insoluble sodium metaphosphate abrasives.[37,40,56,57,60] Although the differences were not always statistically significant, the results suggesed that stannous fluoride-insoluble sodium metaphosphate dentifrices might be slightly more effective than stannous fluoride-calcium pyrophosphate dentifrices.

In the early 1960s, several stannous fluoride-insoluble sodium metaphosphate dentifrices were marketed (Cue, Fact, and Super Stripe) that were very stable and provided clinically proven caries inhibition.[79-81] More recently, another stannous fluoride dentifrice (Aim) has been clinically tested[78] and marketed. This product is a clear gel dentifrice based on a stannous fluoride-silica abrasive system in which the fluoride is more stable than in the stannous fluoride-calcium pyrophosphate system. The single published clinical trial reported 15% caries inhibition over a 3-year period.

During clinical testing of fluoride dentifrices, some investigators[58,63-67,70] noted a greater incidence of tooth pigmentation (staining) in subjects who used stannous fluoride dentifrices. Staining occurred chiefly in thick pellicle or the chalky, porous enamel of incipient lesions.

Sodium monofluorophosphate dentifrices

Perhaps the most widely used fluoride source for dentifrices throughout the world is sodium monofluorophosphate. This fluorine containing salt has advantages over sodium

Table 8-4 Clinical trials of dentifrices containing stannous fluoride

Investigators	Study location	Principal abrasive[*]	Initial age (years) of subjects	Duration of study (years)	Percent caries reduction (DMFS)
Muhler et al[47]	U.S.A.	$Ca_2P_2O_7$	5-15	1	49
Muhler et al.[33]	U.S.A.	$Ca_2P_2O_7$	6-16	1	36
Muhler & Radike[48]	U.S.A.	$Ca_2P_2O_7$	17-36	2	34
Jordan & Peterson[49]	U.S.A.	$Ca_2P_2O_7$	8-11	2	21
Hill[50]	U.S.A.	$Ca_2P_2O_7$	9-16	2	15
Muhler[51]	U.S.A.	$Ca_2P_2O_7$	6-16	2	25
Peffley & Muhler[52]	U.S.A.	$Ca_2P_2O_7$	10-19	0.8	57
Kyes et al.[36]	U.S.A.	$Ca_2P_2O_7$	17-24	2	8
Muhler[53]	U.S.A.	$Ca_2P_2O_7$	6-18	3	21
Bixler & Muhler[54]	U.S.A.	$Ca_2P_2O_7$	11-23	1.6	54
Finn & Jamison[55]	U.S.A.	$Ca_2P_2O_7$	6-17	2	0
Henriques et al.[56]	U.S.A.	$Ca_2P_2O_7$	5-12	2	13
Mergele et al.[57]	U.S.A.	$Ca_2P_2O_7$	8-15	2	9[*]
		IMP[+]	8-15	2	16[*]
Slack & Martin[58]	England	IMP	11-13	2	0
Torell & Ericsson[35]	Sweden	$Ca_2P_2O_7$	10-11	2	23
Bixler & Muhler[59]	U.S.A.	$Ca_2P_2O_7$	11-23	1.6	54
Thomas & Jamison[60]	U.S.A.	$Ca_2P_2O_7$	7-16	2	30
		IMP	7-16	2	31
Brudevold & Chilton[37]	U.S.A.	$Ca_2P_2O_7$	8-17	2	4
		IMP[+]	8-17	2	25
Horowitz et al.[61]	U.S.A.	$Ca_2P_2O_7$	6-10	3	17
Fullmer et al.[62]	U.S.A.	IMP	8-10	3	30
Slack et al.[63]	England	IMP	11-12	3	0
Slack et al.[64]	England	$Ca_2P_2O_7$	11-12	3	5
Jackson & Sutcliffe[65]	England	$Ca_2P_2O_7$	11-12	3	12
James & Anderson[66]	England	$Ca_2P_2O_7$	11-12	3	20
Naylor & Emslie[67]	England	IMP	11-12	3	15
Stiff et al.[68]	U.S.A.	IMP	7-12	3	25
Onishi et al.[69]	Japan	$Ca_2P_2O_7$	Grade 1	2	13
Fanning et al.[70]	Australia	IMP	12-14	2	21
Frankl & Alman[71]	U.S.A.	$Ca_2P_2O_7$	8-14	3	0[**]
Mergele[72]	U.S.A.	IMP	9-14	1.8	10
Mergele[73]	U.S.A.	9-13	9-13	3	13[*]
Peterson & Williamson[38]	U.S.A.	$Ca_2P_2O_7$	9-15	3	25
Zacherl[39]	Canada	$Ca_2P_2O_7$	7-14	1.7	28
Zacherl & McPhail[74]	Canada	$Ca_2P_2O_7$	6-7	2.5	40
Muhler[75]	U.S.A.	$Ca_2P_2O_7$	5-16	1	33
Gish & Muhler[76]	U.S.A.	$Ca_2P_2O_7$	6-13	5	29[*]
Slack et al.[40]	England	IMP	11-12	3	24
		$Ca_2P_2O_7$	11-12	3	18
Zacherl[46]	Canada	$Ca_2P_2O_7$	6-15	2	22[***]
Zacherl[41]	Canada	$Ca_2P_2O_7$	7-14	1.7	28[*]
Zacherl[77]	U.S.A	$Ca_2P_2O_7$	5-12	2	30
Fogels et al.[78]	U.S.A.	SiO_2	5-13	3	15
		$Ca_2P_2O_7$	5-13	3	15

[*]Area with fluoridated drinking water.
[**]Compared to dentifrice containing sodium lauryl sarcosinate.
[***]Aged dentifrice.
[+]IMP = Insoluble sodium metaphosphate.

fluoride and stannous fluoride, including much greater compatibility with common dentifrice abrasives and lack of tooth staining.

When the monofluorophosphate ion reacts with calcium-containing abrasives, it forms relatively soluble calcium monofluorophosphate. When ionic fluoride (F^-) reacts with calcium, it forms calcium fluoride, which is very insoluble and precipitates from solution. Thus, formation of calcium monofluorophosphate does not reduce the amount of soluble fluoride in the dentifrice. The low pH of stannous fluoride solutions also favors reaction of fluoride with calcium abrasives, but this is not a problem with sodium fluoride or monofluorophosphate, which have a pH closer to neutrality. Some ionic fluoride is always present in monofluorophosphate dentifrices. In a fresh dentifrice, this may be 5 to 10%, but it may increase because of slow hydrolysis as the product ages.

The free ionic fluoride "impurities" in monofluorophosphate dentifrices may impart some anticaries benefits to the user in addition to that from the $PO_3F^=$ ion, but they will not account for the major effect unless present in high concentrations. For example, *Ingram*[100] studied caries inhibition in the rat by application of dentifrices containing mixtures of $PO_3F^=$ and F^- and compared the results to caries inhibition from dentifrices containing only the "impurity" level F^-. He found a monofluorophosphate-dicalcium phosphate dentifrice containing 655 ppm F as $PO_3F^=$ and 115 ppm F as F^- inhibited caries 44%, whereas the same dentifrice containing only 143 ppm F^- inhibited caries only 6%. Similarly, a monofluorophosphate-chalk dentifrice containing 800 ppm F as $PO_3F^=$ and 97 ppm F as F^- gave an inhibition of 51%, while the same dentifrice with 354 ppm F^- resulted in a 27% inhibition.

The first commercial dentifrice to be developed containing sodium monofluorophosphate utilized insoluble sodium metaphosphate as the abrasive (Colgate Dental Cream with MFP). Caries reduction in its first clinical trial was 25%.[55] Subsequent clinical trials with this formulation confirmed its efficacy.[67,71-73,88]

Although insoluble sodium metaphosphate has been the most commonly used abrasive for monofluorophosphate dentifrices, the compatibility of monofluorophosphate with other abrasives is clearly shown by the variety of abrasives used in the clinical trials presented in Table 8-5. In addition to insoluble sodium metaphosphate, successful trials were conducted with calcium carbonate, dicalcium phosphate dihydrate, calcium pyrophosphate, silica, and alumina trihydrate. In spite of the great variety in dentifrice products and clinical trial conditions, the frequency distribution of clinical results is less variable than with dentifrices containing sodium fluoride or stannous fluoride (see Fig. 8-5). Seventy-seven percent of the clinical trials found caries inhibition of 11 to 30%, and 50% were between 21 and 30%.

Three clinical trials were conducted in which a sodium monofluorophosphate-insoluble sodium metaphosphate dentifrice was compared to a stannous fluoride-calcium pyrophosphate dentifrice.[55,71,73] The caries inhibitions for monofluorophosphate and stannous fluoride dentifrices respectively were 8% and 0% in Trial 1; 17% and 13% in Trial 2; and 25% and 0% in Trial 3. In Trials 1 and 3, the differences were statistically significant, suggesting that monofluorophosphate dentifrices might be slightly more effective than stannous fluoride dentifrices.

Amine fluoride dentifrice

Based on laboratory studies showing good fluoride uptake, enamel solubility reduction, and antibacterial activity,[101,102] a dentifrice (Elmex) containing amine fluoride compounds was formulated and is marketed in several European countries. Elmex contains

Table 8-5 Clinical trials of dentifrices containing sodium monofluorophosphate

Investigators	Study location	Principal abrasive++	Initial age (years) of subjects	Duration of study (years)	Percent caries reduction (DMFS)
Finn & Jamison[55]	U.S.A.	IMP	6-17	2	25
Torell & Ericsson[35]	Sweden	$CaCO_3$	10-11	2	13
Naylor & Emslie[67]	England	DCPD	11-12	3	18
Møller et al.[82]	Denmark	IMP	10-12	2.5	19
Frankl & Alman[71]	U.S.A.	IMP	8-14	3	8*
Fanning et al.[70]	Australia	IMP	12-14	2	20
Mergele[72]	U.S.A.	IMP	7-21	1.8	21
Mergele[73]	U.S.A.	IMP	8-13	3	17**
Takeuchi et al.[83]	Japan	DCPD	Grades 3–4	1	24
Kinkel & Stolte[84]	Germany	IMP	6-13	2	25-33
Torell[85]	Sweden	$CaCO_3$	Grade 4	1.8	29
Patz & Naujoks[86]	Germany	IMP	18-28	2	8
Onisi & Tani[87]	Japan	DCPD	Schoolchildren	1	16-41
Thomas & Jamison[88]	U.S.A.	IMP	8-16	2	29
Zacherl[41]	Canada	$Ca_2P_2O_7$	7-14	1.7	23**
Kinkel et al.[90]	Germany	DCPD	Schoolchildren	3	17-38
		DCPD	Schoolchildren	3	35-43***
Kinkel et al.[89]	Germany	DCPD	Schoolchildren	7	37
Forsman[91]	Sweden	$CaCO_3$	10-12	2	6+
		SiO_2	10-11	2	7+
Andlaw & Tucker[17]	England	$Al_2O_3 \cdot 3H_2O$	11-12	3	19
Peterson et al.[92]	U.S.A.	$CaCO_3$	8-12	2.7	23**
Niwa et al.[93]	Japan	DCP	Grades 3–5	1	26
Ashley et al.[94]	England	IMP	11-12	2	21
Mainwaring & Naylor[95]	England	$CaCO_3$	11-12	3	16
Glass & Shiere[96]	U.S.A.	$CaCO_3$	6-11	3	28
Howat et al.[97]	England	SiO_2	11-12	3	26
Peterson[98]	U.S.A.	$CaCO_3$	8-12	2.6	20**
		IMP	8-12	2.6	0**
Naylor & Glass[99]	England	$CaCO_3$	11-12	3	23

*Compared to dentifrice containing sodium lauryl sarcosinate.
**Area with fluoridated drinking water.
***Supervised toothbrushing.
+In addition to fortnightly fluoride mouth rinses.
++IMP = insoluble sodium metaphosphate; DCPD = dicalcium phosphate dihydrate; DCP = dicalcium phosphate.

0.125% fluoride, slightly more than other fluoride dentifrices, and insoluble sodium metaphosphate as the abrasive.

Although the amine fluoride dentifrice was developed approximately 20 years ago, only four clinical trials have been conducted. *Marthaler*[103] conducted an unsupervised brushing study in which the dentifrice was sent to the homes of children, initial age 6-8 years. A 32% inhibition was found after 7 years. In another study, *Marthaler*[104] found a 33% inhibition in a small group of subjects, initial age 7.5 years, after 6 years of unsupervised use of the dentifrice.

In contrast to the *Marthaler* studies, *Patz* and *Naujoks*[105] found only a 7% caries inhibition in 15 to 18-year-old subjects after 3 years. The only study conducted in the United States was done by *Ringleberg* and coworkers.[106] They compared the amine fluoride dentifrice and an amine fluoride mouth rinse with a stannous fluoride-calcium pyrophosphate dentifrice and a sodium fluoride mouth rinse. After 30 months' use, the amine fluoride dentifrice provided 18.1% caries inhibition and the stannous fluoride dentifrice 17.8%. Similarly, the amine fluoride mouth rinse provided 22.4% protection and the sodium fluoride mouth rinse 23.4% protection. While these findings suggest that amine fluoride is an effective anticaries agent, they do not support the contention that it is superior to other fluoride sources. Additional studies are required before this can be determined.

Studies with high or low fluoride concentrations

In spite of the rather large number of studies that have been conducted with fluoride dentifrices, very few have been concerned with determining either the optimum or minimum fluoride concentrations required. This is important not only in optimizing treatment benefits, but also in determining the shelf life of a product. Normally, soluble fluoride in a dentifrice decreases with time (see Fig. 8-3). To ensure an efficacious product, manufacturers and distributors must provide that the product reach the consumer before too much of the soluble fluoride has been lost. It can be assumed that less than 1,000 ppm soluble fluoride (or $PO_3F^=$) is still effective, since essentially all positive clinical trials testing dentifrices utilized at least some product that had aged several months or more.

Dentifrices containing 250, 500, and 1,000 ppm F from sodium fluoride in a calcium pyrophosphate base were clinically tested by *Reed*.[43] After 2 years of unsupervised use, caries inhibition (DMFS) of 7.5%, 8.5%, and 20% were found for the 250 ppm F, 500 ppm F, and 1,000 ppm F dentifrices respectively.

A sodium fluoride dentifrice containing 250 ppm F plus manganese chloride has been reported to be slightly better than a dentifrice containing 1,000 ppm F from sodium fluoride.[107] This study, however, did not include a nonfluoride control group.

Another clinical trial where dentifrices with low fluoride concentrations were compared to dentifrices with conventional concentrations was conducted in a community where all the children routinely received 0.2% sodium fluoride mouth rinses every other week. This study[91] included four groups that received sodium monofluorophosphate dentifrices containing either 250 ppm F or 1,000 ppm F and either calcium carbonate or silicon dioxide abrasives. After 2 years of unsupervised use, the clinical (visual-tactile) examination revealed nonsignificant 0-10% differences between the treated and control groups. The radiographic examination, however, showed 25% and 28% inhibitions for the two groups using the 1,000 ppm F dentifrices and 0% and 15% inhibitions for the two groups using the 250 ppm F dentifrices. A fifth group in this study used a sodium fluoride-silicon dioxide dentifrice containing

Table 8-6 Fluoride dentifrices accepted by the American Dental Association

Dentifrice	Manufacturer	Fluoride source	Abrasive
Crest*	Procter & Gamble Co.	SnF_2	$Ca_2P_2O_7$
Colgate with MFP*	Colgate-Palmolive Co.	Na_2PO_3F	IMP
Macleans Fluoride	Beecham Products, Inc.	Na_2PO_3F	$CaCO_3$
Aquafresh	Beecham Products, Inc.	Na_2PO_3F	$CaCO_3/SiO_2$
Aim*	Lever-Brothers Co.	SnF_2	SiO_2

*After preparation of this chapter, the fluoride-abrasive composition of three dentifrices was changed as follows: Crest now contains NaF and silica, Colgate contains Na_2PO_3F and $CaHPO_4 \cdot 2H_2O$, and Aim contains Na_2PO_3F and silica.

250 ppm F and received a 32% inhibition as evaluated with radiographs.

Three clinical trials have evaluated the effect of high concentrations of sodium monofluorophosphate (2,600 ppm F) in an aluminum oxide trihydrate base. Caries inhibitions in the first trial[108] after 3 years were 23% for 5-year-old children, 8% for 8 year-old children, and 23% for 11-year-old children. The second trial[109,110] was in a fluoridated water area where a 32% inhibition after 3 years' use by 7 to 12-year-old children was found. The third trial[111] resulted in a 24% caries inhibition in 11 to 12-year-old children. Examination of radiographs in this study increased this value to 39%.

While these studies were all positive and tended to give caries inhibition scores in the upper range of those reported for dentifrices containing 1,000 ppm F, they do not support the conclusion that dentifrices containing 2,600 ppm F are superior to those containing 1,000 ppm F. This is not to say that 2,600 ppm F is not better than 1,000 ppm, but because of the variability of clinical trials, studies including both concentrations are required before this can be shown.

Studies in areas with fluoridated drinking water

There is little doubt that fluoride dentifrices add some anticaries benefit to that provided by fluoridated drinking water. Tables 8-3 to 8-5 list six studies conducted in areas with fluoridated drinking water. Results of the trials varied from 0 to 29% inhibition with a mean value of 17%. In addition, a seventh study with a high-fluoride dentifrice[109,110] in a fluoridated area reported 32% caries inhibition.

Taken as a group, the caries inhibition scores reported in fluoridated water areas are slightly lower than in nonfluoridated areas; nevertheless, they show a significant and worthwhile benefit.

American Dental Association classification of fluoride dentifrices

The Council on Dental Therapeutics of the American Dental Association evaluates fluoride dentifrices to determine if the evidence concerning the dentifrice is sufficient to warrant its classification as being an effective anticaries formulation. The Council classifies dentifrice products as "accepted," "provisionally accepted," or "unacceptable."[112] Accepted products include those for which there is adequate evidence of safety and effectiveness. Provisionally accepted products include those for which there is reasonable evidence of usefulness and safety, but which lack sufficient evidence to justify being classified as accepted. Unaccepted products are those for which no substantial evidence of usefulness exists or where there is a question of safety. Both laboratory and clinical evidence is considered in making the classification.

Table 8-6 lists fluoride dentifrices currently classified by the Council.[113-117]

Effect of fluoride-containing dentifrices on dental hypersensitivity

The clinical impression that fluoride-containing dentifrices have a beneficial effect on cervical hypersensitivity was studied in several clinical trials. Although the results varied because of the subjective and often transient nature of hypersensitivity, they supported the clinical impression.

Because of its subjective nature and the natural remission of some hypersensitive areas, placebo treatments frequently elicit a favorable response. In four dentifrice studies reported in the literature, the placebo provided an apparent benefit of from 20 to 73%. Sodium monofluorophosphate dentifrices, however, reduced hypersensitivity to a greater degree. *Bolden* and co-workers[118] found a 66% improvement from a sodium monofluorophosphate dentifrice compared to 46% for a placebo. Other comparisons reported were 59% treated, 38% placebo;[119] 61% treated, 20% placebo;[120] and 77% treated, 56% placebo.[121] The placebo group in the last study mentioned improved after an additional toothbrushing period (4 weeks), until it reached the level of the monofluorophosphate dentifrice. Hypersensitivity to heat and cold was measured after 3 months' use of a sodium monofluorophosphate dentifrice by *Kanouse* and *Ash*,[122] who found reduced sensitivity to both stimuli from the dentifrice.

An early study was reported where hypersensitivity was reduced 11% within 6 weeks from a sodium fluoride dentifrice, and 92% if the same dentifrice was applied with an iontophoretic toothbrush.[123] A confirmation of this iontophoretic effect on fluoride dentifrices has not appeared in the literature.

The use of an anhydrous stannous fluoride gel containing the same level of fluoride as dentifrices (1,000 ppm F) and applied by toothbrushing was reported to reduce hypersensitivity in 20 of 23 subjects compared to only 8 of 23 subjects using a placebo gel,[124] but in another study using the same stannous fluoride gel no effect was found.[125] Stannous fluoride dentifrices also have been clinically tested,[118,119] but have not shown significant effects.

Ingestion of fluoride dentifrice

Some dentifrice is unintentionally swallowed during toothbrushing. The amount of fluoride ingested during brushing, particularly by young children and adults, has been studied by a number of investigators using several methods. The most common methods include analysis of the urine for increased fluoride levels and estimation of the dentifrice recovered after brushing.

The ingestion of dentifrice under normal home use conditions varies with the age of the subjects. *Barnhart* and co-workers[126] found that very young children, aged 2 to 4 years, ingested approximately 35% of the amount applied to the toothbrush. This percentage decreased to 14% at age 5 to 7 years, and to 3% in adults (Table 8-7). Other studies have also shown that a rather large percentage of dentifrice is swallowed by young children.[127-130] However, in a study

Table 8-7 Dentifrice ingestion by several age groups during normal toothbrushing

Age (yrs)	Dentifrice used (gm) mean (range)	Dentifrice ingested (gm) mean	%	Mean fluoride ingested (mg)
2–4	0.86 (0.19–2.41)	0.30	34.9	0.30
5–7	0.94 (0.15–2.08)	0.13	13.9	0.13
11–13	1.10 (0.31–2.00)	0.07	6.4	0.07
20–35	1.39 (0.42–3.29)	0.04	2.9	0.04

Data from *Barnhart* et al.[126]

where 24-hour urine fluoride levels of children using a stannous fluoride dentifrice were compared to a similar group using a placebo dentifrice, no difference could be found.[131] The 24-hour urine fluoride levels in both groups (0.22 mg F) were considerably lower than the urine fluoride levels of a similar group using a nonfluoride dentifrice in a fluoridated water area (0.84 mg F). The increase in urine fluoride levels from fluoride dentifrice use by adults also was too low to detect by chemical measurements,[132] but from radioactive tracer measurements[133] it has been estimated to be approximately 3% of the amount used.

The average amount of fluoride accidentally ingested from swallowed dentifrice ranges from 0.3 mg F in young children to 0.04 mg F in adults (see Table 8-7). Because this amount is within the normal variation of dietary intake, it is not of practical significance. The average ingestion of a population, however, may be misleading, since some children may habitually swallow large amounts. This possibility was investigated and, although it was found that some children tend to behave erratically with regard to dentifrice ingestion, none were consistently high swallowers.[129,130,134] Nevertheless, the parent should monitor the toothbrushing of very young children to be assured that they are not using or swallowing excessive amounts of dentifrice. Persistent ingestion of large amounts of fluoride dentifrice may result in mild fluorosis in the permanent teeth, especially if the child is also taking fluoride supplements. Another concern expressed by some people is the possible toxicity from ingestion of a large quantity of dentifrice in a single dose, for example, an entire tube. The quantity of fluoride contained in a large tube of dentifrice (9 oz., 255 g) is approximately 255 mg. While this amount, if fully absorbed, might make a small child temporarily ill (indeed, 9 ounces probably would even if it were a nonfluoride dentifrice), it would not be a serious danger (see Chapter 3). The estimated lethal dose for a 15 kg child is 500 to 1,000 mg fluoride taken rapidly. If the fluoride were absorbed slowly, as might occur from a dentifrice, its toxicity would be lower.

The amount of fluoride actually absorbed from ingested dentifrice is affected by the composition of the dentifrice. When the dentifrice abrasive is a calcium salt, the amount absorbed is decreased significantly. Studies in rats and guinea pigs in which very large doses of fluoride were given in the presence of calcium salts or in calcium-containing dentifrice, showed that only one-half as much fluoride was absorbed compared to calcium-free dentifrices.[135-137] Similar effects have been found in human adults and children even when smaller doses were given.[135] Children aged 6 to 9 years, who ingested 3 g of a dentifrice with a dicalcium phosphate dihydrate abrasive, excreted in the urine less than one-half of the amount that they did when they ingested 3 g of a dentifrice with a plastic abrasive.[135] It can be assumed that the calcium-containing abrasive formed insoluble compounds with the fluoride, thus preventing its absorption.

Summary

The dentifrice is the most widely used form of fluoride treatment for the prevention of dental caries, with the exception of fluoridated drinking water. Dentifrices are manufactured with fluoride sources often selected to capitalize on superior enamel solubility reduction, compatibility with abrasives, or the possession of antibacterial properties.

All dentifrices have both cosmetic and therapeutic functions. Cosmetic functions include removing stains and food debris and freshening the breath. Therapeutic functions include removing cariogenic food substances and the application of fluoride. To be most effective, toothbrushing should be done within minutes after the ingestion of cariogenic food.

The therapeutic activity of a fluoride dentifrice includes deposition of fluoride in enamel, especially enamel with incipient carious lesions, and deposition in plaque, where it can form a reservoir for slow reaction with enamel or for more rapid reaction during a caries attack. Fluoride in plaque may also have an antibacterial effect on plaque microorganisms.

Dentifrices consist of an abrasive suspended in a liquid phase containing a detergent to produce foam, a humectant to prevent moisture loss, a binding agent to hold the paste together, and flavor, preservatives, and fluoride.

Abrasives, the cleaning and polishing agents, must be selected to be compatible with fluoride. Fluoride may be inactivated by reaction with calcium-containing abrasives. Calcium carbonate and calcium phosphate abrasives are not generally compatible with sodium or stannous fluoride; however, calcium pyrophosphate may be used. Sodium monofluorophosphate is more compatible with abrasives than sodium or stannous fluoride, and it can be used with many calcium-containing abrasives. Sodium monofluorophosphate can also be used with an aluminum oxide trihydrate abrasive.

Insoluble sodium metaphosphate and silica are commonly used abrasives that are compatible with all fluorides used in dentifrices. Sodium bicarbonate and plastic particles are also compatible with all dentifrice fluorides, but they are not commonly used.

The initial evaluation of new dentifrice formulations is done using laboratory tests. These tests, which essentially evaluate the compatibility of the dentifrice fluoride-abrasive system, include determination of the amount of soluble fluoride present, the degree to which the dentifrice is able to reduce enamel solubility in acid, and the amount of fluoride that is deposited in the tooth enamel by a treatment. The best laboratory test is a determination of the amount of caries protection obtained when the dentifrice is applied to experimental animals (rodents).

The final determination of the efficacy of a fluoride dentifrice formulation is a clinical trial in humans. This is done by comparing the increments of new decayed, missing, or filled teeth and surfaces within groups of children using a placebo dentifrice or the test dentifrice. Because of ethical considerations of withholding the benefit of a fluoride dentifrice from the control (placebo) group, an active control is sometimes used. In this case, the test dentifrice is compared to a dentifrice with known anticaries activity.

Dentifrices prepared with sodium fluoride, stannous fluoride, and sodium monofluorophosphate have been widely tested in human clinical trials, and benefits of 20 to 30% caries reduction have been found. A dentifrice containing amine fluoride compounds has also been found to be effective.

The usual fluoride concentration in dentifrices is 1,000 ppm F, but higher and lower concentrations have been tested in clinical trials. It has been found that a concentration as low as 250 ppm F has anticaries activity, but not as much as 1,000 ppm F. A concentration of 2,600 ppm F was also tested and found to provide very good caries protection, but it was not clearly superior to dentifrices containing 1,000 ppm F. Further studies are needed to establish the caries response to different fluoride concentrations.

Fluoride dentifrices have been shown to provide an additional anticaries benefit to that obtained from water fluoridation and also to have a beneficial effect on dental hypersensitivity.

During routine toothbrushing, some dentifrice fluoride is ingested accidentally. The amount is greater for young children, who do not have good control over their swallowing reflexes. The average amount ingested varies from about 35% in children aged 2 to 4 years, to only 3% in adults. As a precaution, parents should monitor the toothbrushing of very young children to prevent excessive dentifrice use and ingestion.

References

1. Bibby, B.G. 1945. Test of the effect of fluoride-containing dentifrices on dental caries. *J. Dent. Res.* 24:297-303.
2. Volpe, A.R. 1977. Dentifrices and mouthrinses. In *A textbook of preventive dentistry,* eds. R. C. Caldwell and R. E. Stallard, W. B. Saunders Co.
3. Axelsson, P.; Lindhe, J.; and Wäseby, J. 1976. The effect of various plaque control measures on gingivitis and caries in schoolchildren. *Community Dent. Oral Epidemiol.* 4:232-39.
4. Bibby, B.G. 1966. Do we tell the truth about preventing caries? *J. Dent. Child.* 33:269-79.
5. Stephan, R.M., and Miller, B.F. 1943. A quantitative method for evaluating physical and chemical agents which modify production of acids in bacterial plaques on human teeth. *J. Dent. Res.* 22:45-51.
6. Fosdick, L.S. 1950. The reduction of the incidence of dental caries. I. Immediate toothbrushing with a neutral dentifrice. *J. Amer. Dent. Assoc.* 40:133-43.
7. Jenkens, G.N. Personal communication. Oct. 9, 1979.
8. Koulourides, T. 1977. To what extent is the incipient lesion of dental caries reversible? Proceedings of symposium on incipient caries of enamel. Ann Arbor: University of Michigan, November.
9. Vallotin, C.F. 1945. An acquired pigmented pellicle of the enamel surface. *J. Dent. Res.* 24:161-69.
10. Kitchen, P.C., and Robinson, H.B.G. 1948. How abrasive need a dentifrice be. *J. Dent. Res.* 27:501-6.
11. Manly, R.S. 1943. A structureless recurrent deposit on teeth. *J. Dent. Res.* 22:479-86.
12. Gerdin, P. 1970. Studies in dentifrices. I. Abrasiveness of dentifrices and removal of discoloured stains. *Swed. Dent. J.* 63:275-82.
13. Wright, K.H.R., and Stevenson, J.I. 1967. The measurement and interpretation of dentifrice abrasives. *J. Soc. Cosmet. Chem.* 18:387-411.
14. Mellberg, J.R. 1979. The relative abrasivity of dental prophylactic pastes and abrasives on enamel and dentin. *J. Clin. Prev. Dent.* 6:13-18.
15. Noren, B., and Harse, C. 1974. The stability of the monofluorophosphate and fluoride ions in dentifrice containing calcium carbonate. *J. Soc. Cosmet. Chem.* 25:3-11.
16. Kestenbaum, R.C., and Roberts, D. Personal communication. July, 1980. Colgate-Palmolive Company internal report. Jan., 1970.
17. Andlaw, R.J., and Tucker, G.J. 1975. A three-year clinical trial of a dentifrice containing 0.8% sodium monofluorophosphate in an aluminum oxide trihydrate base. *Brit. Dent. J.* 138:426-32.
18. Koch, G. 1967. Effect of sodium fluoride in dentifrice and mouthwash on incidence of dental caries in schoolchildren. *Odont. Revy* 18 (Suppl. 12):1-125.
19. Koch, G. 1970. Longterm study of effect of supervised toothbrushing with a sodium fluoride dentifrice. *Caries Res.* 4:149-57.
20. Koch, G. 1972. Comparison and estimation of effect on caries of daily supervised toothbrushing with a dentifrice containing sodium fluoride

and a dentifrice containing potassium fluoride and manganese chloride. *Odont. Revy* 23:341-54.

21. Gerdin, P.-O. 1972. Studies in dentifrices, VI: the inhibitory effect of some grinding and non-grinding fluoride dentifrices on dental caries. *Swed. Dent. J.* 65:521-32.
22. Gerdin, P.-O. 1974. Studies in dentifrices, VIII: clinical testing of an acidulated, nongrinding dentifrice with reduced fluorine contents. *Swed. Dent. J.* 67:283-97.
23. Uchida, T.; Kikuchi, T.; Higashi, T.; Yoshiga, J.; and Okamoto, H. 1975. Clinical evaluation of a dentifrice containing aluminum lactate and aluminum fluoride. *J. Hiroshima Univ. Dent. Soc.* 7:60-66.
24. Gray, J.A. 1968. A critique of enamel dissolution testing for anticariogenic agents. Proceedings of conference on clinical testing of cariostatic agents. *Amer. Dent. Assoc.* October.
25. Herd, J.K.; and Overell, B.G. 1964. Effect of toothpaste containing sodium monofluorophosphate on enamel solubility *in vivo*. *Brit. Dent. J.* 117:286-91.
26. Mellberg, J.R. 1968. Use of uptake tests for evaluation of anti-caries agents. Proceedings of conference on clinical testing of cariostatic agents. *Amer. Dent. Assoc.* October.
27. Mellberg, J.R.; Laakso, P.V.; and Nicholson, C.R. 1966. The acquisition and loss of fluoride by topically fluoridated human tooth enamel. *Arch. Oral Biol.* 11:1213-20.
28. American Dental Association. 1968. Proceedings of the conference on the clinical testing of cariostatic agents.
29. Backer-Dirks, O.; Baume, L.J.; Davies, G.N.; and Slack, G.L. 1967. Principal requirements for controlled clinical trials. *Int. Dent. J.* 17:93-103.
30. Zacherl, W.A., and Long, D.M. 1979. Reduction in caries attack rate—non-fluoridated community. *Int. Assoc. Dent. Res.* Preprinted abstr. No. 535.
31. Marthaler, T.M. 1971. Confidence limits of results of clinical tests with fluoride administration. *Caries Res.* 5:343-72.
32. DePaola, P.F. 1974. The interpretation of findings in clinical caries trials. *J. Dent. Child.* 41:1-8.
33. Muhler, J.C.; Radike, A.W.; Nebergall, W.H.; and Day, H.G. 1955. A comparison between the anticariogenic effect of dentifrices containing stannous fluoride and sodium fluoride. *J. Amer. Dent. Assoc.* 51:556-59.
34. Winkler, K.C.; Backer-Dirks, O.; and van Amerogen, J. 1953. A reproducible method for caries evaluation. Test in a therapeutic experiment with a fluoridated dentifrice. *Brit. Dent. J.* 95:119-24.
35. Torell, P.; and Ericsson, Y. 1965. Two year clinical tests with different methods of local caries prevention. Fluoride application in Swedish schoolchildren. *Acta Odont. Scand.* 23:287-322.
36. Kyes, F.; Overton, N.J.; and McKean, T.W. 1961. Clinical trials of caries inhibitory dentifrices. *J. Amer. Dent. Assoc.* 63:189-93.
37. Brudevold, F., and Chilton, N.W. 1966. Comparative study of a fluoride dentifrice containing soluble phosphate and a calcium-free abrasive. Second year report. *J. Amer. Dent. Assoc.* 72:889-94.
38. Peterson, J.K., and Williamson, L. 1968. Three-year caries inhibition of a sodium fluoride acid orthophosphate dentifrice compared with a stannous fluoride and a non-fluoride dentifrice. *Int. Assoc. Dent. Res.* Preprinted abstr. No. 255.
39. Zacherl, W.A. 1968. A clinical evaluation of sodium fluoride and stannous fluoride dentifrices. *Int. Assoc. Dent. Res.* Abstr. No. 253.
40. Slack, G.L.; Bulman, J.S.; and Osborn, J.F. 1971. Clinical testing of fluoride and non-fluoride containing dentifrices in Hounslow schoolchildren. *Brit. Dent. J.* 130:154-58.
41. Zacherl, W.A. 1972. Clinical evaluation of neutral sodium fluoride, stannous fluoride, sodium monofluorophosphate and acid fluoride-phosphate dentifrices. *J. Can. Dent. Assoc.* 38:35-38.
42. Weisenstein, P.R., and Zacherl, W.A. 1972. A multiple-examiner clinical evaluation of a sodium fluoride dentifrice. *J. Amer. Dent. Assoc.* 84:621-23.
43. Reed, M.W. 1973. Clinical evaluation of three concentrations of sodium fluoride in dentifrices. *J. Amer. Dent. Assoc.* 87:1401-3.
44. Stookey, G.K., and Beiswanger, B.B. 1974. Effect of NaF dentifrice on dental caries in children. *Int. Assoc. Dent. Res.* Abstr. No. 715.
45. Reed, M.W., and King, J.D. 1975. A clinical evaluation of a sodium fluoride dentifrice. *Pharm. Ther. Dent.* 2:77-82.
46. Zacherl, W.A. 1972. Clinical evaluation of an aged stannous fluoride-calcium pyrophosphate dentifrice. *J. Can. Dent. Assoc.* 38:155-57.
47. Muhler, J.C.; Radike, A.W.; Nebergall, W.H.; and Day, H.G. 1955. Effect of a stannous fluoride-containing dentifrice on caries reduction in children. II. Caries experience after one year. *J. Amer. Dent. Assoc.* 50:163-66.
48. Muhler, J.C., and Radike, A.W. 1957. Effect of a dentifrice containing stannous fluoride on den-

tal caries in adults. II. Results at the end of two years of unsupervised use. *J. Amer. Dent. Assoc.* 55:196-98.

49. Jordan, W.A., and Peterson, J.K. 1959. Caries inhibiting value of a dentifrice containing stannous fluoride. Final report of a two year study. *J. Amer. Dent. Assoc.* 58:42-44.
50. Hill, T.J. 1959. Fluoride dentifrices. *J. Amer. Dent. Assoc.* 59:1121-27.
51. Muhler, J.C. 1960. Combined anticariogenic effect of a single stannous fluoride solution and the unsupervised use of a stannous fluoride-containing dentifrice, II. Results at the end of two years. *J. Dent. Res.* 39:955-58.
52. Peffley, G.E., and Muhler, J.C. 1960. The effect of a commercial stannous fluoride dentifrice under controlled brushing habits on dental caries incidence in children. Preliminary report. *J. Dent. Res.* 39:871-74.
53. Muhler, J.C. 1962. Effect of a stannous fluoride dentifrice on caries reduction in children during a three year study period. *J. Amer. Dent. Assoc.* 64:216-24.
54. Bixler, D., and Muhler, J.C. 1962. Experimental clinical human caries test design and interpretation. *J. Amer. Dent. Assoc.* 65:482-90.
55. Finn, S.B., and Jamison, H.C. 1963. A comparative clinical study of three dentifrices. *J. Dent. Child.* 30:17-25.
56. Henriques, B.L.; Frankl, S.N.; and Alman, J.E. 1964. Cited in: Evaluation of Cue toothpaste. *J. Amer. Dent. Assoc.* 71:197-98.
57. Mergele, M.; Jennings, R.E.; and Gasser, E.B. 1964. Cited in: Evaluation of Cue toothpaste. *J. Amer. Dent. Assoc.* 69:197-98.
58. Slack, G.L., and Martin, W.J. 1964. The use of a dentifrice containing stannous fluoride in the control of dental caries. *Brit. Dent. J.* 117:275-80.
59. Bixler, D., and Muhler, J.C. 1966. Effectiveness of stannous fluoride-containing dentifrices in reducing dental caries in children in a boarding school environment. *J. Amer. Dent. Assoc.* 72:653-57.
60. Thomas, A.E., and Jamison, H.C. 1966. Effect of stannous fluoride dentifrices on caries in children: two year clinical study of supervised brushing in children's homes. *J. Amer. Dent. Assoc.* 73:844-52.
61. Horowitz, H.S.; Law, F.E.; Thompson, M.B.; and Chamberlain, S.R. 1966. Evaluation of a stannous fluoride dentifrice for use in dental public health programmes—basic findings. *J. Amer. Dent. Assoc.* 72:408-21.
62. Fullmer, J.; Volpe, A.R.; Apperson, L.D.; and Kiraly, J. 1966. (Unpublished data, Colgate-Palmolive Co. 1966.) Cited in: Volpe, A.R. Dentifrices and mouthrinses. In *A textbook of preventive dentistry,* eds. R. C. Caldwell and R. E. Stallard. W. B. Saunders, 1977.
63. Slack, G.L.; Berman, D.S.; Martin, W.J.; and Young, J. 1967. Clinical testing of a stannous fluoride-insoluble metaphosphate dentifrice in Kent schoolgirls. *Brit. Dent. J.* 123:9-16.
64. Slack, G.L.; Berman, D.S.; Martin, W.J.; and Hardie, J.M. 1967. Clinical testing of a stannous fluoride-calcium pyrophosphate dentifrice in Essex schoolgirls. *Brit. Dent. J.* 123:26-33.
65. Jackson, D., and Sutcliffe, P. 1967. Clinical testing of a stannous fluoride-calcium pyrophosphate dentifrice in Yorkshire schoolchildren. *Brit. Dent. J.* 123:40-48.
66. James, P.M.C., and Anderson, R. 1967. Clinical testing of a stannous fluoride-calcium pyrophosphate dentifrice in Buckinghamshire schoolchildren. *Brit. Dent. J.* 123:33-39.
67. Naylor, M.N., and Emslie, R.D. 1967. Clinical testing of stannous fluoride and sodium monofluorophosphate dentifrices in London schoolchildren. *Brit. Dent. J.* 123:17-23.
68. Stiff, R.H., Segal, A.N.; George, W.A.; and Picozzi, A. 1967. Anticaries effectivenss of a stannous fluoride-insoluble sodium metaphosphate (IMP) dentifrice in children following three years of supervised toothbrushing. *Int. Assoc. Dent. Res.* Abstr. No. 271.
69. Onishi, E.; Okada, S.; Hinoide, M.; Akada, H.; Kon, K.; Sugano, N.; Sakakobara, Y.; Morita, J.; and Imamura, Y. 1967. Effect of stannous fluoride dentifrice on the reduction of dental caries in schoolchildren. *Jap. J. Dent. Hlth.* 17:68-74.
70. Fanning, E.A.; Gotjamanos, T.; and Vowles, N.J. 1968. The use of fluoride dentifrice in the control of dental caries: methodology and results of a clinical trial. *Aust. Dent. J.* 13:201-6.
71. Frankl, S.N., and Alman, J.E. 1968. Report of a three year clinical trial comparing a toothpaste containing sodium monofluorophosphate with two marketed products. *J. Oral Ther. Pharm.* 4:443-50.
72. Mergele, M. 1968. Report I. A supervised brushing study in state institution schools. *Bull. Acad. Med. N. J.* 14:247-50.
73. Mergele, M. 1968. Report II. An unsupervised brushing study on subjects residing in a community with fluoride in the water. *Bull. Acad. Med. N. J.* 14:251-55.
74. Zacherl, W.A., and McPhail, C.W.B. 1970. Final report on the efficacy of a stannous fluoride-calcium pyrophosphate dentifrice. *J. Can. Dent. Assoc.* 36:262-64.
75. Muhler, J.C. 1970. A clinical comparison of fluo-

ride and antienzyme dentifrices. *J. Dent. Child.* 37:501-2, 511-14.

76. Gish, C.W., and Muhler, J.C. 1971. Effectiveness of a stannous fluoride dentifrice on dental caries. *J. Dent. Child.* 38:211-14.
77. Zacherl, W.A. 1973. A clinical evaluation of a stannous fluoride and a sarcosinate dentifrice. *J. Dent. Child.* 40:451-53.
78. Fogels, H.R.; Alman, J.E.; Meade, J.J.; and O'Donnell, J.P. 1979. The relative caries-inhibiting effects of a stannous fluoride dentifrice in a silica gel base. *J. Amer. Dent. Assoc.* 99:456-59.
79. American Dental Association, Council on Dental Therapeutics. 1964. Evaluation of Cue toothpaste. *J. Amer. Dent. Assoc.* 69:197.
80. American Dental Association, Council on Dental Therapeutics. 1965. Evaluation of Fact toothpaste. *J. Amer. Dent. Assoc.* 71:930.
81. American Dental Association, Council on Dental Therapeutics. 1966. Evaluation of Super Stripe toothpaste. *J. Amer. Dent. Assoc.* 72:1515, 1966.
82. Møller, I.J.; Holst, J.J.; and Sorensen, E. 1968. Caries reducing effect of a sodium monofluorophosphate dentifrice. *Brit. Dent. J.* 124:209-13.
83. Takeuchi, M.; Schimizu, T.; Kawasaki, T.; and Kizu, T. 1968. A field study on the effect of a dentifrice containing sodium monofluorophosphate in caries prevention. *J. Soc. Oral Hyg.* 18:26-37.
84. Kinkel, H.J., and Stolte, G. 1968. Zur wirkung einer natrium monofluorophosphat-und bromchlorophen-haltigen zahnpasta in chronischen tierexperiment and auf die karies bei kindern wahrend eines zwei jahre langen, unuberwachten gebrauches. *Deutsche Zahnarzteblatt.* 22:455-60.
85. Torell, P. 1969. (The use of fluoride toothpaste combined with fluoride rinsing every two weeks.) (Swe.) *Sveriges Tandlak. Tidning.* 61:873-75.
86. Patz, J., and Naujoks, R. 1969. Clinical investigation of a fluoride-containing dentifrice in adults. Results of a two year unsupervised study. *Dtsch. Zahnaertztl. Z.* 7:614-21.
87. Onisi, M., and Tani, H. 1970. Clinical test on the caries-preventive effect of two kinds of fluoride dentifrices. *Jap. J. Dent. Hlth.* 20:105-11.
88. Thomas, A.E., and Jamison, H.C. 1970. Effect of a combination of two cariostatic agents on caries in children: two-year clinical study of supervised brushing in children's homes. *J. Amer. Dent. Assoc.* 81:118-24.
89. Kinkel, H.J.; Raich, R.; and Muller, M. 1977. Kie Karieshemmung einer Na_2PO_3F—Zahnpasta nach 7 jahren applikation. *Schweiz Mschr. Zahnheilk* 87:1218-20.
90. Kinkel, H.J.; Stolte, G.; and Westrate, J. 1974. (Study of the effect of a toothpaste containing fluorophosphate on the dentition of children.) (Fre.) *Schweiz Mschr. Zahnheilk* 84:577-89.
91. Forsman, B. 1974. Studies on the effect of dentifrices with low fluoride content. *Community Dent. Oral Epidemiol.* 2:166-75.
92. Peterson, J.; Williamson, L.; and Casad, R. 1975. Caries inhibition with MFP-calcium carbonate dentifrice in fluoridated area. *Int. Assoc. Dent. Res.* Abstr. No. L338.
93. Niwa, T.; Baba, K.; and Niwa, N. 1975. The caries preventive effects of dentifrices containing sodium monofluorophosphate, sodium monofluorophosphate plus dextranase and sodium monofluorophosphate plus sodium phosphate. *Jap. J. Dent. Hlth.* 25 (3):30-52.
94. Ashley, F.P.; Mainwaring, P.J.; Emslie, R.D.; and Naylor, M.N. 1977. Clinical testing of a mouthrinse and a dentifrice containing fluoride. A two-year supervised study in school children. *Brit. Dent. J.* 143:333-38.
95. Mainwaring, P.J., and Naylor, M.N. 1978. A three year clinical study to determine the separate and combined caries-inhibiting effects of sodium monofluorophosphate toothpaste and an acidulated phosphate fluoride gel. *Caries Res.* 12:202-12.
96. Glass, R.L., and Shiere, F.R. 1978. A clinical trial of a calcium carbonate base dentifrice containing 0.76% sodium monofluorophosphate. *Caries Res.* 12:284-89.
97. Howat, A.P.; Holloway, P.J.; and Davies, T.G.H. 1978. Caries prevention by daily supervised use of a MFP gel dentifrice. Report of a 3-year clinical trial. *Brit. Dent. J.* 145:233-35.
98. Peterson, J.K. 1979. A supervised brushing trial of sodium monofluorophosphate dentifrices in a fluoridated area. *Caries Res.* 13:68-72.
99. Naylor, M.N., and Glass, R.L. 1979. A 3-year clinical trial of calcium carbonate dentifrice containing calcium glycerophosphate and sodium monofluorophosphate. *Caries Res.* 13:39-46.
100. Ingram, G.S. 1977. Reaction between apatite and monofluorophosphate: modification by fluoride and condensed phosphate. *Caries Res.* 11:30-38.
101. Mühlemann, H.R.; Schmid, H.; and Konig, K.G. 1957. Enamel solubility reduction studies with inorganic and organic fluorides. *Helv. Odont. Acta* 1:23-33.
102. Konig, K.G.; and Mühlemann, H.R. 1961. Caries inhibiting effect of amine fluoride containing dentifrice tested in an animal experiment and a

clinical study. In *The present status of caries prevention by fluorine-containing dentifrices*, eds., H.R. Mühleman and K. G. Konig, pp. 126-30. Berne: Huber.

103. Marthaler, T.M. 1968. Caries-inhibition after seven years of unsupervised use of an amine fluoride dentifrice. *Brit Dent. J.* 124:510-15.

104. Marthaler, T.M. 1974. Caries-inhibition by an amine fluoride dentifrice. Results after 6 years in children with low caries activity. *Helv. Odont. Acta* 18 (Suppl. VIII):35-44.

105. Patz, J., and Naujoks, R. 1970. The prophylactic anticaries effect of an amine fluoride containing dentifrice on adolescents after unsupervised use for 3 years. *Deutsch Zahnaertzl Z.* 25:617-25.

106. Ringleberg, M.L.; Webster, D.B.; Dixon, D.O.; and LaZotte, D.C. 1979. The caries preventive effect of amine fluorides and inorganic fluorides in a mouthrinse or dentifrice after 30 months of use. *J. Amer. Dent. Assoc.* 98:202-8.

107. Gerdin, P.-O. 1974. Studies in dentifrices, VIII: Clinical testing of an acidulated, nongrinding dentifrice with reduced fluorine contents. *Swed. Dent. J.* 67:283-97.

108. Hargreaves, J.A., and Chester, C.G. 1973. Clinical trial among Scottish children of an anticaries dentifrice containing 2% sodium monofluorophosphate. *Community Dent. Oral Epidemiol.* 1:47-57.

109. Lind, O.P.; Møller, I.J.; von der Fehr, F.R.; and Larsen, M.J. 1974. Caries-preventive effect of a dentifrice containing 2% sodium monofluorophosphate in a natural fluoride area in Denmark. *Community Dent. Oral Epidemiol.* 2:104-13.

110. Lind, O.P.; von der Fehr, F.R.; Larsen, M.J.; and Møller, I.J. 1976. Anticaries effect of a 2% Na_2PO_3F–dentrifice in a Danish fluoride area. *Community Dent. Oral Epidemiol.* 4:7-14.

111. James, P.M.C.; Anderson, R.J.; Beal, J.F.; and Brodnock, G. 1977. A 3-year clinical trial of the effect on dental caries of a dentifrice containing 2% sodium monofluorophosphate. *Community Dent. Oral Epidemiol.* 5:67-72.

112. American Dental Association, Council on Dental Therapeutics. 1975. Accepted dental therapeutics. 36th ed. Chicago.

113. American Dental Association, Council on Dental Therapeutics. 1964. Reclassification of Crest toothpaste. *J. Amer. Dent. Assoc.* 69:195-96.

114. American Dental Association, Council on Dental Therapeutics. 1969. Council classifies Colgate with MFP (sodium monofluorophosphate) in group A. *J. Amer. Dent. Assoc.* 79:937.

115. American Dental Association, Council on Dental Therapeutics. 1976. Council accepts Macleans Fluoride dentifrice. *J. Amer. Dent. Assoc.* 92:966-67.

116. American Dental Association, Council on Dental Therapeutics. 1978. Council accepts Aquafresh. *J. Amer. Dent. Assoc.* 97:80.

117. American Dental Association, Council on Dental Therapeutics. 1979. Council accepts Aim. *J. Amer. Dent. Assoc.* 99:699.

118. Bolden, T.E.; Volpe, A.R.; and King, W.J. 1968. The desensitizing effect of a sodium monofluorophosphate dentifrice. *Periodontics* 6:112-14.

119. Hazen, S.P.; Volpe, A.R.; and King, W.J. 1968. Comparative desensitizing effect of dentifrices containing sodium monofluorophosphate, stannous fluoride and formalin. *Periodontics* 6:230-32.

120. Hernandez, F.; Mohammed, C.; Shannon, I.; Volpe, A.; and King, W. 1972. Clinical study evaluating the desensitizing effect and duration of two commercially available dentifrices. *Periodontol.* 43:367-72.

121. Shapiro, W.B.; Koslick, R.S.; Chasens, A.I.; and Weinstein, D. 1970. Controlled clinical comparison between a strontium chloride and a sodium monofluorophosphate toothpaste in diminishing root hypersensitivity. *J. Periodontal.* 41:523-25.

122. Kanouse, M.C., and Ash, M.M., Jr. 1969. The effectiveness of a sodium monofluorophosphate dentifrice on dental hypersensitivity. *J. Periodontal* 40:38-39.

123. Jensen, A.L. 1964. Hypersensitivity controlled by iontophoresis: double blind clinical investigation. *J. Amer. Dent. Assoc.* 68:216-25.

124. Miller, J.T.; Shannon, I.L.; Kilgore, W.S.; and Bookman, J.E. 1969. Use of a water-free stannous fluoride-containing gel in the control of dental hypersensitivity. *J. Periodontal* 40:490-91.

125. Zinner, D.D.; Duany, L.F.; and Lutz, H.J. 1977. A new desensitizing dentifrice: preliminary report. *J. Amer. Dent. Assoc.* 95:982-85.

126. Barnhart, W.E.; Hiller, L.K.; Leonard, G.J.; and Michaels, S.E. 1974. Dentifrice usage and ingestion among four age groups. *J. Dent. Res.* 53:1317-22.

127. Eichler, O. 1961. Cited by Buttner, W.; Schulke, S.; and Soyka, S. in: Toxicity of fluorine-containing dentifrices. In *Caries symposium, Zurich*, eds. H.R. Mühlemann and K.G. Konig, pp. 92-103. Bern: Huber.

128. Ericsson, Y., and Forsman, B. 1969. Fluoride retained from mouthrinses and dentifrices from preschool children. *Caries Res.* 3:290-99.

129. Hargreaves, J.A.; Ingram, G.S.; and Wagg, B.J.

1972. A gravimetric study of the ingestion of toothpaste by children. *Caries Res.* 6:237-43.

130. Hargreaves, J.A.; Ingram, G.S.; and Wagg, B.J. 1970. Excretion studies on the ingestion of a monofluorophosphate toothpaste by children. *Caries Res.* 4:256-68.
131. Schweinsberger, R.A.; and Muhler, J.C. 1956. Urinary fluorine levels in children following the clinical use of a stannous fluoride-containing dentifrice. *J. Dent. Res.* 35:760-62.
132. Buttner, W.; Schulke, S.; and Soyka, S. 1961. Toxicity of fluorine-containing dentifrices. In: *Caries symposium, Zurich,* eds. H.R. Mühlemann and K.G. Konig, pp. 92-103. Bern: Huber.
133. Duckworth, R. 1964. Distribution and excretion of dentifrice fluoride. *Nature (Lond.)* 204:489-90.
134. Naylor, M.N.; Melville, M.; Wilson, R.F.; Ingram, G.S.; and Wagg, B.J. 1971. Ingestion of dentifrice by young children: a pilot study using a fecal marker. *J. Dent. Res.* 50:687.
135. Forsman, B., and Ericsson, Y. 1973. Fluoride absorption from swallowed fluoride toothpaste. *Community Dent. Oral Epidemiol.* 1:115-20.
136. Shaner, E.O., and Smith, R.R. 1946. Clinical and bacteriological studies of the use of a fluoride dentifrice. *J. Dent. Res.* 25:121-26.
137. Despande, S.S.; and Bester, J.F. 1964. Absorption and retention of fluoride from ingested stannous fluoride dentifrice. *J. Pharm. Sci.* 53:803-7.

Chapter 9

Self-applied Topical Fluoride

The traditional application of topical fluoride involves a dentist or dental hygienist treating one patient at a time (see Chapter 7). This one-to-one approach has been recognized as too costly and time-consuming to satisfy the requirements of most public health programs in which large numbers of children are enrolled.

To bring the benefits of topically applied fluoride to more people at a reasonable cost, procedures have been developed for the *self-application* of fluoride. While the investigation of self-application techniques was prompted by their need in public health programs, they can also be used by individual dental patients who will conscientiously apply them regularly in their own homes. In these instances, self-application procedures should be used in conjunction with other caries control methods as part of a total program of caries prevention.

It is the purpose of this chapter to describe the methods of self-application, indicate their levels of effectiveness, and make recommendations for their use.

Self-application methods

The most common method of self-application is brushing the teeth with a fluoride-containing dentifrice. Since most people brush their teeth with a dentifrice, it requires very little additional effort to substitute a fluoride-containing dentifrice for a nontherapeutic one. The use of fluoride dentifrices is specifically discussed in Chapter 8. The three methods of self-application that have been studied in public health programs, and which are described in this chapter, are

Toothbrushing—A fluoride solution, gel, or fluoride-containing prophylaxis paste is applied to a standard toothbrush by the patient, who then brushes his own teeth with the topical fluoride agent.

Mouth rinsing—The patient swishes with a measured amount of fluoride-containing mouth rinse. Depending upon the concentration of the fluoride rinse, the availability of therapeutic levels of systemic fluoride, and the age of the individual, the solution is either swished and swallowed or swished and expectorated.

Use of mouth trays—Several drops of fluoride gel are placed into custom-fitted or disposable mouth trays. The individual then positions the trays in his mouth, allowing the gel to contact the teeth for several minutes.

Each of the methods of self-application has its particular advantages and disadvantages. However, all have the benefit of requiring less professional time than the traditional operator-applied, topical fluoride techniques and, thus, the potential of reaching more children. Additionally, when used by the conscientious patient at home, these techniques provide many more fluoride contacts to the teeth than can be professionally provided in the dental office.

Self-application of topical fluoride by brushing

In the early 1960s, two reports by *Berggren* and *Welander*[1,2] described the results of clinical trials conducted on Swedish schoolchildren, in which different fluoride solutions were applied to the teeth by toothbrushing. In these studies, 1% sodium fluoride, 0.5% sodium fluoride, zirconium fluoride, or ferric fluoride was brushed on the teeth by the children themselves four or ten times during 2 years. Brushing with the 1% sodium fluoride solution produced a 25 to 30% caries reduction in the maxillary arch, but failed to have an effect in the mandibular arch.[1] The investigators felt that salivary dilution of the fluoride solution during brushing might have been responsible for the ineffectiveness of the technique on the mandibular teeth. It was also noticed that more frequent brushing was more effective.[2] *Berggren* and *Welander* emphasized that about 200 children per day could be supervised as they treated themselves by the self-application method; whereas, in the traditional operator-applied technique, less than 30 children could have received treatment in the same amount of time.

Since these initial reports from Sweden, other investigators have clinically evaluated the cariostatic effectiveness of topical fluoride compounds applied by self-brushing.[3-26] Tables 9-1, 9-2, and 9-3 list the caries reductions achieved by this technique when applied to the permanent teeth of children residing in fluoride-deficient communities. Table 9-4 lists the results from optimally fluoridated communities, and Table 9-5 lists the results obtained from primary teeth. While approximately two dozen clinical trials have been reported, scrutiny of the tables reveals little uniformity in either the type of fluoride employed, the fluoride vehicle, or the frequency of application. For instance, neutral sodium fluoride (NaF), acidified sodium fluoride,* stannous fluoride (SnF_2), sodium monofluorophosphate (Na_2PO_3F), amine fluoride, zirconium fluoride (ZrF_2), and ferric fluoride (FeF_3) have all been used in self-application brushing programs. Initially, the fluoride was applied in aqueous solution (Table 9-1).[1,2,5-11] Later, it was incorporated into a prophylaxis paste by combining it with abrasives such as zirconium silicate or silicon dioxide (Table 9-2).[12-21] By the addition of an alkylcellulose, the fluoride solutions were rendered viscous and children brushed with fluoride gels (Table 9-3).[8,9,22] As recorded in these tables, some school-based programs required brushing to be performed only once or twice a year; in others it was performed five or more times a year; while in one program, children were requested to brush daily in their homes.

The results obtained by self-brushing using fluoride solutions, fluoride-containing prophylaxis pastes, and fluoride gels were reviewed in 1974 by *McConchie*[27] as part of an international workshop on fluoride. His assessment that "the results of published studies demonstrate a wide spectrum of degrees of effectiveness" is still valid today. Because of the lack of uniformity among the clinical trials listed in Tables 9-1 through 9-4, it is difficult to predict the potential preventive capabilities of self-brushing programs. Nevertheless, a perusal of the results suggests that only a limited caries inhibition of the permanent

*Chemically acidified NaF preparations may be buffered or unbuffered. If buffered, they are listed in the tables of this chapter as APF (acidulated phosphate fluoride).

Table 9-1 Effect of self-application by brushing of topical fluoride solutions on the permanent teeth of children residing in fluoride-deficient communities

Study	Initial age (years) of subjects	Solution	Brushing frequency (times/year)	Duration of study	Percent reduction DMFT	DMFS
Berggren & Welander[1]	7–13	1% NaF	4–5	2 years	16	
Berggren & Welander[2]	10	0.5% NaF	5	2 years	29	
		0.25% ZrF_2	5	2 years	17	
		0.50% FeF_3	5	2 years	33	
	10	0.5% NaF	2	2 years	17	
		0.25% ZrF_2	2	2 years	0	
		0.50% FeF_3	2	2 years	8	
Bullen et al.[5,6]	6	APF (1.23% F from NaF & HF), pH 3	4–5	1 year		39
	6	APF (1.23% F from NaF & HF), pH 3	4–5	2 years		15
Conchie et al.[7]	11–16	APF (1.23% F from NaF & HF), pH3	4–5	2 years		25
Heifetz et al.[8]	12–14	APF (0.6% F from NaF & HF), pH3	5	2 years	+7	3
	12–14	brushed with non-F prophy paste followed by APF solution (0.6% F from NaF & HF), pH3	5	2 years	8	11
Horowitz et al.[9]	14–17	APF (0.6% F from NaF & HF), pH3	5	3 years		26
	14–17	brushed with non-F prophy paste followed by APF solution (0.6% F from NaF & HF), pH 3	5	3 years		26
Gallagher et al.[10]	10	APF (0.6% F from NaF & HF), pH 3	5	26 months	18	
Marthaler & Muhlemann[11]	6–13	22 mg NaF tablet (10 mg F) chewed, dissolved in saliva, and brushed*	11	1 year	34–23**	24–35**

*After brushing, the children immediately chewed another NaF tablet and swished with the fluoride-impregnated saliva.
**Grades 1 and 3 respectively.

Table 9-2 Effect of self-application by brushing fluoride containing prophylaxis pastes on the permanent teeth of children residing in fluoride-deficient communities

Study	Initial age (years) of subjects	Agent and abrasive	Brushing frequency (times/year)	Duration of study	Percent reduction DMFT	DMFS
Muhler et al.[12]	6–14	9% SnF_2-$ZrSiO_4$*	1	1 year	41	60
Fleming et al.[13]	11–15	9% SnF_2-$ZrSiO_4$	1	2 years	+3	+16
	11–15	9% SnF_2-$ZrSiO_4$	2	2 years	24	5
Horowitz & Bixler[14]	9–14	9% SnF_2-$ZrSiO_4$	2 (for first year) 1 (for second and third years)	3 years	14-20**	15-23**
Gish et al.[15]	6–14	9% SnF_2-$ZrSiO_4$	2	3 years	32	37
Woodhouse[16]	12–13	10% SnF_2-$ZrSiO_4$	2	3 years	19	16
Woods[17]	5–9	10% SnF_2-$ZrSiO_4$	3	2 years	36	50
Muhler[18]	7–13	SnF_2-alkali aluminum silicate	1	1 year	31	33
Mellberg et al.[19]	6–14	APF-SiO_2*** (0.4% F from ammonium silicofluoride), pH 3.2	2	3 years	14	21
Long[20]	10–13	APF-SiO_2 (0.4% F from ammonium silicofluoride), pH 3.2	3	2 years	17	
Trubman & Crellin[21]	8.12****	APF-SiO_2 (0.4% F from ammonium silicofluoride), pH 3.2	4	3 years	4	10
	8.12	APF-SiO_2 (0.4% F from ammonium silicofluoride), pH 3.2 followed by APF gel-tray application	4	3 years	25	22

*Stannous fluoride active agent; zirconium silicate abrasive.
**Two independent examiners.
***Acidulated phosphate fluoride active agent; silicon dioxide abrasive.
****Average age.

teeth of children can be expected from the self-brushing method; nor are the results of self-brushing to the primary teeth consistent (Table 9-5). While *Bullen* and co-workers[5] found no effect to the primary teeth from self-brushing with a fluoride solution, *Woods*[17] reported a 76% reduction when a stannous fluoride-zirconium silicate prophylaxis paste was self-brushed three times a year. However, the latter indicated that the caries reversal rate in the treatment group was high. (Reversals are teeth or surfaces that are diagnosed as carious at one examination and as sound at a subsequent examination.) While a reversal may be due to the therapeutic agent's effect on the carious lesion (see Chapter 1), it may also be due to examiner error. A large number of reversals in the treatment group will inflate the caries reductions obtained.

Table 9-3 Effect of self-application by brushing fluoride gels on the permanent teeth of children residing in fluoride-deficient communities

Study	Initial age (years) of subjects	Gel	Brushing frequency (times/year)	Duration of study	Percent reduction DMFT	Percent reduction DMFS
Heifetz et al.[8]	12–14	brushed with non-F prophy paste followed by APF gel (1.23% F from NaF & HF), pH 3	5	2 years	11	8
Horowitz et al.[9]	14–17	APF gel (1.23% F from NaF & HF), pH 3	5	3 years		19
	14–17	brushed with non-F prophy paste followed by APF gel (1.23% F from NaF & HF), pH 3	5	3 years		33
Marthaler et al.[22]	6–9	1.25% F from NaF & amine fluoride	30 (for first year); 16 (for second and third years)	3 years		34–40*

*Grades 1 and 3 respectively.

Table 9-4 Effect of self-application by brushing topical fluoride on the permanent teeth of children residing in optimally fluoridated communities

Study	Initial age (years) of subjects	Agent	Brushing frequency	Duration of study	Percent reduction DMFT	Percent reduction DMFS
Brushing with topical fluoride solutions						
Goaz et al.[23,24]						
	6–14	6% MFP* solution	1 time/day	14 months		42
	6–14	6% MFP solution	1 time/day	21 months		47
Brushing with fluoride-containing prophylaxis pastes						
Gunz[25]	7–11	9% SnF_2-$ZrSiO_4$**	1 time/year	14 months	11	11
Lang et al.[26]	6–10	9% SnF_2-$ZrSiO_4$	2 times/year	18 months	27***	38***
					41	42
					41	42
Gish et al.[15]	6–14	9% SnF_2-$ZrSiO_4$	2 times/year	3 years	30	25

*MFP = Sodium monofluorophosphate (Na_2PO_3F).
**Stannous fluoride active agent; zirconium silicate abrasive.
***Three independent examiners.

Table 9-5 Effect of self-application by brushing topical fluoride on the primary teeth of children*

Study	Initial age (years) of subjects	Agent	Brushing frequency (times/year)	Duration of study	Percent reduction dft	Percent reduction dfs
Brushing with topical fluoride solutions						
Bullen et al.[5]	6	APF solution (1.23% F from NaF & HF), pH 3	4-5	1 year		4
Brushing with fluoride-containing prophylaxis pastes						
Woods[17]	5-9	10% SnF_2-$ZrSiO_4$**	3	2 years	76	

*All studies in fluoride-deficient communities; no self-application brushing studies to the primary teeth have been conducted in fluoridated communities.
**Stannous fluoride active agent; zirconium silicate abrasive.

Self-application of topical fluoride by mouth rinsing

In the 1940s, *Bibby*[28,29] co-authored two reports in which an acidified sodium fluoride mouth rinse was evaluated for its potential to reduce dental caries. While these studies were negative, they nevertheless introduced the concept of a therapeutically active mouth rinse for the prevention of dental caries. During the next decade, little attention was paid to this caries preventive method in the United States, with the exception of the reported use of a neutral sodium fluoride mouth rinse by *Weisz*[30] for patients in his private pedodontic practice. However, the amount of total fluoride recommended for daily use by *Weisz* was considered too high, and his regimen, though successful in reducing dental caries, was not accepted.

During the 1960s, the use of fluoride-containing mouth rinses was extensively investigated, particularly in the Scandinavian countries.[31-40] The results of most of these studies were positive and established therapeutic mouth rinsing as an effective caries preventive method. The Scandinavian findings were substantiated by numerous other studies instituted in the 1970s in many different countries including the United States.[41-71]

While potassium fluoride (KF),[32,40] ferric fluoride (FeF_3),[31] stannous fluoride (SnF_2)[50,59,72] ammonium fluoride (NH_4F),[60] and amine fluoride[68] have been tested in mouth rinses, most clinical trials have evaluated either neutral or acidified (usually APF) sodium fluoride. In 1975, the Council on Dental Therapeutics of the American Dental Association accepted both neutral sodium fluoride and acidulated phosphate fluoride mouth rinses as effective agents in reducing the incidence of dental decay.[73]

A variety of rinsing solutions and regimens has been tested. In addition to differences in the type of fluoride compound employed and the pH of the solution, other variables have included the frequency with which rinsing is performed and the concentration of fluoride employed. Rinsing frequency has varied from three to four times a year[38] to as much as twice a day.[30,53] However, the most common frequencies employed are once a day, once a week, and once every 2 weeks. A wide range of fluoride ion concentrations has been tested. As seen in Table 9-6, the fluoride ion concentrations have ranged from a low of 45 ppm[28,29] to a high of approximately 3,000 ppm.[46] Because of this range, fluoride mouth rinses have sometimes been categorized as "low potency" or "high potency." While the designation is arbitrary, low potency rinses may be considered to contain 250 ppm fluoride ion (F) or less, and high potency rinses to contain more than 250 ppm F. Generally, the low potency rinses are recommended for daily use, while the high potency rinses are used less often.

Effectiveness of fluoride mouth rinsing

Neutral sodium fluoride mouth rinses

Clinical studies of neutral sodium fluoride rinses (NaF) are listed in Table 9-7. The studies are grouped according to rinsing frequency. (The same report may be cited more than once if different rinsing frequencies were evaluated.)

It can be seen that when rinsing was performed once a week or once every 2 weeks, a high potency rinse, usually employing 0.2% NaF (900 ppm F) was used. Conversely, when rinsing was performed once a day, the rinse concentration used was 0.05% NaF (225 ppm F).

Because of the variability of the fluoride concentrations and of the frequency of rinsing, to say nothing of the variables normally inherent in clinical trials (e.g., patients' ages, baseline caries activity, caries diagnostic criteria, use of radiographs, etc.), it is difficult to generalize the results presented in Table 9-7. However, a review of the table leads to the conclusions that use of a neutral NaF rinse is an effective cariostatic technique and that a reduction of approximately 35% of dental caries in the permanent dentition may be expected when rinsing is routinely performed in a fluoride-deficient community for 2 years or longer.

From the results presented in Table 9-7 it is not possible to determine which of the two basic rinsing regimens, *high potency-low frequency* or *low potency-high frequency,* is the more effective, since, viewed collectively, the results are similar. However, the reports of three independent investigations, in which intrastudy comparisons were performed involving either two or three groups of children on different rinsing regimens, suggest that low potency-high frequency rinsing may be more beneficial.[34,38,45] Especially noteworthy is the study by *Torell* and *Ericsson,*[34] which compared one group of children rinsing daily at home with a 0.05% NaF solution with another group rinsing every 2 weeks at school with a 0.2% NaF solution. After 2 years, the children who rinsed more frequently with the less concentrated solution

Table 9-6 Equivalency table of fluoride concentrations employed in rinsing studies

% NaF*	% SnF_2	% NH_4F	% F	F ppm
.01			.0045	45
.02			.0090	90
.025			.0113	113
.04			.0180	180
.05			.0225	225
.10			.0450	450
.20			.0900	900
.25			.1125	1,125
.40			.1800	1,800
.50			.2250	2,250
.66			.2970	2,970
	.04		.0097	97
	.08		.0194	194
	.10		.0243	243
		.20	.1027	1,027

*Neutral or acidified.

Table 9-7 Effect of neutral sodium fluoride mouth rinses on the permanent teeth of children residing in fluoride-deficient communities

Study	Initial age (years) of subjects	Rinse concentration	Rinsing frequency	Duration of study	Percent reduction* DMFT	DMFS
Koch[38]	9–11	0.5% NaF	3-4 times/year	3 years		18
Padron & Maiwald[48]	6–7	0.2% NaF	once/2 weeks	28 months		47
	8–9					32
	10–11					28
	12–13					11
Torell & Ericsson[34]	11	0.2% NaF	once/2 weeks	2 years		21
Koch[38]	9–11	0.5% NaF	once/2 weeks	3 years		23
Moreira & Tumang[45]	7	0.1% NaF	once/2 weeks	2 years		23
Koch[39]	10	0.5% NaF	once/2 weeks	3 years	20	25
Kann[36]	6–16	0.2% NaF	once/2 weeks	2 years		30
Birkeland[56]	8	0.2% NaF	once/2 weeks	6 years		31**
Lundstam[33]	6–15	0.2% NaF	once/2 weeks	9 months		36
Bennie et al.[66]	6	0.2% NaF	once/2 weeks	5 years	49	42
Fjaestad-Seger et al.[31]	5–9	0.2% NaF	once/2 weeks	1 year		58
Forsman[35]	10–12	0.2% NaF	once/2 weeks	2 years		80
Horowitz et al.[41]	6	0.2% NaF	once/week	20 months	25	16
	11	0.2% NaF	once/week	20 months	52	44
Ripa et al.[65]	5–13	0.2% NaF	once/week	2 years	20	20
Ringelberg et al.[57]	8–12	0.2% NaF	once/week	2 years	21	22
Moreira & Tumang[45]	7	0.1% NaF	once/week	2 years		25
Gallagher et al.[51]	11–13	0.4% NaF	once/week	2 years	34	34
Heifetz et al.[46]	10–12	0.66% NaF	once/week	2 years		38
Petchel & Mello[58]	5–13	0.2% NaF	once/week	2 years	50	
Brandt et al.[43]	11.5***	0.2% NaF	twice/week	2 years		39
Moreira & Tumang[45]	7	0.1% NaF	3 times/week	2 years		47
Ringelberg et al.[68]	11	0.05% NaF	once/day	18 months	11	11
	11	0.05% NaF + SnF_2 dentifrice	once/day	18 months	9	11
Aasenden et al.[42]	8–11	0.05% NaF	once/day****	3 years	26	27
Rugg-Gunn et al.[47]	11–12	0.05% NaF	once/day	34 months	32	36
Torell & Ericsson[34]	11	0.05% NaF	once/day	2 years		49
Kasakura[37]	10–11	0.25% NaF	once/day	2 years		80
Weisz[30]	5–9	0.25% NaF	twice/day	2-10 years		80–90

*Based on caries incidence or prevalence data.
**Compared to self-brushing 4-5 times per year with 0.5% NaF solution.
***Mean age.
****Rinse and swallow.

Table 9-8 Effect of acidified sodium fluoride mouth rinses on the permanent teeth of children residing in fluoride-deficient communities

Study	Initial age (years) of subjects	Rinse concentration and pH	Rinsing frequency	Duration of study	Percent reduction DMFT	DMFS
Heifetz et al.[46]	10–12	0.66% NaF APF*, pH 4	once/week	2 years		28
Packer et al.[54]	8–9	0.25% NaF APF, pH 4	once/week	28 months		41
Ashley et al.[61]	12.3***	0.02% NaF APF, pH 3.5	once/day	2 years		14
	12.3	0.02% NaF APF, pH 3.5 +MFP dentifrice**	once/day	2 years		27
Kani et al.[49]	10	0.1% NaF APF, pH ?	once/day	3 years		20–30
Frankl et al.[44]	14***	0.044% NaF APF, pH 4	once/day	2 years	26	22
Aasenden et al.[42]	8–11	0.044% NaF APF, pH 4	once/day****	3 years	32	30
Packer et al.[54]	8–9	0.044% NaF, APF, pH 4	once/day	28 months		27
Luoma et al.[67]	11–15	0.044% NaF succinic acid/NaOH buffer, pH 5.9	once/day	2 years		31
DePaola et al.[60]	10–12	0.2% NaF APF, pH 4.4	once/day	2 years		47
Finn et al.[53]	8–13	0.02% NaF APF, pH 3.5	twice/day	26 months	16	18
	8–13	0.04% NaF APF, pH 3.5	twice/day	26 months	28	29

*APF = acidulated phosphate fluoride.
**MFP = monofluorophosphate.
***Mean age.
****Rinse and swallow.

experienced a 49% caries reduction, compared to a 21% reduction for the other group. It is interesting to note that the several studies listed in Table 9-7 in which high potency rinses were frequently employed produced superior results, further emphasizing the importance of *frequency* in determining success, and also suggesting that the alternative combination of *high potency, high frequency* may be very beneficial.[30,43,45]

Acidified sodium fluoride mouth rinses

It was mentioned earlier that *Bibby* and coworkers[28,29] were the first to clinically evaluate an acidified sodium fluoride rinse. They employed a 0.01% NaF solution (45 ppm F) acidified to pH 4. While these studies were negative, later studies by other investigators using acidified NaF solutions at higher concentrations produced positive results.

Studies of acidified NaF rinses are listed in Table 9-8. By averaging the results of these studies, a collective 28% reduction (DMFS) is obtained. This is slightly less than the 35% reduction obtained by averaging the results of studies with neutral rinses (see Table 9-7).

Two different reports compared the effects of rinsing with neutral and acidified NaF solutions. *Heifetz* and co-workers[46] evaluated a high potency-low frequency regimen (approximately 3,000 ppm F, once a week). They found a 38% caries reduction from use of the neutral NaF solution and a 28% reduction from the acidified one. *Aasenden* and co-workers[42] evaluated a low potency-high frequency regimen (225 ppm once a day). They reported a 27% caries reduction associated with the neutral rinse and a comparable 30% reduction from the acidified one (see Tables 9-7 and 9-8).

Non-sodium fluoride mouth rinses

Some of the Scandinavian investigations conducted in the 1960s evaluated potassium fluoride,[32] ferric fluoride,[31] and potassium fluoride-manganese chloride[40] mouth rinses. The results of these investigations, though positive, were presented in terms of the reduced restorative needs of the children[31,32] or were evaluated against a therapeutic control rinse[40] and cannot be easily summarized in tabular form. Other studies, in which the results were presented in a more orthodox fashion, tested stannous fluoride[59,72] amine fluoride,[68] and ammonium fluoride.[60] These studies are summarized in Table 9-9.

Three of the four studies presented in Table 9-9 used a low potency-high frequency regimen and posted caries reductions of 17 to 31%.[59,68,72] *DePaola* and co-workers[60] used a high potency ammonium fluoride mouth rinse (1,000 ppm F) with a high frequency (once a day) and obtained a caries reduction of 54%.

Mouth rinsing in different clinical situations

Effectiveness in a fluoridated community—Stannous fluoride,[50] acidified sodium fluoride,[55] and neutral sodium fluoride mouth rinses[70] have been tested in children residing in communities with optimal water fluoridation. The results of these studies, presented in Table 9-10, suggest that an additive effect can be realized from fluoride rinsing by children already benefiting from community water fluoridation. This impression is further substantiated by the findings of *DePaola* and co-workers,[60] who found that children with prior exposure to systemic fluoride had the same percentage of caries reduction when either an acidified sodium fluoride or an ammonium fluoride mouth rinse was used, compared to children with no history of systemic fluoride exposure.

Effectiveness in combination with other fluoride therapy—*Ashley* and co-workers[61] evaluated a program of daily rinsing with acidified NaF and brushing with a monofluorophosphate dentifrice, either alone or in combination. A 14% caries reduction was reported for the group that rinsed, and a 27% reduction was reported for the group with the combined therapy (see Table 9-8). *Ringelberg* and co-workers[68] evaluated the effects of an amine fluoride mouth rinse and a neutral NaF rinse, both alone and with an amine fluoride or stannous fluoride dentifrice respectively. No differences were noted by the addition of the therapeutic dentifrices (see Tables 9-7 and 9-9). While the results of these two studies seem contradictory, a significant difference between them was that in the study by *Ashley* et al., dentifrice use was supervised in the classroom, while in the study by *Ringelberg* et al., the dentifrice was used at home.

Horowitz et al.[63,69] evaluated a school-based program involving daily use of a 1 mg acidulated phosphate fluoride tablet and weekly rinsing with a 0.2% neutral NaF solution. Additionally, the children used either a stannous fluoride or monofluorophosphate dentifrice at home. After 3 years, a 35% reduction in caries prevalence was reported.[69] Although a comparison group that only rinsed was not included, considering the combination of fluoride therapy that was employed, these results cannot be considered dramatic.

Heifetz et al.[70] conducted a school-based program involving weekly rinsing with a neutral 0.2% NaF solution and gel-tray treatments applied 15 times a year in three sets of five applications each. After 30 months, a 30% caries reduction was obtained (see Table 9-10). Since this study was conducted in an optimally fluoridated community, this can be considered a promising result.

Effectiveness on the primary dentition—*Birkeland* and co-workers[64] evaluated the

Table 9-9 Effect of non-sodium fluoride mouth rinses on the permanent teeth of children residing in fluoride-deficient communities

Study	Initial age (years) of subjects	Type of rinse	Rinsing frequency	Duration of study	Percent reduction DMFT	DMFS
McConchie et al.[59]	10*	0.04% SnF_2	once/day	2 years	20	20
	10	0.08% SnF_2	once/day	2 years	20	17
Swerdloff & Shannon[72]	11–15	0.1% SnF_2**	once/day	5 months	33	31
Ringelberg et al.[68]	11	amine fluoride (250 ppm F)	once/day	18 months	11	21
	11	amine fluoride (250 ppm F) + amine F dentifrice	once/day	18 months	19	22
DePaola et al.[60]	10–12	0.2% NH_4F, pH 4.4	once/day	2 years		54

*Mean age.
**Some of study population drinking optimally fluoridated water.

Table 9-10 Effect of fluoride mouth rinses on the permanent teeth of children residing in optimally fluoridated communities

Study	Initial age (years) of subjects	Type of rinse	Rinsing frequency	Duration of study	Percent reduction DMFT	DMFS
Radike et al.[50]	8–13	0.1% SnF_2	once/day	20 months		33–43*
Laswell et al.[55]	8–9	0.044% NaF APF, pH 4	once/day	28 months		23
	8–9	0.25% NaF APF, pH 4	once/week	28 months		46
Heifetz et al.[70]	10–11	0.2% NaF + APF gel-tray**	once/week	30 months		30

*Two examiners.
**Gel-tray application was made on 5 consecutive days, repeated 3 times a year.

effectiveness of fluoride rinsing on the primary dentition based upon changes in dental treatment needs in Norwegian schoolchildren. Although there was a decrease in the number of primary teeth requiring extractions during a 3-year period, the data for the number of teeth requiring fillings were equivocal.

In the only reports of the effect of fluoride rinsing on caries activity in the primary dentition, *Ripa* and *Leske*[71] found a reduction of 20% (dfs/child) in caries prevalence after 2 years of rinsing. However, after 3 years, the reduction was only 17%, while for the permanent dentition in the same aged children, the reduction was 40%.[74] *Ripa* and *Leske* concluded that, like other topical fluoride methods, the benefits to the primary dentition from fluoride rinsing are less than those generally obtained for the permanent dentition.

Table 9-11 Effect of fluoride mouth rinses on different tooth surfaces

Study	Rinse, frequency, and duration	Percent caries reduction—all surfaces	Percent caries reduction by type of surface: Occlusal	Buccolingual	Proximal
Ashley et al.[61]	0.02% NaF, pH 3.5; once/day, 2 years	14	5	22*	24
Koch[39]	0.5% NaF; once/2 weeks, 3 years	25	5	35-38	31
Rugg-Gunn et al.[47]	0.05% NaF; once/day, 34 months	36	32	55	33–56**
Luoma et al.[67]	0.044% NaF, pH 5.9; once/day, 2 years	31	1	9	43
Ripa et al.[65]	0.2% NaF; once/week, 2 years	20	20	15***	40

*Includes proximal surfaces.
**Posterior and anterior proximal surfaces respectively.
***Lesions were mainly of the pit and fissure variety.

Effectiveness on different tooth surfaces—The effectiveness of fluoride rinsing on the caries activity of different tooth surfaces is summarized in Table 9-11. Like other methods of fluoride therapy, fluoride rinsing provides preferential protection to the smooth tooth surfaces, while the least benefit is derived by the pits and fissures of the occlusal surface.

Effectiveness on newly erupted permanent teeth—Studies of other topical fluoride methods have indicated that newly erupting teeth derive more benefit from topical fluoride treatments than teeth that were in the mouth for longer periods of time. Fluoride rinsing is no exception. The results of several studies demonstrate that higher caries reductions are achieved when there is early contact to newly erupting teeth compared to teeth that were in the mouth before rinsing began.[41,42,47,59,60,70]

Effectiveness with increased duration of rinsing—*Birkeland* and *Torell*,[75] in a review of fluoride rinsing studies, concluded that the benefits increased as the duration of the program continued. An example of this effect may be seen in the caries prevalence of a rinsing population as reported by *Ripa* and co-workers after three years.[76] Children in kindergarten through grade 6 rinsed once a week with a 0.2% neutral NaF solution. After 1 year, the reduction in caries prevalence (DMFS) among rinsing participants, compared to children who never rinsed, was 10%; after 2 years of rinsing, it was 20%; and after 3 years, 31%.

Self-application of topical fluoride gels using mouth trays

There have been four reports in which fluoride gels, self-applied to the permanent teeth in mouth trays, have been tested in children residing in fluoride-deficient communities (Table 9-12), and four reports in which this method was evaluated in optimally fluoridated communities (Table 9-13), one of which was on the primary dentition.[82]
In the first program of this type, *Englander*

Table 9-12 Effect of self-application of fluoride gels in mouth trays on the permanent teeth of children residing in fluoride-deficient communities

Study	Initial age (years) of subjects	F-gel with tray	Application frequency	Duration of study	Percent reduction DMFT	DMFS
Englander et al.[77]	11–14	APF gel (0.5% F), pH 4.5	once/day	21 months	75	64
	11–14	NaF gel (0.5% F), pH 7	once/day	21 months	80	67
Englander et al.[78]	11–14	APF gel (0.5% F), pH 4.5	no additional treatment	44 months*	70	70
	11–14	NaF gel (0.5% F), pH 7	no additional treatment	44 months*	69	70
Trubman & Crellin[21]	8.12**	brushed with a non-F prophy paste followed by APF gel (1.23% F from NaF & HF), pH 3	4 times/year	3 years	23	35
	8.12	brushed with APF prophy paste (0.4% F) followed by APF gel (1.23% F from NaF and HF), pH 3	4 times/year	3 years	25	22
Shern et al.[79]	6–13	APF gel (1.23% F from NaF & HF), pH 3.2	once/day for 1 week (total: 5 applications)	2 years		+0.5
	6–13	Amine F gel (1.25% F from organic F & NaF), pH 4.5	once/day for 1 week (total: 5 applications)	2 years		32
	6–13	Amine F gel (1.25% F from organic F and NaF), pH 4.5	once/ week for 5 weeks (total: 5 applications)	2 years		25

*Includes 21 months' treatment and 23 months of no treatment.
**Mean age.

and co-workers[77] reported high caries reductions when children self-applied custom-fitted mouth trays containing either an acidified sodium fluoride gel or a neutral sodium fluoride gel (see Table 9-12). The gels, which remained in contact with the teeth for 6 minutes, were applied daily for 2 school years. Thus, the average participant gave himself 245 topical fluoride treatments. At the conclusion of the program, each treatment group had 75 to 80% less carious teeth compared to a control group of children who received no treatment. Twenty-three months after discontinuing treatment, the children were re-examined to determine if there were a residual effect from the fluoride therapy.[78] Only those teeth that were present during the treatment phase were examined. There were approximately 70% fewer carious teeth in each of the previously treated groups, compared to the control group of children, indicating that the caries protection

Table 9-13 Effect of self-application of fluoride gels in mouth trays on the permanent teeth of children residing in optimally fluoridated communities

Study	Intial age (years) of subjects	F-gel with tray	Application frequency	Duration of study	Percent reduction DMFT	DMFS
Englander et al.[80]	11–15	APF gel (0.5% F), pH 4.5	3 times/week	27–31 months		29
Mellberg et al.[81]	9–12	APF gel (1.23% F from NaF & HF), pH 3.2	once/day for 1 week (total: 5 applications)	1 year		7
	9–12	APF gel (1.23% F from NaF & HF), pH 3.2	once/day for 2 weeks (total: 10 applications)	1 year		30
	9–12	APF gel (1.23% F from NaF & HF), pH 3.2	once/day for 5 weeks (total: 25 applications)	1 year		35
Heifetz et al.[70]	10–11	APF gel (1.23% F from NaF & HF), pH 3.2 + weekly mouth rinsing with 0.2% NaF (0.09% F)	once/day for 1 week; repeated 3 times/year (total: 15 applications per year)	30 months		30

acquired during treatment had been maintained.

Englander and co-workers[80] conducted a similar program in an optimally fluoridated community. Using only the acidified NaF gel, children self-applied fluoride to their teeth in custom-fitted mouth trays three times a week for 3 school years. The mean number of treatments was 255, similar to the 245 treatments achieved in the study conducted in the fluoride-deficient community. At the conclusion of the study, a modest 29% reduction (DMFS) was achieved (Table 9-13).

Trubman and *Crellin*[21] also evaluated gel-tray therapy in a fluoride-deficient community. In their study, the children first brushed their teeth with either a nontherapeutic prophylaxis paste or one that contained fluoride. Applications, however, were made only four times a year, and after 3 years, the caries reductions (Table 9-12) were less dramatic than those achieved by *Englander*'s daily therapy.

In addition to the *high frequency-high duration* gel-tray therapy pioneered by *Englander*, others have evaluated a technique involving a *short, intensive series of fluoride applications* using the gel-tray system.[70,79,81] In this technique, the fluoride gel is usually applied on a daily basis for one, two, or several consecutive weeks. Studies employing this technique have been conducted in both fluoride-deficient[79] and fluoridated communities,[70,81] and generally have posted caries reductions of from 25 to 35%, provided the intensive series is given for more than 1 week (Tables 9-12 and 9-13).

In only one study was the gel-tray method evaluated for its effect on caries activity in the primary dentition. In that study, conducted by *Englander* and co-workers,[82] pre-

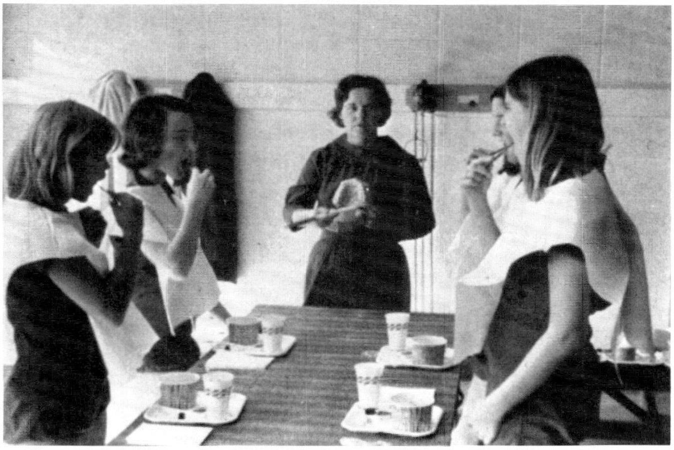

Fig. 9-1 A brush-in being conducted in a school gymnasium. (Compliments of Dr. H. *Horowitz*.)

school children, 2 to 6 years of age, used an acidified NaF gel (1.1% NaF, pH 4.5), which was self-applied three times a week. The children received adult assistance when they placed the custom-fitted trays in their mouths. After 28 months, a statistically non-significant 15% caries reduction (defs) was achieved in this population, who were also receiving the benefits of waterborne fluoride.

Recommendations for the use of self-application methods in public health programs

Self-application of topical fluoride by brushing

Beginning in the mid-1960s, "brush-in" programs were conducted not only in schools but any place where people congregated.[3,4,82-92] These programs were sponsored by public health agencies, local dental societies, and individual dentists. Since this type of mass preventive therapy was especially promoted by dental researchers from Indiana University, it is not surprising that of the 675,000 individuals identified as participating in brush-in programs by 1968, approximately 20% were from the state of Indiana.[87] In these programs, the 9% stannous fluoride-zirconium silicate (SnF_2-$ZrSiO_4$) prophylaxis paste was the agent most often employed.

Brush-ins were conducted in school classrooms and gymnasiums, in school playing areas, in shopping centers, on college campuses, and in community centers.[86] Schools usually offered an ideal setting (Figure 9-1).

The materials required for each child participating in a brush-in included[15]

- a multitufted soft nylon bristle toothbrush
- approximately 5-6 grams of fluoride-containing prophylaxis paste
- a 5-ounce paper cup containing water for rinsing
- an 8-ounce paper cup used to expectorate
- two paper towels or napkins

In addition, a paper or plastic bib to protect the child's clothing was usually desirable.

Generally, approximately 25 to 30 children in

a classroom were treated simultaneously. The children remained seated at their desks with the brushing materials in front of them. Instruction and supervision were provided by two individuals, one of whom was a professional, such as a dentist, dental hygienist, dental assistant, or school nurse. This individual served as an instructor. The other person, who helped supervise during the brushing, was usually the classroom teacher, a teacher's assistant, or a volunteer mother.

The instructor explained the purpose of the procedure and demonstrated the proper brushing technique. Generally, the facial and lingual surfaces of the teeth were brushed with a rolling motion and the occlusal surfaces with a scrubbing motion. Children first practiced the procedure with a dry brush before applying the treatment paste.

Each child was given 5 to 6 grams of the fluoride-containing prophylaxis paste.[3,15] Enough paste was spread on the toothbrush to cover the bristle tips. Children brushed following the lead of the instructor. The teeth were brushed in the following sequence with paste being applied to the toothbrush as each segment of teeth was brushed:

- maxillary right and mandibular right occlusal surfaces
- maxillary left and mandibular left occlusal surfaces
- maxillary facial surfaces
- mandibular facial surfaces
- maxillary lingual surfaces
- mandibular lingual surfaces

While the children brushed, the instructor counted slowly to ten for each segment. At the same time the aid checked that each child was performing the procedure correctly. The children could empty their mouths when necessary, but were instructed to rinse only at the end of each brushing sequence. It was emphasized that the paste should not be swallowed, but should be expectorated into the cup provided for that purpose. A final brushing was performed in which the children again coated the bristle tips of their toothbrushes with the fluoride-containing paste and brushed any area of the teeth that they may have missed. Then they emptied their mouths and thoroughly rinsed with water.

At the conclusion of the brushing session, the children cleaned their brushes, dried them on a paper towel, and replaced them in their original wrappers to take them home. The paper cups and napkins used during the brush-in were collected in a disposable bag and the expectorated saliva was emptied in a partially covered pail and flushed in the restroom.

The time required for the entire brush-in procedure was approximately 20 to 30 minutes. This included the initial arrangements, the demonstration, and the brushing. The actual time for brushing was about 5 minutes.

In 1975, *Gish* and co-workers[15] estimated that the cost of the materials for a brush-in was $0.25 per child and, if the supervisory personnel were paid, this added an additional $0.25 per child. *Heifetz*[93] calculated that the cost-effectiveness of semiannual toothbrushing with a 9% SnF_2-$ZrSiO_4$ paste, including personnel salaries, was $2.50 per tooth surface saved.

Horowitz and *Horowitz*[94] have observed that brush-ins are less frequent today than they were only a few years ago. The reasons for this include the fact that many children disliked the taste of the treatment paste and a large number complained of becoming nauseous.[83] In addition, the results of controlled clinical trials of this procedure were equivocal, with some investigators reporting no benefit (see Tables 9-2 and 9-4). Other disadvantages of this procedure were that it is more difficult to supervise and administer than mouth rinsing (described in the next section), and that waste collection was unsightly. Proponents of this technique have claimed that participation in a brush-in program, which provides toothbrushing instruction, may promote better gingival health. This claim, however, has yet to be proved. In fact, a Norwegian study comparing the oral hygiene and gingival health status of participants in a supervised toothbrushing program found these oral health parameters to be no different from those of participants in a mouth rinsing program.[56]

Recently, the SnF_2-$ZrSiO_4$ prophylaxis paste has been withdrawn from the American market, so that its use is now only of academic interest. However, brush-ins may still be accomplished using other fluoride containing prophylaxis pastes. These programs should be discouraged unless there is unequivocal evidence that use of these pastes will provide a caries reduction.

Self-application of topical fluoride by mouth rinsing

There is convincing evidence that neutral NaF and acidified buffered NaF (acidulated phosphate fluoride) mouth rinses are beneficial in reducing dental decay. The two regimens most frequently used employ a 0.05% NaF solution daily (low potency-high frequency regimen) or a 0.2% NaF solution once a week or once every 2 weeks (high potency-low frequency regimen). As previously discussed, evidence of superior efficacy of one regimen over the other is lacking; therefore, other factors such as cost and convenience determine the choice of which regimen to adopt for a school-based fluoride mouth rinsing program.

Since it is less expensive and involves less classroom time, weekly rinsing with a 0.2% NaF solution is more widely used in schools than daily rinsing with a 0.05% NaF solution. *Horowitz* and *Horowitz* state that weekly fluoride mouth rinsing is "the most extensively adopted school-based self-applied fluoride program in the United States."[94] As of January, 1980, approximately eight million school children nationally are participating in a fluoride mouth rinsing program.

Rinsing should begin in kindergarten and extend to the highest grade level within the school system. While the participation and cooperation of children in the lower grades is usually excellent, *DePaola* and *Soparkar*[95] have emphasized that a rinsing program at the high school level is frequently fraught with logistical problems, poor participation, and indifference on the part of many of the students.

The rinse itself may be purchased already prepared, as a concentrate to which tap water is added, or as a premeasured packet of powder that must be mixed with the appropriate volume of tap water. Other materials needed for rinsing are bottles equipped with pumps calibrated to dispense 5 or 10 ml of solution, disposal bags, and a paper cup and napkin for each participant.

If a prepared rinse is unavailable, the fluoride solution must be mixed. A 0.2% NaF solution is prepared by combining 3 g NaF with 1,500 ml of tap water. If stored in a plastic, rather than a glass container, the fluoride will not become chemically inactivated. However, storage of a fluoride solution prepared from tap water gives it a stale or "flat" taste that is less acceptable to the rinsing participants and more likely to induce nausea. In addition, nonpathogenic airborne fungus can settle in the bottles and pumps when the rinse is alternately stored and reused. It is advisable, therefore, to prepare a fresh solution on each morning that rinsing is scheduled.

The mixed NaF solution can be dispensed into disposable paper cups and taken on carts to the individual classrooms, or one dispensing bottle can be brought to each classroom and the cups filled there. In each classroom, the names of the children whose parents have provided written consent to participate are called. Each child receives a paper cup containing 10 ml of fluoride rinse and a paper napkin. Kindergarten children

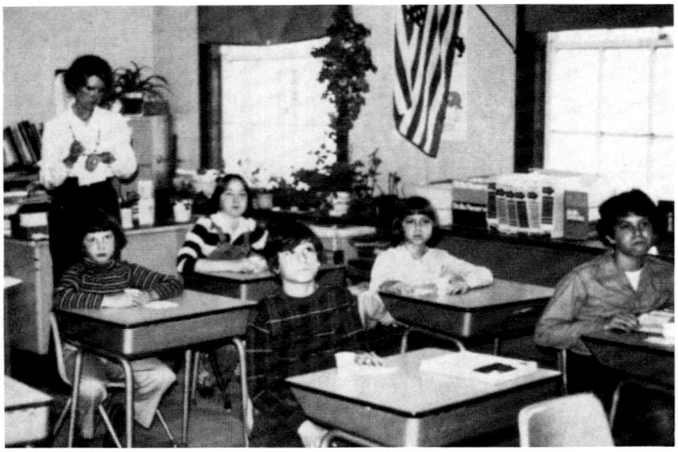

Fig. 9-2 Children participating in a weekly school-based fluoride mouth rinsing program.

receive 5 ml of solution. Rinsing is timed for 60 seconds, usually by the homeroom teacher. The children do *not* brush their teeth prior to rinsing. During rinsing, the teacher reminds the children to swish the solution vigorously between their teeth and not to swallow it (Fig. 9-2). After 60 seconds, the children expectorate back into the paper cups, wipe their mouths with the napkins, and stuff them into the paper cups to absorb the solution and saliva. The cups and napkins are then collected in a disposal bag that is deposited in the classroom wastebasket. The total time for the classroom rinse is approximately 5 minutes.[96-98] Children are asked not to eat, drink, or rinse for one-half hour.

After rinsing, the materials are collected and stored in a *locked* area of the school. Considering such factors as vacations, holidays, and time to initially locate the children in their new homerooms at the beginning of the school year, approximately 30 weekly rinses can be accomplished during an academic year.

Heifetz[93] calculated that the cost of supplies for weekly rinsing with a 0.2% NaF solution was approximately $0.50 per child per school year. If rinsing were performed every school day, the cost for supplies would be expected to increase fivefold to $2.50. In most rinsing programs, teachers, school nurses, or volunteer lay personnel prepare and distribute the rinse and supervise the children. If the rinse personnel are paid by the program, however, the cost per child will obviously increase above that calculated by *Heifetz*. Since the personnel can be trained lay individuals, who would be expected to be compensated at a lower rate than dental professionals, the additional costs are not inordinate. In a school-based rinsing program described by *Levinson* et al.,[99] teachers supervised the weekly rinse sessions and thus were not compensated by the program; however, paid personnel prepared and distributed the rinse, collected the rinse materials, and returned them to the storage areas each week. Additionally, the program employed a half-time coordinator. Inclusion of personnel salaries, as well as some minimal capital expenses, raised the actual cost per child in this program to approximately $2.30 a school year.

A school-based weekly fluoride mouth rinsing program has the following advantages:[94]

— The procedure has been consistently

effective in reducing dental caries.
- The classroom time required each week is minimal (about 5 minutes).
- The technique can be easily accomplished by school-aged children.
- The rinsing supplies are few and inexpensive.
- Nondental personnel can be easily trained to supervise the procedure.
- The solution is generally well accepted by the participants.

School-based mouth rinsing programs should be located in schools where the concentration of fluoride in the local water supply is below therapeutic levels.* The question arises as to whether there is an advantage to institute a mouth rinsing program in an optimally fluoridated community. Although two studies have reported positive findings when NaF mouth rinsing is performed alone[55] or in combination with gel-tray applications,[70] and one study using a SnF_2 mouth rinse also obtained positive results[50] (see Table 9-10), there is still insufficient evidence to unreservedly justify school-based mouth rinsing programs in communities receiving the benefits of water fluoridation. However, schools that are located in communities that have optimally fluoridated water, but which also draw part of their enrollment from contiguous fluoride-deficient communities, may be considered for a rinsing program.

Preschool programs, such as Head Start, offer an excellent opportunity to institute dental preventive therapy to children at an early age. There are, however, several considerations that mitigate against the use of mouth rinsing for this age group. First, the technique is difficult for young children to master, and it has been shown that younger rinse participants tend to swallow more of the rinse solution than older ones (see the section on Safety of Self-applied Topical Fluoride later in this chapter). Second, the effects of topical therapy to the primary teeth are minimal, whereas, in this age group there is the opportunity to provide systemic fluoride therapy to the developing permanent teeth. Third, although the appropriate concentration and amount of fluoride solution could be swished daily and then *swallowed* in order to provide both a topical effect to the erupted primary teeth and a systemic effect to the developing permanent teeth, this therapy can be more economically accomplished with a daily 1 mg fluoride tablet that is chewed, swished, and swallowed.

*Therapeutic fluoride level = 0.7 to 1.2 ppm F, depending upon annual average maximum daily air temperature.

Self-application of topical fluoride gels using mouth trays

As mentioned earlier in this chapter, fluoride gels have been tested in school-based programs on a daily basis or every other day during the school year, or have been provided in a short, intensive series of daily applications lasting from one to several weeks. Most often, an APF gel (1.1% NaF, pH 4.5, or 1.23% NaF, pH 3.2) has been employed in these treatments.

As generally practiced, implementing a gel-tray program involves the taking of impressions of the maxillary and mandibular arches by a dentist or dental hygienist and the construction of custom mouth trays. The trays can be made from thermoplastic polyvinyl sheets, which are vacuum adapted to the children's dental casts, and then trimmed into horseshoe shapes. The mouth trays are stored at the children's school in individual boxes, along with small plastic squeeze bottles of fluoride gel.

Treatment is usually accomplished in the school cafeteria or some other large room where there are adequate sinks for the children to rinse their mouths and clean their trays after the fluoride application (Fig. 9-3). As decribed by *Englander* et al.,[77] the children put about 5 to 10 drops of the gel

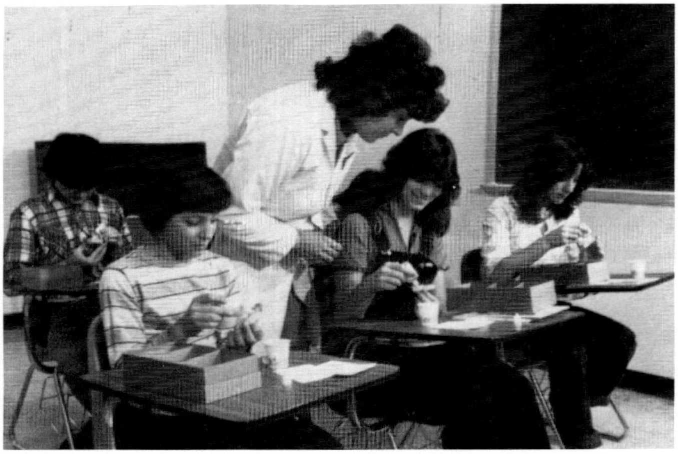

Fig. 9-3 Children participating in a school-based gel-tray program.

(about 1 to 2 mg F) into each mouth tray and, using the nozzle of the fluoride container, spread the gel thinly and evenly along the trays. Both trays are simultaneously placed in the mouth and held with biting pressure for 6 minutes. In the short intensive therapy programs, gel contact has been maintained for as long as 15 minutes.[81] Any excess gel oozing from the periphery of the trays is expectorated into paper towels. The self-application treatment is directed and supervised by dental hygienists or other dental personnel. After the children remove the trays, they rinse their mouths with water, wash the trays and dry them with a paper napkin, and return them to the storage boxes.

Although *Englander*[7] reported very high caries reductions from gel-tray treatments conducted in a fluoride-deficient community, and a strong residual effect 2 years after discontinuing therapy,[78] this method has generally not been used in school programs. *Davies*[100] considered this method too expensive to even perform a cost analysis. *Heifetz*[93] calculated that gel-tray self-applications would cost $21.30 for each tooth surface saved. In addition to the high costs, the technique requires much time, is complex relative to the mouth rinsing procedure, and requires a significant amount of school storage space if many children are to be treated.

Recommendations for the use of self-application methods for individual patients

For individual patients, the advantage of fluoride self-application is that it allows more frequent treatments than are possible by the traditional method of topical application in the dental office. The patient at home can give himself as many as 365 applications of fluoride a year, compared to one or two treatments in the dental office.

Successful use of self-application techniques depends upon the cooperation of the patient, or both the parent and child patient, to faithfully follow the dentist's recommendations. Additionally, the specific method prescribed for individual patients should be based upon considerations of efficacy, practicality, and the ability of the patient to master the technique.

Self-application of topical fluoride by brushing

Most preschool children cannot be expected to rinse properly and may find it difficult to accept custom trays; therefore, for the preschooler, brushing is the preferred self-application technique. There have been only two studies of the effect of self-application brushing methods on the primary teeth; one was successful,[17] the other was not.[5] The dentist who recommends this technique, therefore, should be aware that it is being recommended on an empirical basis. Nevertheless, it is quite possible that a technique that does not demonstrate efficacy when tested on a group of patients who exhibit a range of caries activity may be beneficial for the individual patient who is highly caries susceptible.

Since a gel will best adhere to the toothbrush bristles, a fluoride gel can be recommended for home brushing. One commercial company supplies to dentists a flavored APF gel packaged in small 7 g tubes for individual use.* If a dentist stocks the tubes, they can be dispensed to the parents of young patients for whom this therapy may be indicated; the tubes are not available from a pharmacy. Alternatively, a dentist may purchase 1 ounce (30 ml) plastic dispensing bottles that can be filled two-thirds full with the APF gel used in the dental office. Twenty milliliters of the fluoride gel provide 246 mg fluoride ion, which is below the acute toxic dose and allows a margin of safety in the unlikely event that a child accidently consumes the entire contents of the bottle.

Before bedtime, the parent should brush the child's teeth using a dentifrice in the usual manner. Then, a thin ribbon of gel is squeezed onto the bristles of the child's brush and the parent brushes the child's teeth, using a scrubbing motion, for approximately 4 to 5 minutes. After the fluoride application, the child may expectorate but, preferably, should not rinse. Brushing with the gel should be performed once a month. Used at this frequency, the contents of the tube should last for more than a year.

Self-application of topical fluoride by mouth rinsing

Young school-age children should be able to master either a rinsing technique or the use of custom trays. However, a 6 to 12 year-old child is in the mixed dentition stage of dental development. Exfoliation of primary teeth and eruption of permanent teeth contraindicates the routine use of custom trays in this age group since frequent reconstruction would be required. Consequently, for a school-age child with a mixed dentition, mouth rinsing is recommended.

Dentists have a choice of recommending either a daily low potency or a weekly high potency rinsing regimen. It has already been pointed out that it is not clear which is the more effective; therefore, the choice of rinsing regimen is based upon other considerations. Dentists may write a prescription for the pharmacist to compound either preparation (Fig. 9-4 and 9-5) or may prescribe a 0.2 or 0.05% NaF rinse. In addition, a commercial rinse is available without prescription that has a 0.05% NaF concentration.* An advantage of the daily rinsing regimen is that if the patient misses several sessions, it is probably less critical than if he was on a weekly schedule. Another advantage of the 0.05% NaF concentration is that it can be used to provide both a topical and *systemic* benefit when indicated for the individual patient. Because of these practical considerations, the low potency, high frequency

*Luride topical gel (7 g tubes), Hoyt Laboratories, Norwood, Massachusetts

*Fluoriguard® (0.05 % neutral sodium fluoride), Colgate-Palmolive Company, New York, New York.

℞ *Sodium fluoride* 0.2 gm
Distilled water 100 cc

Sig. Rinse mouth with one teaspoonful for 60 seconds once-a-week after brushing teeth at bedtime. Do not swallow.

Caution: Keep out of reach of young children.
Do not use for preschool children.

Fig. 9-4 Example of a prescription to compound a 0.2% neutral NaF mouth rinse. The rinse may be used once a week as directed on the prescription or once every 2 weeks.

℞ *Sodium fluoride* 0.2 gm
Distilled water 400 cc

Sig. Rinse mouth with one teaspoonful for 60 seconds daily after brushing teeth at bedtime. Do not swallow.

Caution: Keep out of reach of young children.
Do not use for preschool children.

Fig. 9-5 Example of a prescription to compound a 0.05% neutral NaF mouth rinse. The rinse is used daily. In a fluoride-deficient community (F ≦ 0.3 ppm), the patient may be directed to swish and swallow. One teaspoonful will provide the recommended systemic supplement of 1 mg F.

(0.05% NaF daily) rinsing regimen is recommended for home use.

The child is instructed to rinse each evening for 60 seconds after first brushing the teeth, and then to expectorate. One teaspoonful (5 ml) of a 0.05% neutral sodium fluoride or APF solution is used. The solution can be compounded by the pharmacist, prescribed, or purchased over the counter. The rinse-and-expectorate technique can be used for patients in fluoride-deficient communities or for those in optimally fluoridated communities who nevertheless exhibit a high susceptibility.

A teaspoonful of 0.05% NaF solution will, if swallowed, deliver 1 mg of sodium fluoride. A swish-and-swallow technique, as opposed to a swish-and-expectorate technique, should be recommended if the concentration of fluoride in the drinking water is 0.3 ppm or less and if the patient is not already taking a systemic supplement. *Dentists must be aware, however, that the over-the-counter product as well as many of the other commercial rinses are not meant to be swallowed.*

Table 9-14 Recommendations for the self-application of topical fluoride by individual patients

Brushing	Rinsing	Custom trays
For preschool children (primary dentition)	For young school-age children (mixed dentition)	For patients 12 years or older (permanent dentition)
Parent brushes the child's teeth with an APF gel once a month.	Rinse once a day with 1 teaspoonful (5 ml) of 0.05 % NaF solution. Swallow or expectorate depending upon availability of other systemic fluoride.	Use 5 times per week, 5 to 10 drops of APF gel (pH 4.5) or neutral NaF gel placed in each tray and held against dental arches for 5 minutes.

Self-application of topical fluoride gels using mouth trays

For the caries-susceptible patient who is 12 years or older, the use of custom mouth trays is recommended. Not only has this method proven to be highly effective in reducing dental caries,[77] but since all permanent teeth (except third molars) have erupted by this age, frequent changes of the mouth trays to accommodate a changing dentition are not necessary.

Using vacuum equipment, horseshoe-shaped mouth trays for the maxillary and mandibular arches may be constructed from thermoplastic sheets. The mouth trays are adjusted in the patient's mouth and peripheral overextensions are trimmed with scissors and smoothed with a hand-held alcohol torch. The patient is given the custom-fitted trays and an APF or neutral gel* and instructed to place 5 to 10 drops in each tray, which are to be held in contact with the teeth for 5 minutes. Excess gel that may ooze from the periphery of the trays should be expectorated into a paper napkin. The mouth trays may be used five times a week regardless of whether the patient is a resident of a fluoride-deficient or an optimally fluoridated community.

Recommendations for the use of topical fluoride self-application techniques are summarized in Table 9-14.

*Thera-Flur® (pH 4.5) or Thera-Flur-N® (pH 7), Hoyt Laboratories; Norwood, Massachusetts.

Recommendations for the use of self-application methods for special patients

Two groups of patients who are in a heightened state of caries susceptibility are those undergoing orthodontic therapy and those with xerostomia, especially individuals who have recieved radiation therapy to the head and neck. Both groups can benefit from a caries preventive program that includes fluoride self-application.

Patients undergoing orthodontic therapy

Because of the accumulation of food debris and plaque around orthodontic bands, appliances, and direct-bonded attachments, patients undergoing active orthodontic treatment or who are in retention are considered to be expecially caries susceptible.[101,102] While fluoride self-application should not be considered a substitute for good oral hygiene practices, it can be considered an adjunctive caries preventive method during this period of heightened caries susceptibility.[103]

Patients undergoing orthodontic therapy often develop enamel demineralization adjacent to bands, under loose-fitting bands, and in areas of the teeth that are difficult to brush because of the presence of direct-bonded attachments and orthodontic wires. In a series of reports, *Shannon* and his co-workers[104-106] have indicated that treatment with a two-step mouth rinsing procedure using separate solutions of APF (0.31% F) and 0.4% SnF_2 or brushing with a 0.04% SnF_2 gel was effective in reducing the expected number of decalcified areas in orthodontic patients. In another study, *Hirschfield*[107] found that patients who were placed on a daily home rinse program using an APF solution (0.05% NaF) had less decalcified areas than patients not on the home program. Of special interest to the orthodontic situation is the finding of *von der Fehr* and co-workers[108] that experimentally produced demineralized areas in volunteers could be reversed when the cariogenic challenge was altered and the patients rinsed daily with a 0.2% NaF solution.

When patients are identified as needing orthodontic therapy, a program of fluoride self-application should be planned. If self-treatment can be started before banding, the patient can be placed on a short series of intensive fluoride therapy treatments using the gel-tray method. The custom trays can be conveniently constructed at the time pretreatment study models are prepared and the patient placed on daily gel-tray applications for a period of at least 4 weeks. Once the patient is banded or an appliance is inserted, gel-tray procedures may be terminated and daily fluoride rinses started, using a 0.05% neutral NaF or an APF solution. The over-the-counter 0.05% NaF rinse is both economical and convenient for this purpose, especially if systemic fluoride therapy is not indicated. If the patient requires both topical and systemic fluorides, then a rinse should be selected that can be swished and then swallowed and that will deliver 1 mg F daily.

Patients with xerostomia

The important role of the saliva in helping to maintain host resistance against caries and the effect of xerostomia on caries incidence were discussed in Chapter 1. Several investigators have reported the successful use of topical fluoride self-application methods to prevent or control rampant caries in oncology patients who have developed radiation-induced xerostomia.[109-114]

Self-application treatment has included daily brushing with a 0.4% SnF_2 gel[109] or the daily use of neutral NaF or APF gels applied in custom mouth trays.[110,111,114] While most investigators have indicated that the self-application therapy must be continued indefinitely in order to maintain caries protection, *Johanson* and *Olsen*[114] supervised a unique multiple preventive program in which the gel-tray self-applications were discontinued after 4 weeks. Their program included the following procedures:

Oral hygiene—Brushing was done with a fluoride-containing dentifrice. Dental floss and cotton swabs were used to clean hard-to-reach tooth surfaces and cervical areas.

Gel-tray Application—An APF gel (1.23% F)

or a neutral NaF gel (1% F) was used with custom trays twice a day for 2 weeks and once a day for 2 weeks thereafter. The patients rinsed with water following the gel-tray application.

Remineralizing mouth rinse—Rinsing for 2 minutes with a supersaturated solution of calcium, phosphate, and fluoride was performed after each gel-tray application. When the tray applications were discontinued, rinsing was continued twice a day but was performed after toothbrushing.

Salivary gland stimulation—A specially formulated nonsweetened gum was chewed by the patients to stimulate saliva.

While the gel-tray applications were stopped after 4 weeks, the rest of the regimen was continued for periods up to 4 years. *Johanson* and *Olsen* reported that this treatment not only prevented the development of new carious lesions, but also promoted the arrestment and rehardening of lesions that were already in progress at the time the preventive therapy began.

For patients who are about to receive head and neck radiation therapy or for those who already have, a dental preventive program that includes the use of self-applied topical fluorides must be instituted. In addition, the patients must be trained in proper oral hygiene methods, including the use of dental floss. Brushing should be performed with a fluoride-containing dentifrice that has been approved by the American Dental Association. Mouthguards should then be constructed and either a neutral NaF gel or an APF gel should be used by the patient on a daily basis. It may be necessary to train other members of the patient's family to help the patient perform the dental preventive therapy.

All of the reports describing the prevention of dental caries in patients with radiation-induced xerostomia stress that strict oral hygiene must be maintained and that the patient must rigorously comply with the recommended preventive program. The best results were achieved by those patients who conscientiously adhered to the program.

Safety of self-applied topical fluoride

Like other forms of fluoride therapy, the potential for acute or chronic toxic effects must be considered when self-application methods are proposed.

The most frequent adverse effect associated with the brushing technique has been nausea. Nausea has been reported when the stannous fluoride-zirconium silicate paste was used[15,83] and when an APF solution was used.[7] While the amount of fluoride retained from self-applied brushing procedures has never been reported, even if the entire amount used during a single treatment was swallowed, this would not constitute a serious health hazard. For instance, the amount of SnF_2-$ZrSiO_4$ paste used for brushing was generally 5 or 6 g and the acute toxicity of the paste was about 4 g/kg body weight; thus providing a large margin of safety.[15]

Retention of fluoride from the gel-tray treatment was studied by *Englander* and coworkers.[77] The urinary fluoride level of 40 children participating in a school-based program was monitored 2 and 8 hours after self-administration of fluoride gel in trays. Tests were repeated during 3 days of treatment. No increase in the level of urinary fluoride was detected.

Since the most prevalent form of self-application therapy currently practiced is fluoride mouth rinsing, a more detailed review of the safety of this method is indicated.

Safety of fluoride mouth rinses

Since some solution may be inadvertently swallowed during rinsing, the chronic toxicity of repeated retention of small amounts of fluoride must be discussed. Additionally, the potential for an acute episode from the inadvertent or deliberate consumption of a large amount of fluoride rinse must also be considered.

Chronic toxicity

Effect on developing teeth—The enamel organ is particularly sensitive to high concentrations of fluoride. Repeated high doses of systemic fluoride can result in enamel fluorosis, which clinically manifests as unesthetic hypoplastic or hypocalcific defects of the tooth crown (see Chapter 5). For this reason, it is important to evaluate the effect of inadvertent repetitive ingestion of fluoride while mouth rinsing.

Several variables influence the amount of solution that may be retained while rinsing. Among these are the age of the participant, the volume of solution used for rinsing, and the rinsing time.

Ericsson and *Forsman*[115] found that most 2- and 3-year-old children could not perform mouth rinsing without swallowing the solution. They also reported that 3- and 4-year-olds could keep the solution in their mouths for 30 seconds, and 5- and 6-year-olds for 60 seconds and expectorate most of the rinse. The amount of solution retained decreased with age. When rinsing was performed with 7 ml, the average 3-year-old retained 14% of the solution, whereas the average 5- to 6-year-old retained 5 to 7%.

Birkeland[116] studied the amount of retained fluoride from mouth rinsing in 10- and 11-year-old children and in adults using 7 ml and 10 ml of solution. He found that both age groups retained about 14 to 15% of the solution. However, retention was significantly increased when 10 ml, rather than 7 ml, were used. *Hellstrom*[117] reported that 7- to 15-year-old children who rinsed for 60 seconds with 15 ml swallowed an average of 19% of the solution, and *Birkeland* and *Lokken*[118] found that adults swallowed more solution when rinsing was performed for two minutes compared to 30 seconds.

By age 8, all of the permanent teeth, exclusive of third molars, will usually have completed mineralization of the tooth crown. Since fluoride rinsing is not recommended for preschool children, *the period of concern relative to tooth development is from ages 5 or 6 to age 8.*

Rinsing is usually performed for 60 seconds using either 5 or 10 ml of solution. The most common rinsing regimens use either a 0.05% NaF solution daily (low potency, high frequency) or a 0.2% solution weekly or every 2 weeks (high potency, low frequency). Assuming that the maximum amount of solution retained is 20%, as seen in Table 9-15, the amount of fluoride retained with these regimens varies from 0.2 mg to 1.8 mg. The inadvertent ingestion of 0.2 to 0.4 mg fluoride daily (low potency, high frequency technique) by 6- to 8-year-old children, even if they are receiving optimal systemic fluoride from other sources, would not be expected to cause a cosmetic problem to the developing dentition. Likewise, there is no evidence to indicate that the *infrequent* ingestion of 0.9 or 1.8 mg fluoride (high potency-low frequency technique) in this age group would cause cosmetic problems.

Effect on gingival health—Not all of the fluoride retained from mouth rinsing is swallowed. A small amount is retained intraorally, especially in the dental plaque.[119-122] The possibility that this fluoride might be detrimental to the gingiva has been considered by several investigators. In general, it has been found that fluoride rinsing either has no effect on the level of gingivitis,[123-126] or reduces it,[127,128] and that it has no effect on plaque accumulation,[125,126] or reduces

Table 9-15 Fluoride ingestion from common mouth rinses assuming 20 percent retention

Rinse Concentration (% NaF)	Amount of rinse	mg F in rinse	mg F retained at 20% retention level
0.05%*	5 ml	1 mg	.2 mg
	10 ml	2 mg	.4 mg
0.2%**	5 ml	4.5 mg	.9 mg
	10 ml	9.0 mg	1.8 mg

*Used in low potency, high frequency technique.
**Used in high potency, low frequency technique.

it.[123,128-130] Thus, routine fluoride rinsing has not been found to adversely effect gingival health.

Extrinsic staining of teeth—Some staining of the teeth has been associated with the use of stannous fluoride mouth rinses but not with sodium fluoride rinses. *McConchie* and co-workers[59] reported staining in "a very small number of children" who were rinsing daily with a 0.04% or 0.08% SnF_2 solution. The investigators indicated that the children who developed stains exhibited a poor level of oral hygiene.

Acute toxicity

Two deaths have been associated with the dental therapeutic use of fluoride. One involved a medically compromised patient on kidney dialysis in which the level of fluoride in the tap water used in the kidney machine was accidentally raised to about 15 ppm. Unfortunately, the other was a young child who was given a cup of fluoride solution with which to rinse.

In the latter instance, a 3-year-old, who was being examined in a dental clinic, was given a 3-ounce (45 ml) cup containing 4% SnF_2 (10,000 ppm F). The cup thus contained 435 mg of fluoride.[131] Approximately 5 minutes after using the solution, the child vomited and had a convulsive seizure. He died 3 hours later. Not only was the amount and concentration of the rinse incorrect (too much solution; too high a fluoride concentration), the frequency incorrect (once-a-year office application has never been recommended), and the age of the child incorrect (preschool children cannot be expected to master the rinsing technique), but the treatment was not even indicated since the child was free of caries and resided in a fluoridated community!

This episode tragically illustrates the maxim that any therapeutic agent that is incorrectly prescribed or administered is potentially harmful. It is not, however, an indictment of fluoride rinsing, since the treatment administered in this particular case bore no relationship to the types of fluoride rinsing programs discussed in this chapter and advocated by the dental profession.

Since the most frequently used fluoride rinsing regimens are the daily use of a 0.05% NaF solution or the weekly or fortnightly use of a 0.2% NaF solution, the following discussion of acute toxicity is limited to these therapeutic regimens.

If during rinsing a child accidentally swallows 5 or 10 ml of a 0.05% NaF solution, he will have ingested 1 or 2 mg F respectively. This is the equivalent of one or two NaF tablets (a 2.2 mg NaF tablet contains 1 mg F).

Since one NaF tablet is recommended daily for optimum dental health in a fluoride-deficient community, it is obvious that the inadvertent ingestion of this amount of rinse poses no acute health problem.

Five or 10 ml of 0.2% NaF solution contains 4.5 or 9.0 mg F respectively. This amount is the equivalent of four and a half and nine NaF tablets respectively. The American Dental Association recommends that, for safety, no more than 120 NaF tablets be dispensed at any one time. The amount of fluoride contained in the single dose of rinse solution is about 1/14 to 1/28 this amount. While a child may become nauseous if the entire 5 or 10 ml is swallowed, this constitutes no serious health hazard.

Earlier in this chapter the use of fluoride rinses for individual patients in their own homes was discussed. A 0.5% NaF concentration was recommended for daily use. These rinses are commercially available in bottles of 250 and 500 ml. Since 5 ml of rinse contains 1 mg F, these containers are the equivalent of 50 or 100 tablets of NaF and are, therefore, well within the margin of safety recommended by the American Dental Association. (Actually, on a weight basis, the lethal dose for a small preschool child weighing 9 kg (20 lbs.) is approximately 0.7 to 1.5 g sodium fluoride, which is the equivalent of 350 to 700 NaF tablets.) If a child should manage to drink as much as 500 ml of a 0.05% NaF solution, vomiting would probably be spontaneous; if not, it should be induced to avoid stomach cramps. More severe symptoms from this amount of fluoride in an otherwise healthy child are unlikely.

School-based fluoride rinsing programs generally use the higher concentration 0.2% NaF rinse. The rinse is either purchased already prepared or is mixed from premeasured packets of NaF and tap water. The packets of one supplier contain 3,000 mg NaF, or the equivalent of 1,300 tablets of NaF. This small package can be attractive to a young child. If the entire package is consumed, it can be fatal. The prepared solutions are usually stored in containers of 1 or 1.5 liters. One liter of a 0.2% NaF solution contains approximately 2,000 mg NaF, the equivalent of about 900 NaF tablets. In the unlikely event that a young child consumed the entire liter, the consequences could be fatal. It is more likely, however, that the child could not consume that quantity of liquid at once or, if he did, he would immediately vomit most of it.

In the United States alone, there are about eight million children enrolled in school-based fluoride rinsing programs. Attesting to the safety of these programs and the conscientiousness of the individuals in charge is the fact that no fatality or serious accident has ever been reported. Nevertheless, those in charge of such programs should make sure all fluoride supplies are carefully stored in a locked cabinet or closet and that a strict daily inventory is maintained. Additionally, emergency procedures for inadvertent fluoride ingestion should be posted in the school nurse's office and should be familiar to all rinse personnel. Figure 9-6 is an example of an emergency poster used in a school-based fluoride rinsing program in which the 0.2% solution is prepared from NaF packets.

In an international workshop report on fluoride rinses, the committee stated that, "the use of fluoride rinses by individuals age six and above, whether they reside in an optimally water fluoridated or non-fluoridated community, can be safely recommended." Additionally, the committee recommended that, "fluoride rinses, containing up to 120 mg F in a single container, should be available to the public on a non-prescription basis."[132] Since that report, a commercial NaF mouth rinse, discussed previously in this chapter, is available without prescription.

Fluoride Rinsing Program

EMERGENCY PROCEDURES FOR INADVERTENT INGESTION OF SODIUM FLUORIDE

FLUORIDE IN CUPS
The amount of fluoride used in the weekly rinsing sessions is approximately **4.5 mg** for kindergarten children, and **9 mg** for all others. Inadvertent swallowing of this amount of fluoride, while it may cause nausea, does **not** constitute a health hazard.

FLUORIDE IN DISPENSING BOTTLES
The amount of fluoride present in the dispensing bottles (1/3 full = 500 ml) **452 mg**. If the entire contents of the dispensing bottle is inadvertently consumed, the effect **can be serious**, depending upon the size and weight of the child. Immediate attention is required.

FLUORIDE IN PACKETS
The amount of fluoride in the cellophane packets is **1357 mg**. If the entire contents of the packet is inadvertently consumed by a child, the effect can be **very serious**. Immediate action is required.

SYMPTOMS OF FLUORIDE OVER-DOSAGE
SALTY OR SOAPY TASTE
INCREASED SALIVATION
NAUSEA
ABDOMINAL CRAMPS
VOMITING
DIARRHEA
DEHYDRATION AND THIRST

FIRST AID
1. FORCE COPIOUS QUANTITIES OF MILK.
2. INDUCE VOMITING BY PLACING INDEX FINGER AT BACK OF THROAT OR ADMINISTERING AN IPECAC PREPARATION.
3. REPEAT UNTIL VOMITED FLUID IS CLEAR.
4. SEEK PROFESSIONAL EMERGENCY AID **IMMEDIATELY!**

Container	Sodium Fluoride	Fluoride
Packet	3000 mg	1357 mg
Bottle	1000 mg*	452 mg

* bottles delivered 1/3 full; proportionately less depend-upon amount used in class.

Fig. 9-6 An emergency poster used in a school-based rinsing program in which the 0.2% NaF solution is prepared from premeasured NaF packets.

Effect of fluoride compounds on dental restorations

Only a few *in vitro* studies have been conducted to determine the effect of fluoride compounds on the surfaces of dental restorations.[133-136] These studies have found that, under the proper experimental conditions, APF, SnF_2, or NaF can enhance amalgam corrosion or etch porcelain dental restorations. In some instances, the least effects have been observed with SnF_2 and the greatest with acidified NaF. Since self-application techniques employ fluoride compounds on a frequent basis, the condition of the restorations of patients who are on this therapy should be carefully observed for any unusual surface deterioration. As an added precaution, patients with a glazed porcelain restoration should not be placed on a daily regimen that uses an acidified NaF gel.[136]

Summary

The self-application of topical fluorides offers advantages not available with other more traditional forms of fluoride therapy. For instance, compared to operator-applied topical fluoride programs, public health programs that utilize self-application techniques can treat more children in less time, with fewer personnel, and for less cost. When self-application procedures are employed in individual dental preventive programs, conscientious patients can give themselves many more topical fluoride applications than is practical to administer professionally in the dental office.

Three self-application methods have been studied—toothbrushing, mouth rinsing, and the use of mouth trays. For individual patients, each method has its particular indications; although for very young patients in the primary dentition, recommendations must be made on an empirical basis. Patients who are caries prone, are undergoing orthodontic treatment, who have xerostomia caused by head and neck radiation therapy or from other reasons are special candidates for topical fluoride self-application home therapy.

While the highest caries reductions have been reported when fluoride gels have been applied daily in mouth trays, this method has not gained acceptance in public health programs, probably because of the difficulty of implementing the technique in schools. "Brush-ins" were popular during the late 1960s, but use of this method has declined since the efficacy of the technique could not be satisfactorily established. On the other hand, mouth rinsing has consistently proven to be effecitve, is easy to accomplish, and is relatively inexpensive. Today, this is the most popular form of topical fluoride self-application in schools.

Two methods of fluoride mouth rinsing have been most often studied—low potency-high frequency and high potency-low frequency. Generally, the former therapy uses 0.05% NaF (either neutral NaF or APF) once a day while the latter employs a 0.2% NaF solution once a week or once every 2 weeks. Clinical evidence does not lead to the definite conclusion that one technique is superior to the other. Nevertheless, daily applications are generally recommended for home use, while the weekly or fortnightly rinse is more convenient for school-based programs.

All of the topical fluoride self-application methods are safe. Fluoride rinsing offers the greatest potential for swallowing some of the solution. However, the inadvertent ingestion of 5 or 10 ml of either a 0.05% or 0.2% NaF solution will not cause acute problems other than possibly nausea at the higher concentration. Five milliliters of the 0.05% solution provide 1 mg F, which is the equivalent of a standard 2.2 NaF tablet. Thus, in communities with fluoride-deficient water supplies, the 0.05% NaF solution can be rinsed and then swallowed, providing a topical effect to the erupted teeth and a systemic effect to the teeth that are unerupted.

When fluoride rinsing is employed in schools, the supplies must be carefully monitored and kept in locked storage areas when not in use. The fluoride materials used in these programs can be hazardous to children if they are accidentally consumed in unsupervised amounts.

References

1. Berggren, H., and Welander, E. 1960. Supervised toothbrushing with a sodium fluoride solution in 5,000 Swedish school children. Results and analysis of procedures. *Acta Odontol. Scand.* 18:209-34.
2. Berggren, H., and Welander, E. 1964. The caries-inhibiting effect of sodium, ferric, and zirconium fluorides. A comparative study on school children using supervised brushing as the mode of application. *Acta Odontol. Scand.* 22:401-13.
3. Muhler, J.C. 1968. Mass treatment of children with a stannous fluoride-zirconium silicate self-

administered prophylactic paste for partial control of dental caries. *J. Am. Coll. Dent.* 35:45-57.

4. Kelley, G.E. 1970. Mass self-administered stannous fluoride prophylactic paste. *Can. J. Public Health* 61:226-31.
5. Bullen, D.C.T.; McCombie, F.; and Hole, L.W. 1965. One-year effect of supervised toothbrushing with an acidulated fluoride-phosphate solution. *J. Canad. Dent. Assoc.* 31:231-35.
6. Bullen, D.C.T.; McCombie, F.; and Hole, L.W. 1966. Two-year effect of supervised toothbrushing with an acidulated fluoride-phosphate solution. *J. Canad. Dent. Assoc.* 32:89-93.
7. Conchie, J.M.; McCombie, F.; and Hole, L.W. 1969. Three years of supervised toothbrushing with a fluoride-phosphate solution. *J. Public Health Dent.* 29:11-18.
8. Heifetz, S.B.; Horowitz, H.S.; and Driscoll, W.S. 1970. Two year evaluation of self-administered procedure for the topical application of acidulated phosphate fluoride: final report. *J. Public Health Dent.* 30:7-12.
9. Horowitz, H.S.; Heifetz, S.B.; McClendon, B.W.; Viefas, A.R.; Guinaraes, L.O.C.; and Lopes, E.S. 1974. Evaluation of self-administered prophylaxis and supervised toothbrushing with acidulated phosphate-fluoride. *Caries Res.* 8:39-51.
10. Gallagher, S.J.; Maclean, M.W.; Costanzo, A.; and Caldwell, R. 1975. Self-application in a phospho-fluoride brushing study. *J. Canad. Dent. Assoc.* 9:505-8.
11. Marthaler, T.M., and Mühlemann, H.R. 1970. Clinical anticaries effect of supervised toothbrushing with fluoride tablets for topical application. *Helv. Odont. Acta* 14:77-79.
12. Muhler, J.C.; Kelley, G.E.; Stookey, G.K.; Lindo, F.I.; and Harris, N.O. 1970. The clinical evaluation of a patient-administered SnF_2-$ZrSiO_4$ prophylactic paste in children. I. Results after one year in the Virgin Islands. *J. Amer. Dent. Assoc.* 81:142-45.
13. Fleming, W.J.; Burgess, R.C.; and Lewis, D.W. 1976. Effect on caries of self-application of a zirconium silicate paste containing 9 percent stannous fluoride. *Community Dent. Oral Epidemiol.* 4:142-48.
14. Horowitz, H.S., and Bixler, D. 1976. The effect of self-applied SnF_2-$ZrSiO_4$ prophylactic paste on dental caries: Santa Clara County, California. *J. Amer. Dent. Assoc.* 92:369-73.
15. Gish, C.W.; Mercer, V.H.; Stookey, G.K.; and Dahl, L.O. 1975. Self-application of fluoride as a community preventive measure: rationale, procedures, and three-year results. *J. Amer. Dent. Assoc.* 90:388-97.
16. Woodhouse, A.D. 1978. A longitudinal study of the effectiveness of self-applied 10 percent stannous fluoride paste for secondary school children. *Aust. Dent. J.* 23:422-28.
17. Woods, R. 1976. A community dental health project I. Self-applied SnF_2-$ZrSiO_4$ prophylactic paste and dental caries in primary school children. *Aust. Dent. J.* 21:205-10.
18. Muhler, J.C. 1976. A clinical evaluation of the dental caries experience in children receiving a self-applied stannous fluoride-alkali aluminum silicate prophylactic paste during a twelve-month study period. *J. Dent. Child.* 43:345-46.
19. Mellberg, J.R.; Peterson, J.K.; and Nicholson, C.R. 1974. Fluoride uptake and caries inhibition from self-application of an acidulated-phosphate-fluoride prophylaxis paste. *Caries Res.* 8:52-60.
20. Long, J.G. 1972. Self-applied fluoride paste: effect on dental caries. *J. Public Health Dent.* 32:161-64.
21. Trubman, A., and Crellin, J.A. 1973. Effect on dental caries of self-application of acidulated phosphate fluoride paste and gel. *J. Amer. Dent. Assoc.* 86:153-57.
22. Marthaler, T.M.; Konig, K.G.; and Mühlemann, H.R. 1970. The effect of a fluoride gel used for supervised toothbrushing 15 or 30 times per year. *Helv. Odont. Acta* 14:67-77.
23. Goaz, P.W.; McElwaine, L.P.; Biswell, H.A.; and White, W.E. 1963. Effect of daily applications of sodium monofluorophosphate solution on caries rate in children. *J. Dent. Res.* 42:963-72.
24. Goaz, P.W.; McElwaine, L.P.; Biswell, H.A.; and White, W.E. 1966. Anticariogenic effect of a sodium monofluorophosphate solution in children after 21 months of use. *J. Dent. Res.* 45:286-90.
25. Gunz, G.M. 1971. The effect of self-applied fluoride paste. *J. Public Health Dent.* 31:177-81.
26. Lang, L.A.; Thomas, H.G.; Taylor, J.A.; and Rothhaar, R.E. 1970. Clinical efficacy of a self-applied stannous fluoride prophylactic paste. *J. Dent. Child.* 37:211-16.
27. McConchie, J.M. 1974. The potential benefits of "brush-in" programmes as regards prevention of dental caries, dental health education, and public relations. In International workshop on fluorides and dental caries reductions, eds. D.E. Forrester and E.M. Schulze, Jr., pp. 259-304. Baltimore: Univ. of Maryland.
28. Bibby, B.G.; Zander, H.A.; McKelleget, M.; and Labansky, B. 1946. Preliminary reports on the effect on dental caries of the use of sodium fluoride in a prophylactic cleaning mixture and a mouthwash. *J. Dent. Res.* 25:207-11.

29. Roberts, J.F.; Bibby, B.G.; and Wellock, W.D. 1948. The effect of an acidulated fluoride mouthwash on dental caries. *J. Dent. Res.* 27:497-500.
30. Weisz, W.S. 1960. The reduction of dental caries through use of a sodium fluoride mouthwash. *J. Amer. Dent. Assoc.* 60:438-56.
31. Fjaestad-Seger, M.; Norstedt-Larsson, K.; and Torell, P. 1961. Forsok med enkla metoder for klinisk fluorapplikation. *Sverige Tandlak-Forb. Tidn.* 53:169-80.
32. Torell, P., and Siberg, A. 1962. Mouthwash with sodium fluoride and potassium fluoride. *Odont. Revy* 13:62-72.
33. Lundstam, R. 1964. Teachers administering mouthwash with fluorides in Jamtland, Sweden. *Sverige Tandlak-Forb. Tidn.* 56:681-82.
34. Torell, P., and Ericsson, Y. 1965. Two-year clinical tests with different methods of local caries-preventive fluorine application in Swedish school children. *Acta Odontol. Scand.* 23:287-322.
35. Forsman, B. 1965. Effect of mouth rinses with sodium fluoride in schools at Vixjo. *Sverige Tandlak-Forb. Tidn.* 57:705-9.
36. Kann, J. 1965. Systemic controlled fluoride mouth rinses. *Tandleyebladet* 69:638-41.
37. Kasakura, T. 1966. Dental observation on school feeding Part 3. Effect of the dental caries prevention by oral rinsing with sodium fluoride solution after school feeding. *Odontology* 54:22-32.
38. Koch, G. 1967. Effect of sodium fluoride in dentifrice and mouthwash on incidence of dental caries in school children. *Odont. Revy* 18 (Suppl. 12):1-125.
39. Koch, G. 1969. Caries increment in school children during and two years after the end of supervised rinsing of the mouth with sodium fluoride solution. *Odont. Revy* 20:323-30.
40. Gerdin, P.-O., and Torell, P. 1969. Mouth rinses with potassium fluoride solutions containing manganese. *Caries Res.* 3:99-107.
41. Horowitz, H.S.; Creighton, W.E.; and McLendon, B.J. 1971. The effect on human dental caries of weekly oral rinsing with a sodium fluoride mouthwash: a final report. *Arch. Oral Biol.* 16:609-16.
42. Aasenden, R.; DePaola, P.F.; and Brudevold, F. 1972. Effects of daily rinsing and ingestion of fluoride solutions upon dental caries and enamel fluoride. *Arch. Oral Biol.* 17:1705-14.
43. Brandt, R.S.; Slack, G.L.; and Waller, D.F. 1972. The use of a sodium fluoride mouthwash in reducing the dental caries increment in eleven year old English school children. *Proc. Br. Paedod. Soc.* 2 (October):23-25.
44. Frankl, S.N.; Fleisch, S.; and Diodati, R.R. 1972. The topical anticariogenic effect of daily rinsing with an acidulated phosphate fluoride solution. *J. Amer. Dent. Assoc.* 85:882-86.
45. Moreira, B.H., and Tumang, A.J. 1972. Prevencao da carie dentaria atraves de bochechos com solucoes de fluoreto de sodio a 0.1% Resultados apos dois anos de estudos. *Rev. Bras. Odontol.* 29:37-42. Cited in Council classifies fluoride mouthrinses. Council on Dental Therapeutics. *J. Amer. Dent. Assoc.* 91:1250-52, 1975.
46. Heifetz, S.B.; Driscoll, W.S.; and Creighton, W.E. 1973. The effect on dental caries of weekly rinsing with a neutral sodium fluoride or an acidulated phosphate-fluoride mouthwash. *J. Amer. Dent. Assoc.* 87:364-68.
47. Rugg-Gunn, A.J.; Holloway, P.J.; and Davies, T.G.H. 1973. Caries prevention by daily fluoride mouthrinsing. Report of a three-year clinical trial. *Brit. Dent. J.* 135:353-60.
48. Padron, F.S., and Maiwald, H.J. 1973. Analisis de los resultados de las aplicaciones a grupos de poblacion en Cuba. *Rev. Cub. Est.* 10:173-79. Cited in Council classifies fluoride mouthrinses. Council on Dental Therapeutics. *J. Amer. Dent. Assoc.* 91:1250-52, 1975.
49. Kani, M.; Fujioka, M.; Nagamine, Y.; et al. 1973. The effect of mouthwash on human dental caries during three years of regular usage with acidulated sodium fluoride solution. (Jap.) *J. Dent. Health* (Tokyo) 23:244-50. Cited in Council classifies fluoride mouth rinses. Council on Dental Therapeutics. *J. Amer. Dent. Assoc.* 91:1250-52, 1975.
50. Radike, A.W.; Gish, C.W.; Peterson, J.K.; King, J.D.; and Segreto, V.A. 1973. Clinical evaluation of stannous fluoride as an anticaries mouthrinse. *J. Amer. Dent. Assoc.* 86:404-8.
51. Gallagher, S.J.; Glassgow, I.; and Caldwell, R. 1974. Self-application of fluoride by rinsing. *J. Public Health Dent.* 34:13-21.
52. Forsman, B. 1974. The caries preventing effect of mouthrinsing with 0.025 percent sodium fluoride solution in Swedish children. *Community Dent. Oral Epidemiol.* 2:58-65.
53. Finn, S.B.; Moller, P.; Jamison, H.; Regattieri, L.; and Manson-Hing, L. 1975. The clinical cariostatic effectiveness of two concentrations of acidulated phosphate-fluoride mouthwash. *J. Amer. Dent. Assoc.* 90:398-402.
54. Packer, M.W.; Laswell, H.R.; Doyle, J.; Naff, H.H.; and Brown, F. 1975. Cariostatic effects of fluoride mouthrinses in a non-fluoridated community. *J. Tenn. Dent. Assoc.* 55:22-26.

55. Laswell, H.R.; Packer, M.W.; and Wiggs, J.S. 1975. Cariostatic effects of fluoride mouthrinses in a fluoridated community. *J. Tenn. Dent. Assoc.* 55:198-200.
56. Birkeland, J.M., and Jorkjend, L. 1975. Effect of mouthrinsing and toothbrushing with fluoride solutions on caries among Norwegian school children. *Community Dent. Oral Epidemiol.* 3:201-7.
57. Ringelberg, M.L.; Conti, A.J.; and Webster, D.B. 1976. An evaluation of single and combined self-applied fluoride programs in schools. *J. Public Health Dent.* 36:229-36.
58. Petchel, K.A., and Mello, A.F. 1977. A school fluoride mouth rinse program. *J. Sch. Health* 47:557-58.
59. McConchie, J.M.; Richardson, A.S.; Hole, L.W.; McCombie, F.; and Kolthammer, J. 1977. Caries-preventive effect of two concentrations of stannous fluoride mouth rinse. *Community Dent. Oral Epidemiol.* 5:278-83.
60. DePaola, P.F.; Soparker, P.; Foley, S.; Bookstein, F.; and Bakhos, Y. 1977. Effect of high concentration ammonium and sodium fluoride rinses on dental caries in school children. *Community Dent. Oral Epidemiol.* 5:7-14.
61. Ashley, F.P.; Mainwaring, P.J.; Emslie, R.D.; and Naylor, M.N. 1977. Clinical testing of a mouth rinse and a dentifrice containing fluoride. *Brit. Dent. J.* 143:333-38.
62. Torell, P., and Gerdin, P.-O. 1977. Fortnightly fluoride rinsing combined with topical painting of fluoride solutions containing Al^-, Fe^-, and Mn^- ions. *Scand. J. Dent. Res.* 85:38-40.
63. Horowitz, H.S.; Heifetz, S.B.; Meyers, R.J.; Driscoll, W.S.; and Kortz, D.C. 1977. Evaluation of a combination of self-administered fluoride procedures for control of dental caries in a non-fluoride area: findings after two years. *Caries Res.* 11:178-85.
64. Birkeland, J.M.; Broch, L.; and Jorkjend, L. 1977. Benefits and prognoses following ten years of a fluoride mouthrinsing program. *Scand. J. Dent. Res.* 85:31-37.
65. Ripa, L.W.; Leske, G.S.; and Levinson, A. 1978. Supervised weekly rinsing with a 0.2 percent neutral NaF solution: results from a demonstration program after two school years. *J. Amer. Dent. Assoc.* 97:793-98.
66. Bennie, A.M.; Tullis, J.I.; Stephen, K.W.; and MacFadyen, E.E. 1978. Five years of community preventive dentistry and health education in the county of Southerland, Scotland. *Community Dent. Oral Epidemiol.* 6:1-5.
67. Luoma, H.; Murtomaa, H.; Nuuja, T.; Nyman, A.; Nummikoski, P.; Ainamo, J.; and Luoma, A.R. 1978. A simultaneous reduction of caries and gingivitis in a group of school children receiving chlorhexidine-fluoride applications. Results after two years. *Caries Res.* 12:290-98.
68. Ringelberg, M.L.; Webster, D.B., Jr.; and Dixon, D.O. 1978. Effects of an amine fluoride dentifrice and mouth rinse on the dental caries of school children after 18 months. *J. Prev. Dent.* 5 (4):26-30.
69. Horowitz, H.S.; Heifetz, S.B.; Meyers, R.J.; Driscoll, W.S.; and Korts, D.C. 1979. Evaluation of a combination of self-administered fluoride procedures for the control of dental caries in a non-fluoride area: findings after four years. *J. Amer. Dent. Assoc.* 98:219-23.
70. Heifetz, S.B.; Franchi, G.J.; Mosley, G.W.; MacDougall, O.; and Brunelle, J. 1979. Combined anticariogenic effect of fluoride gel-trays and fluoride mouthrinsing in an optimally fluoridated community. *J. Clinical Preventive Dent.* 6 (1):21-23.
71. Ripa, L.W.; and Leske, G.S. 1979. Two years' effect on the primary dentition of mouthrinsing with a 0.2 percent neutral NaF solution. *Community Dent. Oral Epidemiol.* 7:151-53.
72 Swerdloff, G., and Shannon, I.L. 1969. Feasibility of the use of stannous fluoride mouthwash in a school system. *J. Dent. Child.* 36:363-68.
73. Council on Dental Therapeutics. Council classifies fluoride mouth rinses. *J. Amer. Dent. Assoc.* 91:1250-52.
74. Ripa, L.W., and Leske, G.S. 1980. Effect on the primary dentition of mouth rinsing with a 0.2 percent neutral NaF solution: results from a demonstration program after three school years. *Pediatric Dentistry.* 2:184-9.
75. Birkeland, J.M., and Torell, P. 1978. Caries-preventive fluoride mouth rinses. *Caries Res.* 12 (Suppl. 1):38-51.
76. Ripa, L.W.; Levinson, A.; and Leske, G.S. 1980. Supervised weekly rinsing with a 0.2 percent neutral NaF solution: results from a demonstration program after three school years. *J. Amer. Dent. Assoc.* 100:544-46.
77. Englander, H.R.; Keyes, P.H.; Gestwicki, M.; and Sultz, H.A. 1967. Clinical anti-caries effect of repeated topical sodium fluoride applications by mouthpieces. *J. Amer. Dent. Assoc.* 75:638-44.
78. Englander, H.R.; Carlos, J.P.; Senning, R.S.; and Mellberg, J.R. 1969. Residual anti-caries effect of repeated topical sodium fluoride applications by mouthpieces. *J. Amer. Dent. Assoc.* 78:783-87.
79. Shern, R.J.; Duany, L.F.; Senning, R.S.; and Zinner, D.D. 1976. Clinical study of an amine fluoride gel and acidulated phosphate fluoride gel.

Community Dent. Oral Epidemiol. 4:133-36.
80. Englander, H.R.; Sherrill, L.T.; Miller, B.G.; Carlos, J.P.; Mellberg, J.R.; and Senning, R.S. 1971. Incremental rates of dental caries after repeated topical sodium fluoride applications in children with lifelong consumption of fluoridated water. *J. Amer. Dent. Assoc.* 82:354-58.
81. Mellberg, J.R.; Franchi, G.J.; Englander, H.R.; Mosley, G.W.; and Nicholson, C.R. 1978. Short intensive topical APF applications and dental caries in a fluoridated area. *Community Dent. Oral Epidemiol.* 6:117-20.
82. Englander, H.R.; Mellberg, J.R.; and Engler, W.O. 1978. Observations on dental caries in primary teeth after frequent fluoride toplications in a program involving other preventives. *J. Dent. Res.* 57:855-60.
83. Muhler, J.C. 1968. The clinical demonstration of the mass treatment of children with the SnF_2-$ZrSiO_4$ prophylactic paste. Initial observations concerning conduct of the study. *J. Indiana Dent. Assoc.* 47:428-31.
84. Mercer, V.H., and Gish, C.W. 1968. The self-administered stannous fluoride treatment paste for caries prevention in a community. *J. Indiana Dent. Assoc.* 47:432-34.
85. Schimmele, R.G. 1968. A suggested method for mass application of self-administered prophylactic paste using student auxiliary personnel. *J. Indiana Dent. Assoc.* 47:435-36.
86. Kelley, G.E. 1969. The Bloomington "brush-in." A new experience in dental caries prevention for mass treatment. *J. Indiana Dent. Assoc.* 48:72-75.
87. Preventive Dentistry Research Institute, Indiana University. 1969. Progress report concerning the current status of the self-application of the stannous fluoride-zirconium silicate preventive dentistry paste program for the mass control of dental caries. *J. Indiana Dent. Assoc.* 48:317-19.
88. Hoffman, E. 1970. Operation "brush-in." *J. S. Calif. Dent. Hyg. Assoc.* 12:14-15.
89. Foster, M.J. 1970. Let's have a brush-in. *J. Texas Dent. Hyg. Assoc.* 7:19.
90. Story, F.B. 1970. North Carolina's first brush-in. *J. N. Carolina Dent. Soc.* 53:15-17.
91. Smith, C.E. 1970. "Brush-in:" self-applied topical fluorides. *Ohio Dent. J.* 44:188-90.
92. Praven, J.R. 1973. A "brush-in" with the self-administered stannous fluoride treatment paste. *Tex. Dent. J.* 9(June):10.
93. Heifetz, S.B. 1978. Cost-effectiveness of topically applied fluorides. In The relative efficiency of methods of caries prevention in dental public health, ed. Brian A. Burt, pp. 69-104. Ann Arbor: Univ. of Michigan.
94. Horowitz, A.M., and Horowitz, H.S. 1980. School-based fluoride programs: a critique. *J. Prev. Dent.* 6:89-94.
95. DePaola, P.F., and Soparkar, P. 1980. Operational considerations of supervised weekly sodium fluoride rinsing: results from a demonstration program after two school years. *J. Prev. Dent.* 6:95-100.
96. Ripa, L.W.; Leske, G.S.; and Lowey, W.G. 1977. Fluoride rinsing: a school-based dental preventive program. *J. Prev. Dent.* 4(5):25-30.
97. Leske, G.S., and Ripa, L.W. 1977. Guidelines for establishing a fluoride mouthrinsing caries preventive program for school children. *Public Health Rep.* 92:240-44.
98. Preventing tooth decay: a guide to implementing self-applied fluoride programs in schools. 1977. U.S. Department of Health, Education, and Welfare, Public Health Service, Publication No. (NIH)77-1196.
99. Levinson, A.; Leske, G.S.; and Ripa, L.W. 1980. Cost considerations of supervised weekly sodium fluoride rinsing: results from a demonstration program after two school years. *J. Prev. Dent.* 6:101-6.
100. Davies, G.N. 1974. Cost and benefit of fluoride in the prevention of dental caries. Geneva: World Health Organization, Offset Pub. No. 9.
101. Zachrisson, B.U., and Zachrisson, S. 1971. Caries incidence and orthodontic treatment with fixed appliances. *Scand. J. Dent. Res.* 79:183-92.
102. Zachrisson, B.U., and Zachrisson, S. 1971. Caries incidence and oral hygiene during orthodontic treatment. *Scand. J. Dent. Res.* 79:394-401.
103. Zachrisson, B.U. 1975. Fluoride application procedures in orthodontic practice, current concepts. *Am. J. Orthod.* 45:72-81.
104. Stratemann, M.W., and Shannon, I.L. 1974. Control of decalcification in orthodontic patients by daily self-administered application of a water-free 0.4 percent stannous fluoride gel. *Am. J. Orthod.* 66:273-79.
105. Shannon, I.L.; St. Clair, J.R.; Pratt, G.A.,Jr.; and West, D.C. 1977. Stannous fluoride versus sodium fluoride in preventive treatment of orthodontic patients. *Aust. Orthod. J.* 5:18-24.
106. Magness, W.S.; Shannon, I.L.; and West, D.C. 1979. Office-applied fluoride treatments for orthodontic patients. *J. Dent. Res.* 58:1427.
107. Hirschfield, R.E. 1978. Control of decalcification by use of fluoride mouth rinse. *J. Dent. Child.* 45:458-60.
108. von der Fehr, F.R.; Loe, H.; and Theilade, E.

1970. Experimental caries in man. *Caries Res.* 4:131-48.

109. Westcott, W.B.; Starcke, E.N.; and Shannon, I.L. 1975. Chemical protection against postirradiation dental caries. *Oral Surg.* 40:709-19.
110. Daly, T.E., and Drane, J.B. 1976. Prevention and management of dental problems in irradiated patients. *J. Am. Soc. Prev. Dent.* 6:21-25.
111. Dreizen, S.; Brown, L.R.; Daly, T.E.; and Drane, J.B. 1977. Prevention of xerostomia-related dental caries in irradiated cancer patients. *J. Dent. Res.* 56:99-104.
112. Carl, W.; Schaaf, N.G.; and Chen, T.Y. 1972. Oral care of patients irradiated for cancer of the head and neck. *Cancer* 30:448-53.
113. Miller, J.T., and Shannon, I.L. 1972. Water-free stannous fluoride gel and post-irradiation caries: a clinical report. *J. Public Health Dent.* 32:127.
114. Johanson, E., and Olsen, T.O. 1979. Topical fluorides in the prevention and arrest of dental caries. In A.A.A.S. Selected symposia series, No. 11. Continuing evaluation and use of fluorides, eds. E. Johanson and T.O. Olsen, pp. 61-110. Boulder, Colorado: Westview Press.
115. Ericsson, Y., and Forsman, B. 1969. Fluoride retained from mouth rinses and dentifrices in preschool children. *Caries Res.* 3:290-99.
116. Birkeland, J.M. 1973. Intra- and interindividual observations on fluoride ion activity and retained fluoride with sodium fluoride mouth rinses. *Caries Res.* 7:39-55.
117. Hellstrom, I. 1960. Fluorine retention following sodium fluoride mouthwashing. *Acta Odontol. Scand.* 18:263-78.
118. Birkeland, J.M., and Lokken, P. 1972. The pharmacokinetics of fluoride in mouth rinses as indicated by a reference substance (^{51}Cr-EDTA). *Caries Res.* 6:325-33.
119. Flessa, H.J., and Gulzow, H.J. 1970. Uber die verweildauer von natrium fluorid und aminfluoriden inden plaques. *Dtsch. Zahnarztl. Z.* 25:252-59.
120. Birkeland, J.M.; Jorkjend, L.; and von der Fehr, F.R. 1971. The influence of fluoride rinses on the fluoride content of dental plaque of children. *Caries Res.* 5:169-79.
121. Parkins, F.M. 1972. Retention of fluoride with chewable tablets and a mouth rinse. *J. Dent. Res.* 51:1346-49.
122. Silvera, R.S.; Gabathuler, H.; and Mühlemann, H.R. 1974. Salivary fluoride levels after mouthrinsing with inorganic fluoride and amine fluoride. *Helv. Odont. Acta* 18 (Suppl. 8):79-81.
123. Shern, R.J.; Rundell, B.B.; and Defever, C.J. 1974. Effects of an amine fluoride mouth rinse on the formation and microbial content of plaque. *Helv. Odont. Acta* 18 (Suppl. 8):57-62.
124. Birkeland, J.M.; Jorkjend, L.; and von der Fehr, F.R. 1973. The influence of fluoride mouthrinsing on the incidence of gingivitis in Norwegian children. *Community Dent. Oral Epidemiol.* 1:17-21.
125. Frandsen, A.M.; McClendon, B.J.; Chang, J.J.; and Creighton, W.E. 1972. The effect of oral rinsing with sodium fluoride on the gingiva of children. *Scand. J. Dent. Res.* 80:445-48.
126. Ringelberg, M.L., and Webster, D.B. 1977. Effects of an amine fluoride mouth rinse and dentifrice on the gingival health and the extent of plaque of school children. *J. Periodontol.* 48:350-53.
127. Stoller, N.H.; Cohen, D.W.; and Yankell, S.L. 1977. Clinical evaluations of an amine fluoride mouth rinse on gingival inflammation and plaque accumulation. *J. Periodontol.* 48:650-53.
128. Brayer, L.; Mor, H.; Anaise, J.; and Gedalia, I. 1977. Effect of sodium fluoride rinsing on dental plaque accumulation. *Isr. J. Dent. Med.* 26(4):45-47.
129. Birkeland, J.M. 1972. Effect of fluoride on the amount of dental plaque in children. *Scand. J. Dent. Res.* 80:82-84.
130. Luoma, H.; Ainamo, J.; Soderholm, S.; Meurman, J.; and Helminen, S. 1973. Reduction of enamel solubility and plaque development with chlorhexidine-fluoride solutions. *Scand. J. Dent. Res.* 81:523-27.
131. Horowitz, H. 1977. Editorial: abusive use of fluoride. *J. Public Health Dent.* 37:106-7.
132. Torell, P., and Ericsson, Y. 1974. The potential benefits to be derived from fluoride mouth rinses. In International workshop on fluorides and dental caries reductions, eds. D.E. Forrester and E.M. Schulze, Jr., pp. 113-77. Baltimore: Univ. of Maryland.
133. Stoner, G.E.; Senti, S.E.; and Gileadi, E. 1971. Effect of sodium fluoride and stannous fluoride on the rate of corrosion of dental amalgams. *J. Dent. Res.* 50:1647-53.
134. Gau, D.J., and Krause, E.A. 1973. Etching effect of topical fluorides on dental porcelains: a preliminary study. *J. Canad. Dent. Assoc.* 6:410-15.
135. Darvell, B.W. 1977. The effect of topical fluoride on amalgam. *Brit. Dent. J.* 142:47-51.
136. Schlissel, E.R.; Melnick, D.R.; and Ripa, L.W. 1980. *In vitro* effect of topical fluorides on porcelain surfaces (Abst. 910). *J. Dent. Res.* 59 (Spec. Issue A): 495.

Appendix

Table A-1 Commonly available forms of fluoride products

Form	Fluoride source	Fluoride content
Topical treatment		
For office use		
Gel	APF	1.2%
Solution	APF	1.2%
	2% NaF	0.9%
	8% SnF_2	2.0%
	Amine F	1.0%
Prophylaxis Paste	APF	1.2%
	NaF	1-2%
	$(NH_4)_2SiF_6$	0.4%-1%
Varnishes	NaF	2.2%
	Amine F	0.7%
For home use		
Gels (tray)	APF	0.5%
	NaF	0.5%
	SnF_2	0.1%
Mouthrinses	APF	0.02%
	NaF	0.02%
	NaF	0.1%
Dentifrices	NaF	0.1%
	MFP	0.1%
	SnF_2	0.1%
	Amine F	0.125%
Systemic treatment		
Tablets/lozenges	NaF	0.25–1.0 mg/tablet
Rinse supplement	NaF	1.0 mg/5 ml
Drops	NaF	0.125–0.5 mg/drop
Vitamin F tablets	NaF	0.5–1.0 mg/tablet
Vitamin F liquid	NaF	0.25–0.5 mg/ml
		0.5 mg/0.6 ml

Table A-2 Fluoride exposure from different treatments

Treatment		Fluoride exposure	
Type	F concentration	Usual amount used	mg F
Dietary F supplements			
Tablets	1 mg/tablet	1 tablet	1.0
Drops	0.125 mg/drop*	2-4 drops	0.25-0.5
Liquid F—vitamin	0.25 mg/ml*	1-2 ml	0.25-0.5
Rinse supplement	1.0 mg/5 ml	1 teaspoonful	1.0
Mouth rinses			
Daily	0.02%	1 teaspoonful	1.0
Weekly	0.09%	2 teaspoonsful	9.0
Dentifrices	0.1%*	1 gm	1.0
Topical solutions			
APF	1.2%	5 ml	62
8% SnF_2	2.0%	5 ml	100
2% NaF	1.0%	5 ml	50
Topical gels			
Self-applied (APF)	0.5%	1 ml	5
Professionally applied (APF)	1.2%	8 ml	98
Prophylaxis pastes	1.0%*	3 gm	30

*Other concentrations commercially available.

Table A-3 Fluoride treatment recommendations—Caries free individuals

Water F concentration	Birth—24 months	25—36 months	37 months—13 years	14 years and older
0.0 to 0.3 ppm F	Dietary F supplement—0.25 mg F daily; parent brushes child's teeth daily with ADA-approved F-dentifrice.	Dietary F supplement—0.5 mg F daily; parent brushes child's teeth daily with ADA-approved F-dentifrice.	Dietary F supplement—1.0 mg F daily; parent brushes child's teeth daily with ADA-approved F-dentifrice until child can master technique. Encourage brushing up to three times daily. Professionally applied topical F twice a year.	Patient brushes with ADA-approved F-dentifrice up to three times daily. Professionally applied topical F twice a year. Evaluate need to continue this regimen beyond age 16.
Greater than 0.3 to 0.7 ppm F	Parent brushes child's teeth daily with ADA-approved F-dentifrice.	Dietary F supplement—0.25 mg F daily; parent brushes child's teeth daily with ADA-approved F-dentifrice.	Dietary F supplement—0.5 mg F daily; parent brushes child's teeth daily with ADA-approved F-dentifrice until child can master technique. Encourage brushing up to three times daily. Professionally applied topical F twice a year.	Patient brushes with ADA-approved F-dentifrice up to three times daily. Professionally applied topical F twice a year. Evaluate need to continue this regimen beyond age 16.
Greater than 0.7 ppm F	Parent brushes child's teeth daily with ADA-approved F-dentifrice.	Parent brushes child's teeth daily with ADA-approved F-dentifrice.	Parent brushes child's teeth with ADA-approved F-dentifrice until child can master technique. Encourage brushing up to three times daily.	Patient brushes with ADA-approved F-dentifrice up to three times daily.

Table A-4 Fluoride treatment recommendations—Caries positive inidividuals

Water F concentration	Birth—24 months	25—36 months	37 months—13 years	14 years and older
0.0 to 0.3 ppm F	Dietary F supplement—0.25 mg F daily; parent brushes child's teeth daily with ADA-approved F-dentifrice. Parent applies APF gel (1.2% F) once a month; minimal amount of gel applied to child-size toothbrush.	Dietary F supplement—0.5 mg F daily; parent brushes child's teeth daily with ADA-approved F-dentifrice. Professionally applied topical F twice a year.* Parent applies APF gel (1.2% F) once a month; minimal amount of gel applied to child-size toothbrush.	Dietary F supplement—1.0 mg F daily; parent brushes child's teeth daily with ADA-approved F-dentifrice until child can master technique. Encourage brushing up to three times daily. Professionally applied topical F twice a year.* Parent applies APF gel (1.2% F) once a month until age 6. At age 6, stop *both* parent-administered APF gel and 1.0 mg daily F supplement and place child on a daily oral rinse supplement (0.05% NaF, rinse and swallow).	Patient brushes with ADA-approved F-dentifrice up to three times daily. Professionally applied topical F twice a year.* Daily APF (0.5% F) gel tray self-administration.
Greater than 0.3 to 0.7 ppm F	Parent brushes child's teeth daily with ADA-approved F-dentifrice. Parent applies APF gel (1.2% F) once a month; minimal amount of gel applied to child-size toothbrush.	Dietary F supplement—0.25 mg F daily; parent brushes child's teeth daily with ADA-approved F-dentifrice. Professionally applied topical F twice a year.* Parent applies APF gel (1.2% F) once a month; minimal amount of gel applied to child-size toothbrush.	Dietary F supplement—0.5 mg F daily; parent brushes child's teeth with ADA-approved F-dentifrice until child can master technique. Encourage brushing up to three times daily. Professionally applied topical F twice a year.* Parent applies APF gel (1.2% F) once a month until age 6. At age 6, change to daily rinse (0.05% NaF) and expectorate.	Patient brushes with ADA-approved F-dentifrice up to three times daily. Professionally applied topical F twice a year.* Daily APF (0.5% F) gel tray self-administration.

*For patients with rampant caries, professionally applied topical F should be performed three or four times a year.

Table A-4 (Continued)

Water F concentration	Birth—24 months	25—36 months	37 months—13 years	14 years and older
Greater than 0.7 ppm F	Parent brushes child's teeth daily with ADA-approved F-dentifrice. Parent applies APF gel (1.2% F) once a month; minimal amount of gel applied to child-size toothbrush.	Parent brushes child's teeth daily with ADA-approved F-dentifrice. Professionally applied topical F twice a year.* Parent applies APF gel (1.2% F) once a month; minimal amount of gel applied to child-size toothbrush.	Parent brushes child's teeth daily with ADA-approved F-dentifrice until child can master technique. Encourage brushing up to three times daily. Professionally applied topical F twice a year.* Parent applies APF gel (1.2% F) once a month until age 6. At age 6, change to daily rinse (0.05% NaF) and expectorate.	Patient brushes with ADA-approved F-dentifrice up to three times daily. Professionally applied topical F twice a year.* Daily APF (0.5% F) gel tray self-administration.

*For patients with rampant caries, professionally applied topical F should be performed three or four times a year.

Index

R

S

T

U

V

W

X